Baillière's
CLINICAL
PAEDIATRICS
INTERNATIONAL PRACTICE AND RESEARCH

Baillière's

CLINICAL PAEDIATRICS

INTERNATIONAL PRACTICE AND RESEARCH

Volume 2/Number 4
November 1994

Paediatric Gastroenterology

B. S. KIRSCHNER MD, FAAP
J. A. WALKER-SMITH MD(Sydney), FRCP(Edin), FRCP(Lond), FRACP
Guest Editors

Baillière Tindall
London Philadelphia Sydney Tokyo Toronto

This book is printed on acid-free paper.

Baillière Tindall   24–28 Oval Road,
W.B. Saunders   London NW1 7DX

The Curtis Center, Independence Square West,
Philadelphia, PA 19106–3399, USA

55 Horner Avenue
Toronto, Ontario M8Z 4X6, Canada

Harcourt Brace & Company
Australia
30–52 Smidmore Street, Marrickville, NSW 2204, Australia

Harcourt Brace & Company
Japan Inc,
Ichibancho Central Building, 22–1
Ichibancho, Chiyoda-ku, Tokyo 102, Japan

ISSN 0963–6714

ISBN 0–7020–1866–X (single copy)

Baillière's Clinical Paediatrics is published four times each year by Baillière Tindall. Prices for Volume 2 (1994) are:

TERRITORY	ANNUAL SUBSCRIPTION	SINGLE ISSUE
Europe including UK	£80.00 (Institutional) post free	£27.50 post free
	£70.00 (Individual) post free	
All other countries	Consult your local Harcourt Brace & Company office for dollar price	

The editor of this publication is Catriona Byres, Baillière Tindall, 24–28 Oval Road, London NW1 7DX.

Typeset by Phoenix Photosetting, Chatham.
Printed and bound in Great Britain by the University Printing House, Cambridge.

Contributors to this issue

WILLIAM M. BISSET BSc, MBChB, DCH, MRCP, MSc, MD, Senior Lecturer in Child Health & Honorary Consultant Paediatric Gastroenterologist, University of Aberdeen, Foresterhill, Aberdeen AB9 2ZD, UK.

J. TIMOTHY BOYLE MD, FAAP, Associate Professor of Pediatrics, Case Western Reserve University; Chief, Division of Pediatrics, Gastroenterology & Nutrition, Rainbow Babies & Children's Hospital, 11100 Euclid Avenue, Suite 706, Cleveland, OH 44106, USA.

GRAHAM S. CLAYDEN MBBS, MRCP, MD, Department of Paediatrics, St. Thomas' Hospital, London SE1 7EH, UK.

DEIRDRE A. KELLY MD, FRCPI, Consultant Paediatric Hepatologist, The Childrens Hospital, Birmingham B16 8ET; Senior Clinical Lecturer, University of Birmingham, UK.

BARBARA S. KIRSCHNER MD, FAAP, Professor, Departments of Pediatrics and Medicine, Pritzker School of Medicine, The University of Chicago, Wyler Children's Hospital, 5825 S. Maryland Avenue, Chicago, IL 60637, USA.

NIGEL J. MEADOWS MBBS, MRCP, MD, Consultant Paediatrician, Queen Elizabeth Hospital for Children, London E2 8PS, UK.

PETER J. MILLA MSc, MBBS, FRCP, Reader in Paediatric Gastroenterology: Honorary Consultant Paediatric Gastroenterologist, Institute of Child Health, London WC1N 1EH and Hospital for Sick Children, Great Ormond St., London, UK.

JEAN F. PERRAULT MD, MSc, Associate Professor, Pediatrics, Mayo Foundation, Consultant in Internal Medicine and Gastroenterology: Consultant in Pediatric Gastroenterology, Mayo Foundation, 200 First Street, SW, Rochester, MN 55905, USA.

ALAN D. PHILLIPS BA, PhD, Electron Microscopist and Honorary Lecturer in Paediatric Gastroenterology (EM Department), Academic Department of Paediatric Gastroenterology, Queen Elizabeth Hospital for Children, London E2 8PS, UK.

MAMUN SHAHRIER MBBS, PhD, Research Fellow, Academic Department of Paediatric Gastroenterology, Queen Elizabeth Hospital for Children, London E2 8PS, UK.

EBERHARD SCHMIDT-SOMMERFELD MD, Associate Professor of Pediatrics, Louisiana State University Medical Center, 1542 Tulane Avenue, New Orleans, LA 70112, USA.

MARTIN STERN MD, Professor of Paediatrics, University Children's Hospital, Ruemelinstrasse 23, D-72070 Tuebingen, Germany.

JOHN A. WALKER-SMITH MD(Sydney), FRCP(Edin), FRCP(Lond), FRACP, Professor of Paediatric Gastroenterology, Medical College of St. Bartholomew's Hospital & Queen Elizabeth Hospital for Children, London E2 8PS, UK.

NIZAR N. ZIEN MD, Fellow in Pediatric Gastroenterology, Mayo Foundation, 200 First Street, SW, Rochester, MN 55905, USA.

Table of contents

Preface/B. S. KIRSCHNER & J. A. WALKER-SMITH ix

1 Oral rehydration therapy and its under-utilization 611
M. SHAHRIER

2 Optimal management of chronic constipation 625
G. S. CLAYDEN

3 Role of small bowel biopsy in diagnosis 645
A. D. PHILLIPS & J. A. WALKER-SMITH

4 When to transplant the liver in children 667
D. A. KELLY

5 The role of gastrointestinal motility studies 689
P. J. MILLA

6 Home parenteral nutrition in children 705
W. M. BISSET & N. J. MEADOWS

7 Gastrointestinal food allergy 723
M. STERN

8 Recognizing inflammatory bowel disease 747
B. S. KIRSCHNER

9 Gastro-oesophageal reflux: presentation, evaluation
and management 767
E. SCHMIDT-SOMMERFELD

10 A new look at recurrent abdominal pain in children by
subdivision of patients into symptomatic subgroups:
simplifying the role of endoscopy in the diagnostic evaluation 787
J. TIMOTHY BOYLE

11 Gastrointestinal bleeding 807
N. N. ZIEN & J. F. PERRAULT

Index 833

PREVIOUS ISSUE

Vol. 1, No. 1 1993
Child Abuse
C. J. Hobbs & J. M. Wynne

Vol. 1, No. 2 1993
The New Genetics
I. D. Young

Vol. 1, No. 3 1993
Arthritis in Children and Adolescents
T. R. Southwood & P. N. Malleson

Vol. 1, No. 4 1993
Transplantation
M. Broyer

Vol. 2, No. 1 1994
Coma
J. A. Eyre

Vol. 2, No. 2 1994
Current Issues in the Adolescent Patient
R. S. Tonkin

Vol. 2, No. 3 1994
Epilepsy
E. M. Ross & R. C. Woody

FORTHCOMING ISSUE

Vol. 3, No. 1 1995
Pulmonary Problems in the Perinatal Period and their Sequelae
V. Y. H. Yu

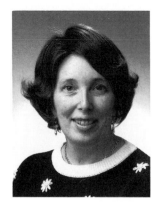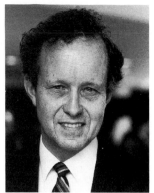

Preface

There are several comprehensive textbooks which cover a broad range of topics within the field of paediatric gastroenterology. Our goal in organizing this edition of *Baillière's Clinical Paediatrics* on Paediatric Gastroenterology was to select specific areas which would be of particular interest and importance to practitioners who care for children and adolescents. Some of the chapters are concerned with specific diseases or categories of disease (chronic inflammatory bowel diseases, gastro-oesophageal reflux, food intolerance, gastro-oesophageal bleeding, recurrent abdominal pain or constipation). Other sections emphasize diagnostic studies (role of small bowel biopsy or motility studies) or therapeutic intervention (oral rehydration therapy, liver transplantation).

Each of the participating authors has extensive clinical expertise and has made significant contributions to the literature in the area they discuss in this text. It is our hope that the reader will gain an appreciation not only of the breath of the clinical entities we have chosen but also for the new advances which have influenced our understanding and current approaches to therapeutic intervention. Depending on the specific chapter, recently developed concepts in genetics, immunology, physiology and surgery are included in the discussion.

The disorders we have chosen are, for the most part, not rare but their presentations may be subtle and varied. It is our desire that the information we have provided is sufficiently comprehensive to enable the reader to recognize these conditions and gain facility in evaluating and managing them. In many instances, the involvement of a paediatric gastroenterologist is necessary and beneficial because of the experience required to perform invasive diagnostic tests and guide complex therapy which may vary substantially in individual patients.

We are grateful to the contributing authors who have donated their time and effort into making this monograph as readable and thorough as it is. As editors, we hope that we have provided sufficient information in each of the areas discussed to meet the expectations and needs of the readers.

B. S. KIRSCHNER
J. A. WALKER-SMITH

1

Oral rehydration therapy and its under-utilization

MAMUN SHAHRIER

The development of oral rehydration therapy (ORT), rehydration and maintenance of hydration of a diarrhoeal patient with solutions given by mouth, is one of the major achievements in the history of medical research in the twentieth century. Very few other therapeutic agents have had such an enormous impact on the survival of man, especially young children. It has been recognized by the World Health Organization (WHO) as 'the single most important in the development programme to manage diarrhoeal disease as well as a key to the reduction of infant and child morbidity and mortality' (Editorial, 1981). Hirschhorn (1980) hailed it as 'potentially the most important achievement of this century since the discovery of penicillin'. Involving simple, inexpensive technology oral rehydration salts are now mass produced, mostly in the developing countries of the world where they are most needed (WHO, 1992).

Access to, and use of oral rehydration solutions, ORS (reconstituted from the oral rehydration salts) have increased dramatically over the last decade. This has brought about a drastic reduction in childhood mortality from diarrhoeal diseases which has been highlighted in a recent report of the United Nations Childrens Emergency Fund (Grant, 1993). According to this report diarrhoeal diseases have been demoted to second place, below upper respiratory tract infections, in the list of major causes of childhood mortality and this has been achieved solely because of the increased use of ORS.

Incidence of diarrhoeal diseases remains high among children of the developing countries (Grant, 1993). It is also a common illness in the children in developed countries (Conway et al, 1990; Guerrant et al, 1990). Each year children in different parts of the world still suffer from more than a billion diarrhoeal episodes. However, despite its tremendous success in the treatment of childhood diarrhoea, oral rehydration therapy is still under-utilized in many parts of the world (Walker-Smith, 1990; Snyder, 1991; WHO, 1992).

Baillière's Clinical Paediatrics—
Vol. 2, No. 4, November 1994
ISBN 0–7020–1866–X

PHYSIOLOGICAL BASIS OF ORT

Water and electrolyte transport in the intestine

The understanding of basic mechanisms of water and solute transport in the intestinal mucosa, under normal and disease conditions, has been translated into the formulation of ORT with unprecedented success (Greenough, 1989).

Transport of water and solutes across the intestinal epithelium is a complex process involving several mechanisms. Water is transported across the intestinal mucosa secondary to the movement of both electrolyte and nonelectrolyte solutes (Bridges and Rummel, 1986).

Absorption of solutes from the lumen by the epithelium involves three basic mechanisms: (i) passive diffusion along the chemical or electrical gradient; (ii) convection or solvent drag (is the movement of solutes secondary to water flow?); and (iii) active transport (Binder, 1983). Sodium absorption involves three active, energy-requiring processes: (i) 'electrogenic' transport in which Na^+ enters the cell following the electrochemical gradient, through selective channels, uncoupled to any other substrate; (ii) 'neutral' transport involving two ion exchangers which allow entry of Na^+ in exchange of H^+ (cation exchanger), and the other Cl^- in exchange of HCO_3^- (anion exchanger); (iii) Na-cotransporter by which Na^+ is absorbed coupled to organic solutes, such as, glucose, amino acids. Chloride transport involves both active and passive processes. It is mostly actively transported from the lumen to the intestinal epithelium coupled to Na^+, as described above. It is also transported through intercellular space in response to the electrical gradient. Potassium is transported only by passive diffusion through the tight junction in between cells (Guandilini, 1988).

Water and electrolytes are also secreted in the intestine. These include K^+ secretion by the colon, Cl^- secretion by both the small intestine and the colon, and HCO_3^- secretion by the colon (Bridges and Rummel, 1986). In normal human small intestine, Cl^- is mainly secreted by the crypt cells (Halm and Frizzell, 1990).

Among enterotoxins, i.e. bacterial toxins which produce secretory diarrhoea without invading the intestinal epithelium, the cholera toxin (CT) of *Vibrio cholerae* has been studied most extensively and the understanding of the mechanism of action of this toxin has been the key to the development of ORS used today.

Oral electrolyte solutions have been in use for the treatment of diarrhoeal patients for almost 50 years (Finberg, 1980). But it was during the late 1950s and 1960s that the key role of glucose in the solutions was established and the foundation of modern oral rehydration therapy laid (Farthing, 1988).

Since then the discovery of other toxins and similarities in their mechanisms of action in producing intestinal secretion has provided the scientific basis of the usefulness of ORT in infectious secretory diarrhoea (Greenough, 1989).

Pathophysiology of infectious diarrhoea

In this section, the three commonest forms of acute, infectious diarrhoea in the world—cholera, enterotoxigenic *E. coli* (ETEC), and rotaviral diarrhoea—will be discussed.

Both *V. cholerae* and ETEC produce secretory diarrhoea by elaborating toxins, enterotoxins, in the intestinal lumen which attach to, but do not invade, intestinal epithelium. The cholera toxin (CT) has two components, a binding and an active component (Kurosky et al, 1976; Fishman, 1980). The active component enters into the cell and stimulates enzyme adenylate cyclase. Stimulation of adenylate cyclase results in the inhibition of NaCl transport and secretion of Cl^- into the intestinal lumen by opening the Cl^- specific apical channels in the epithelial cells. The Na-organic solute co-transporter, however, remains intact and it is this transport mechanism which is utilized for oral rehydration therapy.

The structure and mechanism of action of the heat labile toxin (LT) of ETEC is similar to CT (Hyun and Kimmich, 1984). The heat stable toxin (ST), the other enterotoxin of ETEC, produces secretion which is less dramatic than CT or LT. It has been proposed that its secretory effect is due to inhibition of NaCl absorption only and it does not, in addition, stimulate secretion of Cl^- ions as in the case of CT and LT (Giannella and Drake, 1979).

Studies on water and electrolyte transport in rotaviral diarrhoea have to be performed in animal models as ethical reasons preclude such studies in children. Davidson et al (1977) reported from their study of jejunal tissues of human rotavirus infected piglets in an Ussing chamber, that both the electroneutral NaCl absorption and the Na-glucose cotransporter are abolished during diarrhoea. They also proposed that carbohydrate mal-absorption plays a significant role in the pathophysiology of diarrhoea. Later Graham et al (1984) from their in vivo perfusion study of rotaviral-infected piglet small intestine showed that although there is a depression of water and Na^+ absorption, and Na-glucose cotransporter in the jejunum, these processes remain unaffected in the ileum of the diarrhoeic piglets. By measuring stool electrolyte and osmolality they showed that this diarrhoea is mainly osmotic diarrhoea due to unabsorbed lactose. However, they did not rule out the role of unopposed Cl^- and water secretion from the crypts of the mucosa in which villi are preferentially damaged by the virus. Another group of investigators from Birmingham, England showed from in vitro perfusion studies of intestinal segments that in mice rotavirus produces a secretory diarrhoea (Collins et al, 1988; Starkey et al, 1990a,b). There is impaired water absorption, and also secretion of Na^+, Cl^-, and water by infected small intestine at the peak of diarrhoea (Starkey et al, 1990b). Earlier they also showed that malabsorption of lactose does not occur in rotaviral diarrhoea of mice and thus ruled out any osmotic component (Collins et al, 1988). In a recent study of a neonatal rat model of group-B rotaviral diarrhoea, water secretion had been observed at the peak of diarrhoea during an in vivo whole gut perfusion of the small intestine. Net solute movements paralleled net water movement (Salim, 1990). In rota-viral diarrhoea of both mice and rats, ORS reverse water secretion (Starkey et al, 1990b; Hunt et al, 1992) which indicates that there is a significant secretory component in the pathophysiology of rotaviral diarrhoea.

Experience with children with rotaviral diarrhoea strongly supports these observations on the pathophysiology of rotaviral diarrhoea.

HISTORICAL ASPECTS OF ORT

'Grandmother solutions' have been in use for treatment of diarrhoeal disease for thousands of years (Greenough, 1989). These home solutions of salt, water, and certain solutes, unwittingly and partially used the co-transporters which remain intact during diarrhoeal disease.

The scientific basis of ORT was laid down between the 1940s and 1960s. Scientists studying the mechanisms of intestinal water and electrolyte transport in laboratories, and clinicians with their careful studies of diarrhoeal patients went hand in hand in formulating ORT. In the 1940s, Darrow from his balance studies emphasized the need for replacing sodium and potassium, and correcting acidosis with bases (Darrow, 1946; Darrow et al, 1949). They were the first to start ORT in diarrhoeal patients with solutions which had a composition similar to today's ORS. The observation by Fisher and Parsons (1953), that glucose enhances water absorption in vitro in rat small intestine, was a significant step towards formulating an effective ORS. Later, the Na-glucose cotransport mechanism was established (Schultz and Zalusky, 1964). Concurrent with these laboratory investigations, studies of patients in Egypt and Thailand led to the understanding of the pathophysiology of cholera (Phillips, 1964). With the success in rehydrating and maintaining hydration in cholera patients by oral solutions with well-defined composition in infusion studies, and their success in rural field hospitals and in epidemics, the foundation of modern ORT had been laid (Hirschhorn et al, 1968; Pierce et al, 1968; Cash et al, 1970; Mahalanabis et al, 1971).

COMPOSITION OF ORS

The WHO-ORS is the most widely used ORS at present. It contains in one litre, 90 mmol Na, 80 mmol Cl, 20 mmol K, 10 mmol citrate (base), and 111 mmol glucose. The sodium content is calculated to match the loss in cholera stools (Molla et al, 1981). In infusion studies this concentration improves Na balance in cholera patients (Hirschhorn et al, 1968; Pierce et al, 1968). Sladen and Dawson (1969) from their intestinal perfusion studies showed that maximum glucose absorption from ORS occurs with glucose concentration between 80 and 140 mmol/l. Later clinical studies showed that higher glucose concentrations, as had been common in many formulations available in developed countries at that time, impose osmotic penalty, impair the efficacy of the ORS, and may also increase stool volume (Finberg, 1980). Citrate has replaced bicarbonate as the base in the WHO-ORS in 1984. In the solution, one mole of citrate gives three moles of bicarbonate. In addition to correcting acidosis commonly associated with dehydrating diarrhoeal diseases (Elliot et al, 1987), bicarbonate in mammalian intestine gives the added benefit of promoting water and sodium absorption (Elliot et al, 1987; Rolston et al, 1986). Potassium is essential to replace the substantial loss in diarrhoeal stools, especially in children (Molla et al, 1981). In early days of ORS, Darrow (1946) showed that a concentration between 20 and 30 mmol/l is required to prevent hypokalaemia. This is especially important for malnourished children in developing countries.

RECENT IMPROVEMENTS IN THE FORMULATION OF ORS

The formulation of WHO-ORS and its tremendous success in preventing death from dehydrating diarrhoeas stimulated investigators throughout the world to search for a better ORS. An ORS that would, in addition to enhancing its primary role in preventing dehydration with improved water and sodium absorption and thereby reducing requirement of ORS, would also reduce duration of diarrhoea, provide nutrition, be safer in relation to complications in electrolyte balance sometimes reported in children. Major research efforts have been directed towards the use of new, more effective substrates, optimization of the Na content and osmolality, and re-evaluation of the role of the base in the ORS.

Substrate

The use of glucose as a substrate has the limitation of a maximum concentration of ~200 mmol/l beyond which the efficacy of the ORS is reduced (Finberg, 1980; Elliot et al, 1991). Use of glucose polymers should avoid this problem as these exert less osmolality in the intestinal lumen due to their polymeric structure. Based on this concept the development of rice-based ORS has been a major achievement in improving ORS (Molla et al, 1982; Patra et al, 1982; El-Mougi et al, 1988; Pizarro et al, 1991). A recent meta-analysis of 13 studies has clearly shown that rice-ORS is superior to WHO-ORS in rehydrating and reducing stool volume and ORS requirement in severe diarrhoea like cholera (Gore et al, 1992). From a very recent study from Egypt, WHO-ORS has been reported to be more effective than rice-ORS in reducing stool volume, requirement of ORS, and duration of diarrhoea (Fayad et al, 1993). However, the use of older children and a pre-cooked rice plus vegetable mix refeeding regime has been questioned (Bang, 1993). The role of other shorter chain glucose polymers in ORS, however, remains controversial. Although both in animal models (Daum et al, 1978; Kertzner et al, 1981; Thillainayagam et al, 1993) and in children with diarrhoea (Klish et al, 1980) ORS with glucose polymers have been shown to be superior to glucose containing ORS, most clinical studies in children contradict this (Sandhu et al, 1982; Akbar et al, 1991; Santos Ocampo et al, 1993; Thillainayagam, personal communication).

Experimental evidence that L-alanine is highly effective in transporting sodium across the brush border membrane, and the superiority of L-alanine containing ORS, to standard ORS in reducing stool output and ORS requirement in adults (Patra, 1989) stimulated further clinical trials. However, subsequent studies in children did not show any advantage of

adding L-alanine to standard ORS (Sazawal et al, 1991). Earlier observations that glycyl–glycine improves water absorption and reduces stool
volume in patients with cholera and ETEC diarrhoea (Nalin et al, 1970;
Patra et al, 1984) and some experimental evidence that addition of this to
glucose enhances sodium absorption independent of glycine (Matthews,
1975) stimulated several clinical trials. Although better reduction in stool
output in adult cholera patients has been reported from one study, further
studies showed that it does not have any advantage over standard ORS
(Mahalanabis, 1991). Recently in a pig model of rotavirus diarrhoea,
L-glutamine enhanced water and NaCl absorption (Rhoads et al, 1991). This
may be a good substrate for ORS, as experimental evidence shows that
glutamine improves mucosal repair.

Na content and osmolality

WHO-ORS has a sodium content of 90 mmol/l, and osmolality of
331 mOsm/kg. WHO recommends the use of additional free water in a ratio
of two parts ORS : one part water in children once rehydration has been
achieved, i.e. during the maintenance phase. There have been reports of
hypernatraemia in young children treated with WHO-ORS without
additional free water during maintenance (Chatterjee et al, 1978; Bhargava
et al, 1984; Pizarro, 1986). An effective ORS with lower Na concentration
and osmolality should eliminate the risk of hypernatraemia in children and
can be used for both rehydration and maintenance. In search of such an
ORS, studies have been conducted in both animal models and children with
diarrhoea using hypotonic, i.e. lower sodium containing solutions
(Bhargava et al, 1986; Elliot et al, 1991; Salim, 1990; Rautanen et al, 1993).
These studies have shown that ORS with lower Na content (60 mmol/l) and
osmolality (224–280 mOsm/kg) are more effective than isotonic ORS, i.e.
WHO-ORS. From in vivo whole gut perfusion studies of animal models of
cholera and rotavirus it has been proposed that net positive sodium balance
is not required for efficacy of an ORS, and solvent drag from an hypotonic
solution is more important (Hunt et al, 1992). This is supported by findings
of very recent in vivo whole gut perfusion studies in rat model cholera and
rotaviral diarrhoea (Hunt et al, 1992). In these studies rice powder, and
shorter glucose polymer containing ORS with much lower osmolality have
been found to be more effective than 240–280 mOsm/kg, 60 mmol/l Na
ORS. Results from ongoing clinical trials (WHO, 1992) are awaited before
the universal use of hypotonic ORS can be recommended.

Base and base precursors

WHO recommended the use of citrate to obviate the problems of bicarbonate
containing formulas, i.e. short shelf-life and brown discoloration of the
reconstituted solution due to formation of furfural compounds with glucose.
Citrate has been shown to be effective in the treatment of cholera and other
types of diarrhoea (Islam, 1986). However, with proven efficacy of ORS
without bicarbonate in diarrhoea of children from both developed (Elliot et

al, 1988) and developing countries (Islam and Ahmed, 1984), the need for the re-evaluation of the role of the base in the ORS for children of developed countries has been proposed (Farthing, 1988).

SUCCESS OF ORT

Oral rehydration therapy has been established as one of the cornerstones of the management of diarrhoeal diseases of varied aetiologies. Successful promotion of ORT in developing countries has had a profound impact on the survival of children in these countries. With increased access to, and use of ORT childhood mortality has been reduced to half compared to a decade ago (Grant, 1993). This has been achieved mainly due to drastic reduction of deaths from acute dehydrating diarrhoea. In many developing countries, such as, Bangladesh, Burma, India, Indonesia, Nepal, Nicaragua and Sri Lanka, thousands of volunteers now teach parents the use of ORT. Efforts like these have resulted in the use of ORT by 12% of world's families in the 1980s, which was unknown beyond the specialist circle even at the beginning of that decade (Grant, 1993). In Egypt, the percentage of mothers using ORT has increased from 17 to 79% in ten years between 1980 and 1990 (Miller, 1992). In Bangladesh, school children are now made aware of the life-saving property of ORS (Chowdhury and Cash, 1993). Recently a massive programme of educating 25 million mothers on the home management of diarrhoea and the importance of immunization against childhood killer diseases has also been started in that country (WHO, 1992). Programmes like these will undoubtedly have a major impact on the increased use of ORT in developing countries. Concurrent with the successful promotion, ORS production has also increased dramatically—300% in 7 years between 1983 and 1990—in developing countries. During the last decade, production of ORS has shifted from developed to developing countries where they are most needed. Eighty per cent of the world's ORS are now produced in the developing countries (WHO, 1992).

Ironically, the acceptance of ORT in developed countries has been slow, including those where the basic studies were conducted on the development of this therapy. There were reservations on the appropriateness of this therapy for the treatment of diarrhoea of children of developed countries (Nichols and Soriano, 1977). Also the anxieties about the reported incidence of hypernatraemia due to inappropriate administration of Na-90 ORS, added to the delayed acceptance of the physiological ORS in these countries. Even up to early 1980s most of the ORS available in the UK and USA had inappropriate electrolyte and glucose content, and these contributed to the failure of ORT in many cases (Hutchins et al, 1980; Jalili et al, 1982; Trounce and Walker-Smith, 1985). However, since then there has been a major improvement in this situation. ORT has been promoted for treating children of developed countries (Swedberg and Steiner, 1983; Watkinson, 1983) and study after study conducted in both USA and Europe has shown convincingly that it is an effective therapy in children of developed countries (Santosham et al, 1982; Kumar and Little, 1985;

Santosham et al, 1985; Herzog et al, 1987; Marin et al, 1987). Concern has been expressed about the safety of using WHO-ORS in young children of developed countries (Walker, 1981; Walker-Smith, 1989) although many studies from these countries have shown that WHO-ORS is also safe for neonates and young children of developed countries when it is used appropriately, i.e. with additional free water once rehydration has been achieved (Nalin et al, 1980; Santosham et al, 1985; Herzog et al, 1987; Marin et al, 1987; Cutting et al, 1989). Studies from the USA (Santosham et al, 1982), Finland (Vesikari et al, 1987), UK (Cutting et al, 1989), and Australia (Mackenzie and Barnes, 1991) have shown that ORT drastically reduces the requirement of i.v. hydration for treating dehydrated children with diarrhoea by up to 90%. A study from the USA has shown that the cost of treating a dehydrated child in an urban hospital can be reduced by ten-fold with proper use of ORT (Listernick et al, 1986).

The American Academy of Pediatrics (AAP) in 1985 recommended the use of two solutions for ORT of North American children—a 75–90 mmol/l of Na containing solution for rehydration, and a 40–60 mmol/l solution for maintenance. The recent guideline from the European Society of Paediatric Gastroenterology and Nutrition (ESPGAN) recommends the use of a single 60 mmol/l of Na containing solution for both rehydration and maintenance (ESPGAN, 1992). The recommendation of ESPGAN is based on the predominance of viral diarrhoea in those parts of the world which are associated with less sodium loss in stools, compared to those of bacterial diarrhoeal stools predominantly seen in developing countries, and the proven efficacy of Na-60 ORS in the treatment of children of Europe.

UNDER-UTILIZATION OF ORT

Despite its remarkable success in preventing morbidity and mortality from diarrhoeal diseases, ORT remains under-utilized even today both in developing and developed countries (Conway et al, 1990; Snyder, 1991; WHO, 1992). The factors responsible for the under-utilization of ORT, however, are not the same in these two parts of the world.

In developing countries multiple factors are responsible for the under-utilization of this therapy. The recent estimate by WHO is that 68% of the population of these countries have access to ORS. This is impressive compared to the situation a decade ago. However, when the extent of the problem of diarrhoeal disease is considered, i.e., 1.2 billion episodes worldwide mostly in children under 5 years of developing countries according to a recent estimate of WHO (WHO, 1992), it shows that there is a long way to go before achieving satisfactory utilization of ORT in these countries. According to WHO, even today only 25% of clinics and health centres in developing countries have stocks of ORS and people trained in ORT (Grant, 1993). Even those who have access to it may not always use it—a fact reflected in WHO's recent estimate of a rate of use of 38% which means almost half of those with access to ORT do not use it (WHO, 1992). Parents' wrong perception of the use and efficacy of ORT also lead to the lack of its use in many diarrhoeal episodes (Fauveau et al, 1992). The fact that ORT does not stop diarrhoea may concern some parents (Bari et al, 1989). Ignorance on the part of the health professionals also contribute to the under-utilization of ORT in developing countries. Studies from India and Indonesia show that expensive, ineffective and sometimes harmful drugs are prescribed more often than ORS (Nahar et al, 1988; Gani et al, 1991).

In developed countries the problem is different from that of developing countries. Underestimation of the incidence of diarrhoeal disease by the doctors of these countries contribute to the lack of interest in recent developments and recommendations on ORT (Snyder, 1991). The recent report of a child with gastroenteritis and mild dehydration kept nil by mouth, and on i.v. hydration for 2 days is an extreme example of that (Rhoads, 1993). In a recent survey conducted in the USA, the majority of the physicians who participated would use ORT only in mild or no dehydration despite a clear guidance from the AAP that it can be safely used in most children with moderate dehydration (Snyder, 1991), while another study in the UK showed that less than a third of the children with diarrhoea receive ORT, although 60% of them saw their GPs (Conway et al, 1990). In a survey of pharmacists in the UK, the majority recommended or prescribed an 'antidiarrhoeal' along with ORS (Goodburn et al, 1991). Also, many unphysiological solutions are available and recommended in developed countries (Snyder, 1982; Walker, 1981; Nichols and Soriano, 1977; Snyder, 1991). In the survey by Snyder (1991) only 30% of the physicians recommended physiological solutions. It is depressing to know that even in the USA, the country which is still the major donor to the ORT programmes in the developing countries, parents may not always have access to ORS (Myers et al, 1991). The reluctance of the insurers to reimburse hospitalization due to diarrhoeal dehydration, but not requiring i.v. fluid, also contribute to the under-utilization of ORT in the USA (Kleinman, 1992). The unavailability of parents or time of busy hospital staff may also contribute to the under-utilization of ORT in developed countries (Avery and Snyder, 1990).

RECOMMENDATIONS

The following recommendations are made.

1. Oral rehydration should be used in all cases, including mild and moderate dehydration. Nasogastric feeding may be used if there is strong resistance from the child. Both Na-90 and Na-60 containing ORS are safe for use in children. When a Na-90 ORS is used additional free water must be used through breast feeding, and additional free water at a ratio of 2 (ORS) : 1 (water).
2. So called 'antidiarrhoeals', i.e. adsorbents, spasmolytics should not be used.
3. Antibiotics should only be used when there is strong clinical suspicion or bacteriological evidence of infectious aetiology, i.e. cholera, shigellosis, salmonellosis, enteropathogenic E. coli diarrhoea, and giardiasis.

4. Refeeding should be started as soon as rehydration has been achieved.

SUMMARY

Oral rehydration therapy is one of the major achievements in the history of medical research in the last 50 years. The therapy utilizes the Na-cotransporter which remains intact during infectious secretory diarrhoea. The presence of glucose, either in monomeric or polymeric form, enhances Na and water absorption from the solution by the small intestine and thus prevents dehydration which can be life threatening.

Studies of laboratory animals enabled the understanding of the basic mechanisms of water and electrolyte transport in the intestine. The establishment of pathophysiology of cholera, and the efficacy of glucose–electrolyte solutions in cholera patients have laid the foundation of ORT.

The efficacy of ORT in preventing dehydration in a severe form of secretory diarrhoea, such as cholera, stimulated further studies in formulating more effective and safer ORS, which are still going on in both developing and developed countries of the world. These efforts have resulted in improved formulations, such as rice-based, and hypotonic ORS.

During the last decade the drastic reduction in childhood mortality from diarrhoeal diseases in the developing world has been the direct result of increased use of ORS. Everyday ORT saves thousands of lives and prevents suffering of many more children from diarrhoeal disease worldwide. It has become the cornerstone of the management of diarrhoeal diseases in both developing and developed countries. In the last decade use and production of ORS have increased several-fold especially in the developing countries.

Despite its tremendous success, the utilization ORT remains suboptimal in both developing and developed countries. Logistical problems still restrict access to ORT in developing countries where they are most needed. Under-utilization also results from ignorance of both health care providers and parents, and in many cases lead to use of expensive, ineffective and often harmful 'antidiarrhoeals'. In developed countries the lack of awareness of the extent of the problem of diarrhoeal diseases, recent developments and recommendations contribute to the under-utilization of ORT in these countries. In many cases unphysiological solutions and unnecessary intravenous fluids may be used for the treatment of diarrhoea.

Increased use of ORT will benefit children all over the world. For developing countries this means saving a million lives, and the alleviation of suffering of many more. In developed countries, increased utilization of ORT will drastically reduce the time and costs involved in the hospital treatment of children with diarrhoeal diseases.

REFERENCES

Akbar MS, Baker KM, Aziz MA et al (1991) A randomised, double-blind clinical trial of a maltodextrin containing oral rehydration solution in acute infantile diarrhoea. *Journal of Diarrhoeal Diseases Research* **9:** 33–37.

American Academy of Pediatrics (1985) Use of oral fluid therapy and posttreatment feeding following enteritis in children in a developed country. *Pediatrics* **75**: 358–361.

Avery ME & Snyder TD (1990) Oral therapy for acute diarrhea. The underused simple solution. *New England Journal of Medicine* **323**: 891–894.

Bang A (1993) Towards better oral rehydration. *Lancet* **342**: 755–756.

Bari A, Rahman A, Molla A & Greenough W (1989) Rice-based oral rehydration solution shown to be better than glucose-ORS as treatment of non-dysenteric diarrhoea in children in rural Bangladesh. *Journal of Diarrhoeal Diseases Research* **7**: 1–7.

Bhargava SK, Sachdev HP, Das Gupta B et al (1984) Oral rehydration of neonates and young infants with dehydrating diarrhea: comparison of low and standard sodium content in oral rehydration solutions. *Journal of Pediatric Gastroenterology and Nutrition* **3**: 500–505.

Bhargava SK, Sachdev HP, Das Gupta B et al (1986) Oral therapy of neonates and young infants with World Health Organization rehydration packets: a controlled trial of two sets of instructions. *Journal of Pediatric Gastroenterology and Nutrition* **5**: 416–422.

Binder HJ (1983) Absorption and secretion of water and electrolytes by small and large intestine. In Sleisenger MH & Fordtran JS (eds) *Gastrointestinal Disease*, 3rd edn, pp 811–829. London: W.B. Saunders Co.

Bridges RJ & Rummel W (1986) Mechanistic basis of alterations in mucosal water and electrolyte transport. In Krejs GJ (ed.) *Clinics in Gastroenterology: Diarrhoea*, pp 491–506. London: W.B. Saunders Co.

Cash RA, Nalin DR, Rochat R et al (1970) A clinical trial of oral therapy in rural cholera treatment centre. *American Journal of Tropical Medicine and Hygiene* **19**: 653–656.

Chatterjee A, Mahalanabis D, Jalan KN et al (1978) Oral rehydration in infantile diarrhea. Controlled trial of a low sodium glucose electrolyte solution. *Archives of Disease in Childhood* **53(4)**: 284–289.

Chowdhury AMR & Cash RA (1993) Cultural incorporation of the ORT message. *Lancet* **341**: 1591.

Collins J, Starkey WG, Wallis TS et al (1988) Intestinal enzyme profile in normal and rotavirus-infected mice. *Journal of Pediatric Gastroenterology and Nutrition* **7(2)**: 264–272.

Conway SP, Phillips RR & Panday S (1990) Admission to hospital with gastroenteritis. *Archives of Disease in Childhood* **65**: 579–584.

Cutting WA, Belton NR, Gray JA et al (1989) Safety and efficacy of three oral rehydration solutions for children with diarrhoea (Edinburgh 1984–85). *Acta Paediatrica Scandinavica* **78**: 253–258.

Darrow DC (1946) The retention of electrolyte during recovery from severe dehydration due to diarrhea. *Journal of Pediatrics* **28**: 515.

Darrow DC, Pratt EL, Gamble AH & Wiese HF (1949) Disturbances of water and electrolytes in infantile diarrhea. *Pediatrics* **3**: 129–156.

Daum F, Cohen MI, McNamara H & Finberg L (1978) Intestinal osmolality and carbohydrate absorption in rats treated with polymerised glucose. *Pediatric Research* **12**: 24.

Davidson GP, Gall DG, Petric M et al (1977) Human rotavirus enteritis induced in conventional piglets. Intestinal structure and transport. *Gastroenterology* **60**: 1402–1409.

Editorial (1981) Oral therapy for acute diarrhea. *Lancet* **ii**: 615–617.

El-Mougi M, Hegazi E, Galal O et al (1988) Controlled clinical trial on the efficacy of rice powder-based oral rehydration solution on the outcome of acute diarrhea in infants. *Journal of Pediatric Gastroenterology and Nutrition* **7**: 572–576.

Elliot EJ, Armistead JC, Farthing MJ & Walker-Smith JA (1988) Oral rehydration therapy without bicarbonate for prevention and treatment of dehydration: a double-blind controlled trial. *Alimentary Pharmacology and Therapeutics* **2**: 253–262.

Elliot EJ, Walker-Smith JA & Farthing MJG (1987) The role of bicarbonate and base precursors in the treatment of acute gastroenteritis. *Archives of Disease in Childhood* **62**: 91–95.

Elliot EJ, Watson AJM, Walker-Smith JA & Farthing MJG (1991) Search for the ideal oral rehydration solution: studies in a model of secretory diarrhoea. *Gut* **32**: 1314–1320.

European Society for Paediatric Gastroenterology and Nutrition (1992) Recommendations for composition of oral rehydration solutions for the children of Europe. *Journal of Pediatric Gastroenterology and Nutrition* **14**: 113–115.

Farthing MJG (1988) History and rationale of oral rehydration and recent developments in formulating an optimal solution. *Drugs* **(36 (supplement 4)**): 80–90.

Fauveau V, Yunus M, Islam MS et al (1992) Does ORT reduce diarrhoeal mortality? *Health Policy and Planning* **7**: 243–250.

Fayad IM, Hashem M, Duggan C et al (1993) Comparative efficacy of rice-based and glucose-based oral rehydration salts plus early reintroduction of food. *Lancet* **342:** 772–775.

Finberg L (1980) The role of oral electrolyte–glucose solutions in hydration for children—international and domestic aspects. *Journal of Pediatrics* **96(1):** 51–54.

Fisher RB & Parsons DS (1953) Glucose movements across the wall of the rat small intestine. *Journal of Physiology* **119:** 210–223.

Fishman PH (1980) Mechanism of action of cholera toxin: events on the cell surface. In Field M, Fordtran JS & Schultz SG (eds) *Secretory Diarrhea*, pp 85–106. Bethesda, MD, USA: American Physiological Society.

Gani L, Arif H, Widjaja SK et al (1991) Physicians' prescribing practice for treatment of acute diarrhoea in young children in Jakarta. *Journal of Diarrhoeal Diseases Research* **9:** 194–199.

Giannella RA & Drake KW (1979) Effect of purified *Escherichia coli* heat-stable enterotoxin on intestinal cyclic nucleotides metabolism and fluid secretion. *Infection and Immunity* **24:** 19–23.

Goodburn E, Mattosinho S, Mongi P & Waterston T (1991) Management of childhood diarrhoea by pharmacists and parents: is Britain lagging behind the Third World. *British Medical Journal* **302:** 440–443.

Gore SM, Fontaine O & Pearce (1992) Impact of rice based oral rehydration solution on stool output and duration of diarrhoea: metanalysis of 13 clinical trials. *British Medical Journal* **304:** 287–291.

Graham DY, Sackman JW & Estes MK (1984) Pathogenesis of rotavirus-induced diarrhea. Preliminary studies in miniature swine piglet. *Digestive Diseases and Sciences* **29:** 1028–1035.

Grant JP (1993) *The State of the World's Children*. Oxford, UK: Oxford University Press.

Greenough III WB (1989) Oral rehydration therapy: an epithelial transport success story. *Archives of Disease in Childhood* **64:** 419–422.

Guandilini S (1988) Intestinal water and nutrient transport in health and infectious diarrhoeal diseases. *Drugs* **36 (supplement 4):** 26–38.

Guerrant RL, Hughes JM, Lima NL & Crane J (1990) Diarrhea in developed and developing countries: magnitude, special settings, and etiologies. *Review of Infectious Disease* **12(supplement 1):** S41–S50.

Halm DR & Frizzell RA (1990) Intestinal chloride secretion. In Lobenthal E & Duffy M (eds) *Textbook of Secretory Diarrhea*, pp 47–58. New York: Raven Press.

Herzog LW, Bithoney WG & Grand RJ (1987) High sodium rehydration solutions in well-nourished outpatients. *Acta Paediatrica Scandinavica* **76:** 306–310.

Hirschhorn N (1980) The treatment of acute diarrhea in children. An historical and physiological perspective. *American Journal of Clinical Nutrition* **33(3):** 637–663.

Hirschhorn N, Kinzie JL, Sachar DB et al (1968) Decrease in net stool output in cholera during intestinal perfusion with glucose containing solutions. *New England Journal of Medicine* **279:** 176–181.

Hunt JB, Thillainayagam AV, Salim AFM et al (1992) Water and solute absorption from a new hypotonic oral rehydration solution: evaluation in human and animal perfusion models. *Gut* **33:** 1652–1659.

Hunt JB, Thillainayagam AV, Carnaby S et al (1993) Absorption of a hypotonic oral rehydration solution in a human model of cholera. *Gut* **35(2):** 211–214.

Hutchins P, Wilson C, Manly JA & Walker-Smith JA (1980) Oral solutions for infantile gastroenteritis—variations in composition. *Archives of Disease in Childhood* **55:** 616–618.

Hyun CS & Kimmich GA (1984) Interaction of cholera toxin and *Escherichia coli* enterotoxin with isolated intestinal epithelial cells. *American Journal of Physiology* **247:** G623–G631.

Islam MR (1986) Citrate can effectively replace bicarbonate in oral rehydration salts for cholera and infantile diarrhoea. *Bulletin of the World Health Organization* **64:** 145–150.

Islam MR & Ahmed SM (1984) Oral rehydration solution without bicarbonate. *Archives of Disease in Childhood* **59:** 59: 1072–1075.

Jalili F, Smith EO, Nichols VN et al (1982) Comparison of acquired monosaccharide intolerance and acute diarrheal syndrome. *Journal of Pediatric Gastroenterology and Nutrition* **1:** 81–89.

Kertzner B, Sloan HR, Juhling H & Ailabouni A (1981) Jejunal absorption of short and long chain glucose oligomers in the absence of pancreatic amylase. *Pediatric Research* **15:** 536.

Kleinman RE (1992) We have the solution: now what's the problem? *Pediatrics* **88:** 113–114.

Klish WJ, Udall JN, Calvin RT & Nichols BL (1980) The effect of intestinal solute load on water secretion in infants with acquired monosaccharide intolerance. *Pediatric Research* **14**: 1343–1346.

Kumar GA & Little TM (1985) Has treatment for childhood gastroenteritis changed? *British Medical Journal* **1321**: 1322.

Kurosky A (1976) Chemical characterization of the structure of cholera toxin and its natural toxoid. *Journal of Infectious Diseases* **133 (supplement)**: 14–22.

Kurosky A, Markel DE, Touchstone B & Peterson W (1976) Chemical characterization of the structure of cholera toxin and its natural toxoid. *Journal of Infectious Diseases* **133 (supplement)**: 14–22.

Listernick R, Zieserl E & Davis AT (1986) Outpatient oral rehydration in the United States. *American Journal of Diseases of Children* **140**: 211–215.

Mackenzie A & Barnes G (1991) Randomised controlled trial comparing oral and intravenous rehydration therapy in children with diarrhoea. *British Medical Journal* **303**: 393–396.

Mahalanabis D (1991) Fluid therapy of diarrhea. In Walker WA, Durie PR, Hamilton JR et al (eds) *Pediatric Gastrointestinal Disease*, pp 1561–1567. Philadelphia, Toronto: B.C. Dekker.

Mahalanabis D, Choudhuri AB, Bagchi NG et al (1971) Oral fluid therapy of cholera among Bangladesh refugees. *Johns Hopkins Medical Journal* **132**: 197–205.

Marin L, Saner G, Sokuci S et al (1987) Oral rehydration therapy in neonates and young infants with infectious diarrhoea. *Acta Paediatrica Scandinavica* **76**: 431–437.

Matthews DM (1975) In Matthews DM & Payne JW (eds) *Peptide Transport in Protein Nutrition*, p 61. Amsterdam: North Holland/American Elsevier.

Miller PC (1992) Trends in the management of childhood diarrhoea in Egypt: 1979–1990. *Journal of Diarrhoeal Diseases Research* **10**: 193–200.

Molla AM, Rahman M, Sarker SA et al (1981) Stool electrolyte content and purging rates in diarrhoea caused by rotavirus, *E. coli* and *V. cholerae*. *Journal of Pediatrics* **98**: 835–838.

Molla AM, Sarker SA, Hossain M et al (1982) Rice-powder electrolyte solution as oral-therapy in diarrhoea due to *V. cholerae* and *Escherichia coli*. *Lancet* **i**: 1317–1319.

Myers A, Siegel B & Vinci R (1991) Economic barriers to the use of diarrhoea: a case report. *Journal of American Medical Association* **265**: 1724–1725.

Nahar S, Uppal R, Mehta S & Singh PL (1988) Prescribing for diarrheal diseases. *Indian Pediatrics* **25**: 754–756.

Nalin DR, Cash RA & Rahman M (1970) Effect of glycine and glucose on sodium and water absorption in patients with cholera. *Gut* **11**: 768–772.

Nalin DR, Harland E, Ramlal A et al (1980) Comparison of low and high sodium and potassium content in oral rehydration solutions. *Journal of Pediatrics* **97**: 848–853.

Nichols BL & Soriano HA (1977) A critique of oral therapy of dehydration due to diarrheal syndromes. *American Journal of Clinical Nutrition* **30**: 1457–1472.

Patra FC, Mahalanabis D, Jalan KN et al (1982) Is oral rice electrolyte solution superior to glucose electrolyte solution in infantile diarrhoea? *Archives of Disease in Childhood* **57**: 910–912.

Patra FC, Mahalanabis D, Jalan KN et al (1984) In search of a super solution: controlled trial of glycine–glucose oral rehydration solution in infantile diarrhoea. *Acta Paediatrica Scandinavica* **73**: 18–21.

Patra FC, Sack DA, Islam A et al (1989) Oral rehydration formula containing alanine and glucose for treatment of diarrhoea: a controlled trial. *British Medical Journal* **298**: 1353–1356.

Phillips RA (1964) Water and electrolyte losses in cholera. *Federation Proceedings* **23**: 705–712.

Pierce NF, Banwell JG, Mitra JC et al (1968) Effect of intragastric glucose-electrolyte infusion upon water and electrolyte balance in Asiatic cholera. *Gastroenterology* **55**: 333–343.

Pizarro D (1986) Oral rehydration therapy: its use in neonates and young infants. *Journal of Pediatric Gastroenterology and Nutrition* **5**: 6–7.

Pizarro D, Posada G, Sandi L & Moran JR (1991) Rice-based oral electrolyte solutions for the management of infantile diarrhea. *New England Journal of Medicine* **324**: 517–521.

Rautanen T, El-Radhi S & Vesikari T (1993) Clinical experience with a hypotonic oral rehydration solution in acute diarrhoea. *Acta Paediatrica* **82**: 52–54.

Rhoads FA (1993) Oral rehydration therapy for viral gastroenteritis. *Journal of American Medical Association* **270**: 578–579.

Rhoads JM, Keku EO, Quinn J et al (1991) L-glutamine stimulates jejunal sodium and chloride absorption in pig rotavirus enteritis. *Gastroenterology* **100:** 683–691.

Rolston DDK, Borodo MM, Kelly MJ et al (1986) Efficacy of oral rehydration solutions in a rat model of secretory diarrhoea. *Journal of Pediatric Gastroenterology and Nutrition* **6:** 624–630.

Salim AFM (1990) *Characterization of rotavirus infection in neonatal rats and its use in the evaluation of oral rehydration solutions.* PhD thesis, University of London.

Sandhu BK, Jones BJ, Brook DB (1982) Oral rehydration in acute infantile diarrhoea with a glucose-polymer electrolyte solution. *Archives of Disease in Childhood* **57(2):** 152–154.

Santos Ocampo PD, Bravo LC et al (1993) A randomized double-blind clinical trial of a maltodextrin-containing oral rehydration solution in acute infantile diarrhea. *Journal of Pediatric Gastroenterology and Nutrition* **16:** 23–28.

Santosham M, Burns B, Nadkarni V et al (1985) Oral rehydration therapy for acute diarrhea in ambulatory children in the United States: a double-blind comparison of four different solutions. *Pediatrics* **76:** 159–166.

Santosham M, Daum RS, Dillman L et al (1982) Oral rehydration therapy of infantile diarrhea: a controlled study of well-nourished children hospitalized in the United States and Panama. *New England Journal of Medicine* **306:** 1070–1076.

Sazawal S, Bhatnagar S, Bhan MK et al (1991) Alanine-based oral rehydration solution: assessment of efficacy in acute noncholera diarrhea among children. *Journal of Pediatric Gastroenterology and Nutrition* **12:** 461–468.

Schultz SG & Zalusky R (1964) Ion transport in isolated rabbit ileum II: the interaction between active sodium and active sugar transport. *Journal of General Physiology* **47:** 1043–1059.

Sladen GE & Dawson AM (1969) Interrelationships between the absorptions of glucose, sodium and water by the normal human jejunum. *Clinical Science* **36:** 119–132.

Snyder JD (1982) Pedialyte to popsicles: a look at oral rehydration therapy used in the United States and Canada. *American Journal of Clinical Nutrition* **35:** 157–161.

Snyder JD (1991) Use and misuse of oral therapy for diarrhea: comparison of US practices with American Academy of Pediatrics recommendations. *Pediatrics* **87:** 28–33.

Starkey WG, Candy DCA, Thornber D et al (1990a) An in vitro model to study aspects of the pathophysiology of murine rotavirus-induced diarrhoea. *Journal of Pediatric Gastroenterology and Nutrition* **10:** 361–370.

Starkey WG, Collins J, Candy DCA et al (1990b) Transport of water and electrolytes by rotavirus-infected mouse intestine: a time course study. *Journal of Pediatric Gastroenterology and Nutrition* **11:** 254–260.

Sullivan SK et al (1990) Epithelial K channel expressed in xenopus oocytes is inactivated by protein kinase C. *Proceedings of the National Academy of Sciences of the USA* **87:** 4553–4556.

Swedberg J & Steiner JF (1983) Oral rehydration therapy in diarrhea. Not just for Third World children. *Postgraduate Medicine* **74:** 335–341.

Thillainayagam AV, Dias JA, Salim AFM et al (1994) Glucose polymer in the fluid therapy of acute diarrhoea: studies in a model of rotavirus infection of neonatal rats. *Clinical Science* **86(4):** 469–477.

Trounce JQ & Walker-Smith JA (1985) Sugar intolerance complicating acute gastroenteritis. *Archives of Disease in Childhood* **60:** 986–990.

Vesikari T, Isolauri E & Baer M (1987) A comparative trial of rapid oral and intravenous rehydration in acute diarrhoea. *Acta Paediatrica Scandinavica* **76:** 300–305.

Walker SH (1981) Hypernatremia from oral electrolyte solution in infantile diarrhea. *New England Journal of Medicine* **304:** 1238.

Walker-Smith JA (1989) The role of oral rehydration solutions in the children of Europe: continuing controversies. *Acta Paediatrica Scandinavica* **364 (supplement):** 13–16.

Walker-Smith JA (1990) Management of infantile gastroenteritis. *Archives of Disease in Childhood* **65:** 917–918.

Watkinson M (1983) Oral rehydration: too high a price to pay? *British Medical Journal—Clinical Research* **287:** 618.

World Health Organization (1992) *Programme for control of diarrhoeal diseases. Eighth annual report 1990–1991.* Geneva: World Health Organization.

2

Optimal management of chronic constipation

G. S. CLAYDEN

An essential step in the optimal management of constipation in children is to develop a clear understanding of what the child and family mean by the term. Extremes in the normal variation in stool frequency (Weaver and Steiner, 1984) may cause parental anxiety. The word constipation can be used as a description of the hardness of the stool, of the length of interval between defaecation episodes, or of the distress caused to the child during the passage of the stool. It is essential, therefore, to clarify which meaning is used in the history obtained. A number of children suffer from all these problems within the definition.

FACTORS INVOLVED IN CONSTIPATION

When the clinician is clear about the degree and type of constipation, the next task is to discover the main factors involved. These may be connected with the predisposition to, initial onset of, and persistence of the constipation as in a number of illnesses in childhood (Lask and Fosson, 1989).

Details of the management of the problem at different ages will be set out in this chapter. Firstly, it is worth reviewing the developing pathophysiology of constipation, the clinical features, the relevant investigations and the pharmacology of the commonly used medications. In this way, it should be possible to explain the rationale of various treatments. It is important to recognize that there has been a great deal of controversy over the balance of structural versus psychological factors in the persistence of constipation in childhood (Richmond et al, 1954; Pinkerton, 1958; Coekin and Gairdner, 1960; Berg and Vernon-Jones, 1964; Levin, 1975; Clayden and Lawson, 1976).

As will be demonstrated in this chapter, the most effective management can only be carried out in a multidisciplinary manner where all the factors can be recognized and treated in an integrated fashion by the most appropriate professional and in the most effective order (Clayden, 1992).

Baillière's Clinical Paediatrics—
Vol. 2, No. 4, November 1994
ISBN 0–7020–1866–X

THE DEVELOPMENT OF CHRONIC CONSTIPATION IN CHILDHOOD

Problems arising in the neonatal period or early infancy

A number of children who later present with intractable chronic constipation give a history of an onset soon after birth. Any delay in the passage of meconium should alert the clinician to the possibility of Hirschsprung's disease or another obstructive anal anomaly (Doig, 1992). A classic association of delayed defaecation, abdominal distension, vomiting, failure to thrive and a characteristic gush of flatus and faeces on the withdrawal of the examining finger from the anus, will all increase the suspicion of Hirschsprung's disease (Clayden, 1990).

A high index of suspicion appears to be the safest policy as delay in diagnosis may lead to the complications of necrotising enterocolitis, bowel perforation and Gram-negative septicaemias. A number of children with short segment Hirschsprung's disease may be delayed in their diagnosis as a result of a temporary improvement following a rectal examination. This may be the case particularly when regular digital dilatations of the anus are recommended as is the case when a degree of anal stenosis is diagnosed. Perhaps the discovery of the RET proto-oncogene on chromosome 10 in patients with familial Hirschsprung's disease will lead to a greater refinement in diagnosis.

Anal stenosis or anal stricture is a controversial subject in early infancy (Kiely et al, 1979). A number of babies have a tightness of the anus on digital examination, some of them to the degree that a tight thread is felt when rectal examination is attempted. The presence of a remnant of the anorectal membrane has been suggested as an important cause of illness or disturbance in early infancy, even as long ago as the first century. Soranus recommended that as part of the routine examination of the newborn, a rectal examination should be performed with the fifth finger (with carefully pared fingernail) so as to divide the anorectal membrane remnant (Soranus, 1965). The incidence of 17% in boys and 25% in girls of a palpable anal stricture has been reported (Harris et al, 1953). There is also considerable opinion that anal stenosis or an anal stricture may contribute to the episodes of colic in babies of this age. The recommended regular digital dilatation appears to be effective but has two important drawbacks. Often the mother is shown the technique and persuaded to continue it for a series of days or weeks. This clearly put a major strain on her and can lead to intense anxiety. Another complication is in the delay in the diagnosis of Hirschsprung's disease if the anal tightness was due to aganglionosis rather than just a mere stricture. It could be argued that a number of children who later present with megarectum have developed this megarectum primarily as a response to the obstructive anal stenosis. By the time they come to examination, the passage of large hard stools may well have sufficiently dilated the original stricture or stenosis. It is difficult to imagine how this controversy could be further investigated within ethical limits.

The anus itself may not be obstructive but the stool of the young infant may be of such a nature as to obstruct a relatively normal anorectum. Stools which become so dry that they cannot easily traverse the normal bends of the anorectum may cause considerable difficulty. The usual cause of this is a relative deficiency of fluid in the baby or even evidence of general under-feeding. It is obvious how an over-diagnosis of a surgical cause may be made in a child who has both difficulty in passing stools, delay in defaecation and failure to thrive as a result of poor feeding. Another group of babies who produce a confusing clinical picture are breast-fed babies who may have many days delay in passing stools.

Problems in later infancy

An important cause of constipation in the older infant is a relative lack of fibre in the diet. A number of obligate milk drinkers will produce very dry and hard stools which lead to pain on defaecation. If this pain is perceived and remembered by the infant, then a spasm of the external sphincter muscles and probably the levator ani occur when the child has the sensation of imminent defaecation. Many children will then cry and the parents become confused about whether their child is straining hard to defaecate or in fact, straining to avoid defaecation. It is understandable that the greater the anal discomfort the more likely the child is to discover ways of avoiding that discomfort by delaying defaecation. There may well be a selective process involved at this stage related most closely to the size of the rectum. In those babies with relatively high capacity rectums, it would be possible to retain faeces for several days. In those who have smaller capacities, the babies will inevitably open their bowels each day but with a great deal of pain and upset. In those babies with a larger than average sized rectum, the faeces may accumulate, become dry and because of the continual activity of the rectum, be moulded into a ball of hardening stool which in itself may be virtually impossible to pass. Thus, the anorectum becomes obstructed, more by the stool than by any other factor, even if the child has no longer any clear motivation to withhold the stool. It can then be debated whether the rectum housing this hard, large stool actually develops a larger and larger capacity. There are plenty of other precedents in the body for an obstructed hollow viscus to show the ability to enlarge greatly. This is clearly seen in the stomach when the pylorus is obstructed in the case of congenital hypertrophic pyloric stenosis. It is also clearly seen in the size of the bladder in those boys with posterior urethral valves. It is therefore not too surprising if the rectum should grow in capacity if it becomes obstructed by a faecal ball. Eventually, the mass is passed either intact or in sections, but nearly always with a great deal of pain and fear. Anal fissures are sometimes caused as a result. The situation is aggravated by anal treatments which may increase the fear.

Problems of the toddler

As the child becomes more aware of the imminence of defaecation and of their ability to withhold the stool as they approach their second birthday, then the problem becomes intensified. What started as a purely physical obstruction to the anorectum gradually becomes complicated by the child's emotional response to the memory of painful defaecation. This is further compounded by the family's response to seeing their toddler making every attempt to avoid defaecation. Naturally, the parents are keen to accelerate the passage of the stool so as to avoid their child passing a very large, hard and possibly damaging stool. The child on the other hand, has a clear concept of avoiding the pain associated with the urge to defaecate by immediately taking up a retentive posture. Many parents will report their child with straight or crossed legs straining during episodes throughout the day. Many children learn that if they are disturbed doing this retentive straining, defaecation may occur. This leads them to hide or resist any human contact during the periods when they have the urge to defaecate. This also leads to a number of children defaecating as they wake up in the morning or when they are in the bath.

Problems in older children

As the constipated child grows older, the ability to retain faeces appears to become easier and their physiological ability to defaecate becomes more difficult (Loening-Baucke, 1984; Clayden, 1988a). The increasingly large megarectum and the retained faecal mass produce another, and perhaps more socially devastating problem of overflow faecal incontinence (Buchanan, 1992). Even if the parents have managed to weather the difficulty related to painful defaecation, they will very soon present because of the overflow faecal soiling. This situation disrupts the timing of pot-training which is an essential stage of their integrating into their particular society (Whiting, 1963).

The next stage in the evolution of this difficult problem is that the child may become subjected to more and more vigorous treatments which is found to be both painful and frightening especially if the rectal route is used (Pinkerton, 1958; Levin, 1975). The relationship with the parents often deteriorates and when the child starts school, then further psychological problems will dominate as peer pressure and ridicule about soiling intensify the child's overall feeling of poor self esteem. As the rectum, by this time, may be of incredibly large dimensions, it is not surprising that even if effective methods are found to promote regular defaecation, the child's sensation of the need to defaecate may well be diminished. This relative lack of the sensation of filling of the rectum is compounded by a degree of denial related to the child's feelings of despair about their defaecation habit.

This gradual evolution from a possible minor physical anomaly of the anus through the dietary hard stools on to the retentive anorectum through to the faecally loaded megarectum with overflow faecal soiling and associated psychological problems, is a major challenge to the managing clinician.

CLINICAL FEATURES OF THE CHILD WITH MEGARECTUM

The history of the age of onset and of early feeding or defaecation difficulties will help to determine whether there were mainly dietary or structural problems initially. Details of the length of delays between stools and the pattern of any overflow soiling will help in gauging the severity of the problem. The description of the child's behaviour when defaecation becomes imminent will help to define some psychological factors. Observation of the interaction of the child and family in the consulting room can confirm some of these factors and indicate the degree of urgency of expert child psychiatry input.

Clinical examination should include a general assessment of the child's growth and development as this may indicate failure to thrive if the constipation has a major obstructive component. Poor height velocity (with associated delayed bone age with eventual delayed puberty) is often seen during the child's years of severe constipation. Inspection of the abdomen may sometimes provide a more accurate assessment of faecal loading than palpation especially when the stools are soft or the abdominal muscle tense. Usually palpation demonstrates the presence of faecal 'rocks'.

In a survey of 488 children referred with severe constipation (Clayden 1981, 1992), the findings on abdominal palpation were as follows: 25% had stool palpable but to a point below umbilicus; 20% to the umbilicus; 21% to a point between the umbilicus and the xiphisternum; and 33% who had no stools palpable per abdomen had either recently passed a 'megastool' or had soft faecal loading of their megarectum where the upper limit was not possible to define with ease.

Inspection of the anus is helpful in checking for any degree of ectopia (Reisner et al, 1984; Merlob and Reisner, 1988), the presence of any skin problems (such as group A streptococcal infection, lichen sclerosus et atrophicus, epidermolysis bullosa), any evidence of anal fissure, the presence and type of soiling, whether the anal sphincter is tightly closed or relaxed (as seen in the constipated child with a neuropathic bowel, dystrophia myotonica or in an otherwise neurologically normal child as a consequence of severe rectal loading). A great deal of controversy has ranged over the sign of reflex anal dilatation which may be seen in both the child with a loaded megarectum (Clayden, 1988b) and a child who has been anally abused (Hobbs and Wynne, 1986). It is essential that both possibilities are considered when this appearance is seen (Cleveland Report, 1988) but that psychosocial action is not taken on this as an isolated sign in the absence of any form of verbal disclosure of abuse.

Examination of the spine and sacrum and eliciting the leg reflexes will help to avoid missing the cause of a child's neuropathic bowel.

Investigations

Investigations are helpful to demonstrate the degree of megarectum both to confirm the diagnois for the doctor and to give the child and the family a very clear idea of the structural difficulties, so that these can be balanced against the behavioural and emotional factors. Only when there is a clear communication and a development of a model which is shared by the child, the family and the doctors alike, is there likely to be success in the management. The number and timing of investigations will depend on the severity of the condition and the child's age.

Abdominal X-ray

If faeces are easily palpable per abdomen, then an abdominal X-ray may not be necessary. However, if the faecal retention is soft, especially if a child has been pre-treated with laxative, a plain abdominal X-ray may give useful information about the degree and distribution of the faecal loading. A refinement on the plain abdominal X-ray is to give the child radio-opaque markers on three consecutive days before the X-ray which is taken on the fifth day after the first set of markers are swallowed (Arhan et al, 1981; Bautista Casasnovas et al, 1991). Ten small pieces of radio-opaque tubing, cut into different shapes (about the size of rice grains) one shape for each day, are swallowed by the child and are clearly seen on the abdominal X-ray if there is significant faecal retention. This is easily tolerated by the child who is as fascinated as the parents in seeing the position of these 'armies' of markers as they appear to have chased each other through the bowel. The

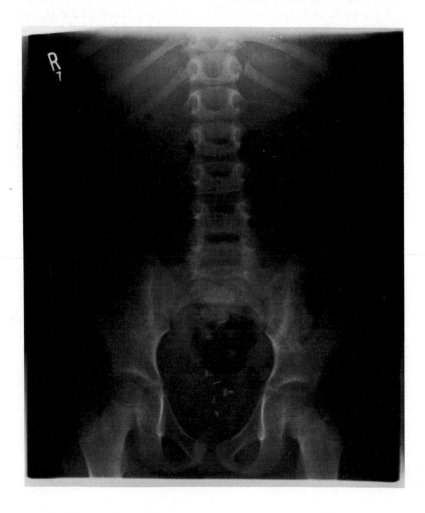

results help to give a clear and concrete concept of the physical nature of the retained stool. This helps to dispel the confusion over the guilt associated with the inevitable overflow soiling in the presence of massive faecal retention. Even when more invasive radioisotope studies of colonic function

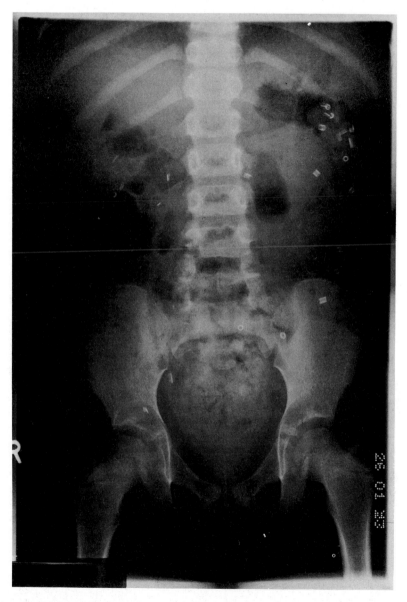

Figure 1. Comparison of abdominal radiographs following ingestion of radio-opaque markers in a child with encopresis (a) and constipation with overflow incontinence (b).

are available for intestinal transit measurement, these simple marker tests are still recommended (Jameson and Misiewicz 1993). Figure 1 shows two abdominal radiographs.

Other forms of imaging such as barium enema are rarely of value in childhood beyond infancy although may be necessary if histochemistry suggests Hirschsprung's disease to enable the surgeon to have a clearer view of the length of the aganglionic segment when choosing the most appropriate operation.

Imaging for urinary tract abnormalities will be indicated if the child has a history of urinary tract infections. This is a common finding in children with constipation (13% in my series) and constipation is commonly associated with recurrent urinary tract infections which improved when the constipation is treated effectively (O'Regan et al, 1985).

Rectal biopsy and histochemical examination

This form of examination of the specimen for the distribution of acetyl-cholinesterase positive enteric nerve fibres is the standard investigation for Hirschsprung's disease (Meier-Ruge, 1972). A superficial mucosal suction biopsy can give valuable evidence of aganglionosis, where the highly acetyl-cholinesterase positive preganglionic fibres appear to have grown chaotically throughout the mucosa and submucosa in a vain attempt to find their ganglion cells. There is considerable debate on the existence of neuronal intestinal dysplasia. This is suggested by seeing excessive numbers of acetyl-cholinesterase positive fibres in the presence of normal or excessive numbers of ganglion cells. Its association with Hirschsprung's disease is less controversial than its presence as an isolated finding as a cause of megarectum/megacolon (Scharli and Meier-Ruge, 1981). Perhaps it is not surprising that the migrating ganglion cells in a 6-week-old embryo fail to reach the anus as these neuroblasts appear to enter the rapidly lengthening gut from the cervical neural crest (Okamoto and Ueda, 1967). Whether neuronal intestinal dysplasia represents the area in the bowel where the migrating neuroblasts become entangled, thus failing to reach the anus, or just as a consequence of the junction between ganglionic and ganglionic bowel is still left to the imagination rather than subject to rigorous scientific proof. Even the existence of ultra-short segment of Hirschsprung's disease is controversial (Neilson and Yazbeck, 1990). It is also likely that a very short segment of Hirschsprung's disease could be present with a much longer zone of neuronal intestinal dysplasia or even no aganglionic zone and only neuronal intestinal dysplasia (Rintala et al, 1989; Simpser et al, 1991). Sometimes there is evidence from the clinical features, imaging and anorectal manometry of Hirschsprung's disease but there is apparently normal histochemistry. These pseudo-Hirschsprung diseases are encouraging a search for the deficiency of putative inhibitory neurotransmitters, such as nitric oxide, which is already implicated in Hirschprung's disease (O'Kelly et al, 1993).

It is essential that the histochemical diagnoses are clarified as a number of children are having major surgical interventions based on the biopsy results.

This dilemma is intensified by the major role that psychological factors have in the persistence of childhood constipation.

Anorectal manometry

This is not required as a routine investigation for childhood constipation but can be very useful in descriminating between obstructive, neuropathic or mainly sensory deficiency problems (Cucchiara et al, 1984). Hirschsprung's disease can be diagnosed confidently using anorectal manometry (Yokoyama et al, 1989). When histochemistry is inconclusive as described above, a failure of the internal anal sphincter to relax in response to rectal distension (the rectoanal reflex) supports a diagnosis of a variant of Hirschsprung's disease. Manometry can help the surgeon discover the effective length of non-propulsive or obstructive gut. In children who have neurological problems, especially spinal cord lesions such as spina bifida, evidence of a neuropathic bowel can be shown (Agnarsson et al, 1993). This is seen as a rapid and complete inhibition of the internal anal sphincter tone with relatively small volumes of rectal distension. Sensory problems can also be identified by anorectal manometry if this can be performed in an unanaesthetized child. This is rarely possible between the ages of 1 and 6 years, but later the sensation caused by inflating the rectal balloon can be accurately assessed. This may also provide a valuable biofeedback for the older child (Loening-Baucke et al, 1988; Benninga et al, 1993). Otherwise ketamine anaesthesia may be used as this preserves the autonomic reflexes. Anorectal manometry has provided valuable research evidence of the pathophysiology of megarectum in children. There is a demonstrable high rectal capacity, reduced anal inhibition in spite of a higher capacity for rectal distension with the manometry balloon, and a poverty of sensation (Molnar et al, 1983; Loening-Baucke, 1984; Clayden, 1988a). Some of these abnormalities persist even when there is clinical improvement (Loening-Baucke, 1989).

Endoanal sonography is becoming a valuable tool for the investigation of the internal anal sphincter. It has been used mainly to demonstrate the anatomy of the anorectum in children who have had operations for imperforate anus and other major malformations. It promises to become a useful imaging technique in children with chronic constipation. It may help in the debate on what degree of internal anal sphincter hypertrophy exists in children with non-Hirschsprung's disease megarectum. This in turn will help to confirm or refute the evidence for this hypertrophy suggested by anorectal manometry and observations during surgery. It may put the decision to perform vigorous anal dilatation under anaesthetic onto a more than empirical basis.

TREATMENTS

Dietary manipulation

Alterations in the diet will have a profound effect on the stool volume consistency which in turn will decrease the transit time. One of the functions of the colon is to reabsorb water from the stool and so it is not surprising that retained stools tend to dry and harden. The hard stool will be more difficult to pass and dietary changes which influence the stool water content will inevitably help to some degree. Many foods which are rich in dietary fibre may be less tolerable to small children than their favourite high fat and carbohydrate snacks and drinks. There is good evidence that intestinal transit is slowed by lipids and caffeine. The constipation in obligate milk-drinking 1-year-olds or exclusive tea, coffee or cola drinkers can be helped by advice on fibre content. However, care should be taken that the relatively low nutrition content, high fibre foods may displace essential calorie and protein sources from the diet of these growing children. Fruits contain natural stimulant laxatives as well as their valuable fibre content. For example, rhubarb contains an anthracene chemically very similar to that in senna. However, the volume of stewed rhubarb for a child with a significant megarectum would be so large that a refined chemical laxative would be easier to administer. Dietary advice is both helpful and hazardous in psychological as well as nutritional areas. There are enough causes of conflict between the child and parents as a result of the bowel problem without adding battles over meals.

Fluid intake is relatively easy to increase although there is no definite evidence of its effectiveness in constipation. Many parents will report an improvement in the effectiveness of the bulking agents if attention is paid to fluid intake.

Laxatives

The timing of the introduction of the laxatives and their most effective order will be considered chronologically later. The medications will be considered individually but will be grouped into their functional categories rather than the traditional pharmacological classes.

At any age the drug treatment of constipation will involve: softening retained stools; evacuating retained stools; increasing the bulk (and water content) of the intestinal contents; and reducing the transit time to reduce the risk of reaccumulation.

Stool softeners

Docusate sodium (Dioctyl paediatric syrup 12.5 mg/5 ml or Dioctyl 1% Solution 50 mg/5 ml or 100 mg tablets) acts like a detergent by reducing the surface tension and so allows the stool to absorb water and its surface progressively to soften. It has a useful role in children where a three times a day dose of 5 or 10 ml, depending on size (not more than 2 ml/kg/day in young children) may soften the stool sufficiently for their next spontaneous stool to evacuate completely the rectum. If complete evacuation is not achieved but the stool is effectively softened it paves the way for more dramatic orally administered evacuants.

Evacuants

Sodium picosulphate elixir or Picolax act as a stimulant and yields an osmotic load which combined with liberal oral water intake leads to excess fluid flushing through the intestine. The softened but retained stool is then evacuated from the colon after a period of 3–6 hours after administration.

In childhood it is best used only when spontaneous evacuation of the megarectum is not achieved, as a weekly dose when maintenance laxatives have produced little output or as a rapid response to the first signs of a relapse. Parents should be warned that the reconstituted Picolax from its sachet may become hot as it dissolves. It appears that Picolax with its magnesium content may produce a more aggressive purge than the picosulphate elixir and it is worth converting in this direction if the child does not tolerate Picolax.

Stronger osmotic cathartics such as polyethylene glycol 3350 or 4000 (Klenprep or Golytely) (Tolia et al,1984) require the child to drink such large volumes of fluid that it is often recommended to be given by nasogastric tube in the younger child. It can then be argued whether an enema is less stressful than the passing of a nasogastric tube. If both are equally distressing for the child then the more humane option is an evacuation manually under anaesthetic, even though this adds the small but important risk of the anaesthetic.

Maintenance laxatives

Senna is a standardized mixture of the anthroquinone sennosides derived from the plant senna. The flowers and their 'megarectum-shaped' pods of this plant have been used for centuries. The dosage is based on the sennoside B concentration and comes in 7.5 mg tablets or as a syrup of 7.5 mg/5 ml. As the purpose of giving the laxative is to prevent the reaccumulation of faeces in the megarectum, a sufficiently large dose must be given. Fortunately it is virtually colon-specific and is inactive in the upper bowel because the sennoside is conjugated with a sugar until this is broken off by colonic bacteria. It is best to give senna in a once daily dosage at a time which promotes peristalsis 12–14 hours later at the most convenient time. Parents should be advised to monitor the timing of administration and the timing of its effect so as to avoid their child having to defaecate at school or during periods of other social activity. They should also be counselled on the avoidance of starting on a high dose but advised to increment the dose daily until the most effective one is found. This dose may be as high as 25 ml once per day but this should be reduced if there is colic or precipitate defaecation.

In those children who are withholding stools with all their ability, the dose which overrides this attempt may produce some abdominal pain because of the stimulation of peristalsis which is, however, relieved by defaecation. The perception of relief from defaecation may go some way towards extinguishing their fear of defaecation. It is vital that the child does not connect the administration of the senna dose with their inability to withhold the stool at a time when they are psychologically most keen to avoid defaecation. This may lead to rejection of the senna syrup which is otherwise quite acceptable because of its sucrose content. As in other medications which are taken for many months which contain sugar, care must be taken to avoid dental caries. A common error in the use of senna is to reduce or stop the medication too soon. Various weaning methods have been tried but too rapid a reduction before the megarectum has had a chance to reduce in capacity or before the child's confidence in defaecation has become established, will lead to disappointing relapses of faecal retention. One of the pressures on parents to stop senna is the belief that prolonged use may lead to abnormalities in the myenteric plexus (Smith, 1968; Cummings, 1974; Rutter and Maxwell, 1976) but prolonged exposure to Senokot in the animal model produced no abnormalities (Douthwaite and Goulding, 1957). It can be argued that administration of stimulant laxatives for a year or two in childhood which prevents the persistence of an abnormally capacious bowel into adulthood may avoid the patient requiring 60–80 years of laxatives as an adult.

Another stimulant laxative which may be preferred by some children is bisacodyl (chemically similar to phenolphthalein which is still used in products such as 'Ex-Lax' chocolate) in spite of its side-effects.

Maintenance stool softeners

Increasing the frequency of defaecation is helpful because of the familiarity of routines especially in those children where fear is a major factor. Avoiding hard stools is also important, so the bulk or softening laxatives have a role in addition to the senna. They may supplement the dietary fibre for a while when stimulant laxatives are discontinued as some insurance against relapse.

Lactulose acts partly as an osmotic laxative and partly by producing fibre. Some of the bacteria of the gut thrive in the presence of Lactulose and they add to the fibre content of the stool thus keeping them soft. The dose is 5–10 ml three times per day limited by excessive looseness of the stool or flatulence. Even small doses may be associated with too wet a stool and so other bulking agents may be more acceptable.

Methyl Cellulose works in a similar way by holding water in the stool, preventing the drying effect of the colon and allowing a larger stool to enter the rectum. It is available in tablet form as Celevac Tablets although its more valuable liquid form is only available through some hospital pharmacies and special medicine suppliers for commercial reasons. Other bulking agents are available and could be tried in children who find the above unpalatable; however they all share that feature.

Anorectal procedures

It may seem reasonable to treat the faecal retention directly with suppositories or enemas. Unfortunately in the child with intact anal sensation a great deal of fear will feed into the vicious cycles built up on the anal pain already experienced as a result of fissure, inflammation or excessive large, hard stools. A phosphate enema given to a child under deep and effective sedation with a drug such as temazepam may be effective. Some parents are gently able to insert a microenema into their sleeping child but if the child awakens during their surreptitious act they may find that a major sleep problem develops to add to their family misery.

Surgical treatments

If the faecal evacuation methods fail or the children are frequent relapsers, they may benefit from an anal dilatation or partial internal anal sphincter-otomy (Bentley, 1966; Clayden and Lawson, 1976; Freeman, 1984) when there is evidence of internal anal overactivity. Table 1 shows data from 230 children with severe protracted constipation and previous failure to respond to standard laxative regimes referred to a specialist clinic and treated over a 4 year period.

Table 1. Response of 230 children with severe constipation.

Current treatment	Response to surgery	Number
Off laxatives	No anal dilatation	47 (20%)
	Rapid response to anal dilatation	32 (14%)
	Slow response to anal dilatation	58 (25%)
	Rapid response to sphincterotomy	7 (3%)
	Slow response to sphincterotomy	6 (3%)
	Needed anal dilatation after sphincterotomy	5 (2%)
Still on laxatives after 4 years		35 (15%)
Failed to attend to complete regime		40 (17%)

Other forms of surgery, such as extended sphincterotomy, partial colectomy and colostomy may be necessary especially when abnormalities of the myenteric plexus are seen. For children with major anorectal anomalies and poor residual internal sphincter function or with major neuropathic conditions, the bowel may be kept free from faecal accumulation by using antegrade continence enemas. This procedure involves using a fine catheter passed into the ascending colon via a continent stoma formed by using the inverted appendix (Malone et al, 1990). This is now being used in children with extreme capacity megarecta where medical treatment has failed and any anal obstruction excluded. Success depends on the completeness of evacuation but may allow the child to avoid overflow faecal soiling by ensuring an empty rectum for the greater part of most days.

These extreme treatments for children with severe constipation should only be considered when every other avenue has been explored. There are two main reasons why a child may fail to respond to treatment: the treatment is being used at an inappropriate stage or that the underlying psychological factors have not been properly addressed.

Psychological factors may interfere directly in the child refusing to co-operate with toilet routines or compliance with medication. Alternatively, feelings of low self esteem, family stress secondary to the stigma of the incontinence, and complicated illness behaviour reactions may have a sub-conscious effect. As in other areas of paediatrics there must be vigilance for the Munchausen's syndrome by proxy, whether by sabotage of essential treatment or falsification of the degree of constipation (effectively extended by radio-opaque marker transit test).

Psychological treatments

It should be recognized by the family and all the professionals working with the child that fear, confusion, shame, guilt, anger, despair, withdrawal, dissociation and abdication from responsibility are likely to develop in a child who has suffered from the effects of chronic constipation and secondary faecal incontinence. Some individual children appear to have amazing resilience to their suffering whereas others are more vulnerable probably as a result of other forms of instability in their lives. This is why it is very difficult to predict the emotional impact of any form of investigation or treatment. Some of the most needy children are denied expert child psychiatric help because of anxieties in their parents. Sometimes the paediatrician or family doctor has to take on some of these roles preferably with the support of the child psychiatry team. It is essential at the onset of the discussion of the child's physical problems that the paediatrician or paediatric surgeon should indicate that extra help may be necessary to overcome some of the associated emotional difficulties. Psychiatric involvement should not be presented as a last ditch treatment when all else fails. The multidisciplinary approach is the only way of avoiding escalating treatments in inappropriate directions when managing children with chronic constipation.

Range of psychological interventions

The following list is in an ascending order of intensity. It ranges from those activities which every clinician should include in their management strategy through to the interventions which require expert assessment and decision making involving external agencies such as the courts of law.

- Careful pathophysiological explanation (demystification)
- Assessment of child's (and family's) perception of the condition
- Child and family support during the chronicity of the problem
- Team support to overcome professional frustration at relapses and slow progress
- Behaviour-modification methods
- Toilet-training contracts and incentives
- Family meetings and involvement in therapy
- Two to three week in-patient training programmes
- Individual psychotherapy using play, art, music etc
- Longer term in-patient training/therapy programmes
- Separating the child from adverse family effects

Psychological treatments from this cascade are more likely to be acceptable to the child and family and more likely to be effective if they are carried out in parallel with and subject to the same respect for timing as the physical treatments.

Every treatment should be understood by the child and family as much as possible depending on the level of maturity. To this end it is useful to provide them with written information as well as careful explanation (Clayden and Agnarsson, 1991).

PATTERNS OF USE OF TREATMENT FOR CONSTIPATION

The individual investigations and treatments have already been described but the importance of using them in a correct order cannot be over-emphasized. Figure 2 illustrates the rationale for these treatments.

It is convenient to group the treatments according to the age of the child but obviously there are no absolute divisions between these stages.

Neonatal

The previously unused anus may be obstructed as a result of its shape, size, position (Leape and Ramenofsky, 1978) or myenteric nerve arrangement. Any suspicion of Hirschsprung's disease must lead to rectal biopsy and appropriate surgery if positive.

If detailed examination (including digital rectal examination) fails to show any evidence of maldevelopment or stricture then a dietary cause is most likely. Usually an increase in properly reconstituted milk intake is sufficient to improve the constipation. However, if this persists extra water should be given. Occasionally lactulose is necessary for a short period. Delays in healthy breast-fed babies are normal and active treatment should be avoided. The characteristic pattern is that the baby may take 7–10 days and appear to be in some discomfort only to pass a large, very soft stool characteristic of a breast-fed baby after this time. A number of parents report that the baby's general mood and alertness improve after the passage of the stool. However, it is difficult to separate this improvement from the overall anxiety which is relieved in the family when the stool is finally passed. Occasionally, constipation may be caused by hypercalcaemia, hypothyroidism or chronic idiopathic intestinal pseudo-obstruction (Glassman et al, 1989).

Infancy

Weaning and the introduction of solid foods may be associated with relative water deprivation. The resulting constipation can be greatly helped by dietary improvement alone. However, a small but regular dose of lactulose may accelerate improvement. Older infants may be obligate milk drinkers to the exclusion of their fibre intake. Constipation will ensue especially because of the lipid effect on intestinal transit. If the older infant begins to associate imminent defaecation with pain due to the hardness of the stool, anal spasm may occur as a forerunner of the more voluntary retention of the

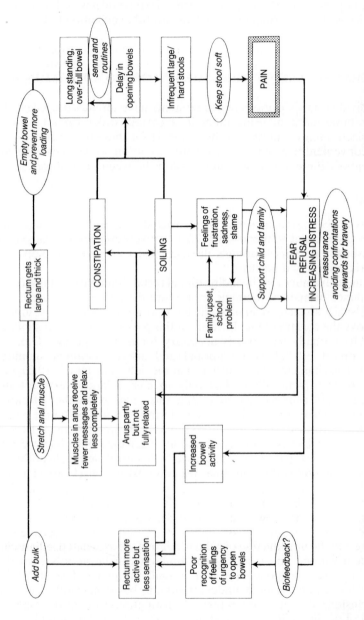

Figure 2. Relationship of aetiological factors and treatments in chronic constipation in childhood. From Clayden and Agnarsson (1991). Reproduced with kind permission of Oxford University Press.

toddler. Lactulose may be necessary if dietary modification is insufficiently helpful.

Toddlers

As the child begins to achieve more voluntary control over the continence muscles (external anal sphincter and levator ani muscles) constipation may ensue in response to painful defaecation. Evidence from the history of straining in an upright posture, the appearance of the perianal region showing evidence of fissure or streptococcal infection and faeces palpable per abdomen will confirm the presence and degree of the problem.

Usually stimulant laxatives are necessary to overcome the attempts at retention. Once daily senna in a high enough dose to guarantee a daily stool will help the child to avoid having to pass very large accumulated stools with the associated pain and fear. Local anal examinations and treatments should be avoided as the fear will become intensified. By increasing the frequency of defaecation the 'great event' nature of defaecation can be avoided and repetition extinguish the fear. The parents may need considerable support through these difficult times (Berg and Vernon Jones, 1964) and occasionally hospital admission and even evacuation of retained faeces under anaesthetic is necessary.

Preschool child

The constipation which started around birth or around pot-training has usually become entrenched by this age. This is partly due to the established megarectum and partly due to the child and family reactions to fears of anal pain and the failure to achieve continence or even fear of lavatories (Pilapil, 1990). Usually when the child is seen there is clear evidence of faecal retention and so the laxatives should be used to soften (docusate) and evacuate (picosulphate) the stool followed by maintenance with senna and bulking agent such as methyl cellulose or lactulose. This age group may frequently relapse or run into problems with compliance. Here a combined admission for evacuation of faeces either surgically under general anaesthetic (combined with anal dilatation) or with polyethylene glycol (Klenprep or Golytely) with a psychological input to establish the compliance with regular lavatory visits and taking the maintenance laxatives is likely to be successful. Regular follow-up and professional access is necessary to modify laxative doses and maintain morale. This can be shared very effectively with specially experienced nurses supported by psychologists and paediatricians.

School-age children

If the problem still persists at this age the extra stress generated at school in response to the overflow soiling indicates an increasing need for parallel psychological help. A vicious cycle of stress and increased soiling secondary to increased intestinal motility may occur (Chaudhary and Truelove, 1961).

It will depend on the previous intensity of laxative treatment whether daily senna and bulking agent will be sufficient.

Quite often children at this age appear to evacuate incompletely their megarecta and need an extra boost with picosulphate or Klenprep at weekends. The feelings of confusion, blame and hopelessness build up progressively and further investigations such as intestinal radio-opaque marker transit studies and anorectal manometry may be helpful. If there is clear evidence of massive megarectum and internal anal sphincter hypertrophy, anal dilatation or partial internal anal sphincterotomy may help as well as providing valuable histopathological specimens to exclude unusual variants of Hirschsprung's disease.

Teenagers

Usually the persistence of the problem into teenage indicates the severity of the megarectum, the poverty of sensation of the urge to defaecate and/or deepening feelings of hopelessness, denial and dissociation. They usually have delayed puberty and a bone age to match. This is one factor which may stimulate them to improve their compliance with treatment. A number of teenagers cast off their battles with parents over their bowels as an independence issue. They are very keen to achieve reliable continence and will often accept the idea of giving themselves regular enemata provided they have not been terrified by them in the past. Individual counselling both for the psychological responses to their problem and to help them utilize aids for continence are useful. Many manage to enter their pubertal growth spurt with strategies of keeping their rectums empty for most of the day. This allows a differential growth of their body from that of their rectum so reducing their pathophysiological disadvantage when fully grown. Unfortunately this does not occur in all and some pass on to adult gastroenterologists and proctological surgeons where the options for further surgery are considered again. As it seems important that they keep their megarectums empty during this growth phase it can be argued that they might benefit in the long term by using more intensive surgical methods in their teens. Colostomy is very difficult to accept at this age although some claim that it is better than coping with the soiling. The antegrade continence enema may provide a middle stage when ordinary enemas are unacceptable or ineffective. These newer methods are being evaluated at present.

SUMMARY

Throughout childhood constipation is a troublesome and distressing condition leading to feelings of desperation in children, families and professionals alike. Slow response to treatment, interwoven physical and psychological factors and the relative lack of hard facts may dissuade professionals from taking this problem as seriously as deserved by the degree of suffering it provokes. A multidisciplinary approach which is tailored to the individual child's combination of needs is the only one likely to succeed.

REFERENCES

Agnarsson U, Warde C, McCarthy G et al (1993) Anorectal function of children with neurological problems. I: spina bifida II: cerebral palsy. *Developmental Medicine and Child Neurology* **35:** 893–902.

Arhan P, Devroede G & Hehannin B (1981) Segmental colonic transit time. *Diseases of the Colon and Rectum* **24:** 625–629.

Bautista Casasnovas A, Varela Vices R, Villanueva Jeremias A et al (1991) Measurement of colonic transit time in children. *Journal of Pediatric Gastroenterology and Nutrition* **13:** 42–45.

Benninga MA, Buller HA & Taminiau JA (1993) Biofeedback training in chronic constipation. *Archives of Disease in Childhood* **68:** 126–129.

Bentley JFRC (1966) Posterior excisional anorectal myotomy in management of chronic faecal accumulation. *Archives of Disease in Childhood* **41:** 144–147.

Berg I & Vernon-Jones K (1964) Functional faecal incontinence in children. *Archives of Disease in Childhood* **39:** 465–472.

Buchanan A (1992) *Children who soil: Assessment and Treatment.* Chichester: John Wiley and Sons.

Chaudhary NA & Truelove SC (1961) Human colonic motility: part III: Emotions. *Gastroenterology* **40:** 27–36.

Clayden GS (1981) *Chronic constipation in childhood.* MD thesis, University of London.

Clayden GS (1988a) Is constipation in childhood a neurodevelopmental abnormality. In Milla PJ (ed.) *Disorders of Gastrointestinal Motility in Childhood,* pp 111–121. Chichester: John Wiley and Sons Ltd.

Clayden GS (1988b) The reflex anal dilatation associated with severe chronic constipation in childhood. *Archives of Disease in Childhood* **63:** 832–836.

Clayden GS (1990) Constipation. In David T (ed.) *Recent Advances in Paediatrics,* pp 41–59. Churchill Livingstone.

Clayden GS (1992) Personal practice: Management of chronic constipation. *Archives of Disease in Childhood* **67:** 340–344.

Clayden GS & Agnarsson U (1991) Appendix. Information booklet for children and parents. In *Constipation in Childhood.* Oxford: Oxford University Press.

Clayden GS & Lawson JON (1976) Investigation and management of long standing chronic constipation in childhood. *Archives of Disease in Childhood* **51:** 918–923.

Cleveland Report (1988) *Summary of Findings.* London: HMSO.

Coekin M & Gairdner D (1960) Faecal incontinence in children. *British Medical Journal* **ii:** 1175–1180.

Cucchiara S, Coremans G, Staiano A et al (1984) Gastrointestinal transit time and anorectal manometry in children with fecal soiling. *Journal of Pediatric Gastroenterology and Nutrition* **3:** 545–550.

Cummings JH (1974) Laxative abuse. *Gut* **15:** 758–766.

Doig CM (1992) ABC of colorectal diseases. Paediatric problems—I (review). *British Medical Journal* **305:** 462–464.

Douthwaite AH & Goulding R (1957) Action of senna. *British Medical Journal* **ii:** 1414–1415.

Freeman NV (1984) Intractable constipation in children treated by forceful anal stretch or anorectal myectomy: preliminary communication. *Journal of the Royal Society of Medicine* **77 (supplement):** 36–38.

Glassman M, Spivac W, Mininberg D & Madara J (1989) Chronic idiopathic intestinal pseudo-obstruction: a commonly misdiagnosed disease in infants and children. *Pediatrics* **83:** 603–608.

Harris LE, Corbin PF & Hill JR (1953) Anorectal rings in infancy: incidence and significance. *Pediatrics* **13:** 59–63.

Hobbs CJ & Wynne JM (1986) Buggery in childhood: A common syndrome of child abuse. *Lancet* **ii:** 762–796.

Jameson JS & Misiewicz JJ (1993) Colonic motility: practice or research. *Gut* **34:** 1009–1012.

Kiely EM, Chopra R & Corkery JJ (1979) Delayed diagnosis of congenital anal stenosis. *Archives of Disease in Childhood* **54:** 68–70.

Lask B & Fosson A (1989) *Childhood Illness: The Psychosomatic Approach. Children Talking with their Bodies*. Chichester: John Wiley and Sons.

Leape LL & Ramenofsky ML (1978) Anterior ectopic anus: a common cause of constipation in children. *Journal of Pediatric Surgery* **13:** 627–630.

Levin MD (1975) Children with encopresis: a descriptive analysis. *Pediatrics* **56:** 412–416.

Loening-Baucke VA (1984) Abnormal rectoanal function in children recovered from constipation and encopresis. *Gastroenterology* **87:** 1299–1304.

Loening-Baucke V (1989) Factors determining outcome in children with chronic constipation and faecal soiling. *Gut* **30:** 999–1006.

Loening-Baucke V, Desch L & Wopfraich M (1988) Biofeedback training for patients with myelomeningocele and fecal incontinence. *Developmental Medicine and Child Neurology* **30:** 781–790.

Malone PS, Ransley PG & Kiely EM (1990) Preliminary report: the antegrade continence enema. *The Lancet* **336:** 1217–1218.

Meier-Ruge W (1972) Hirschsprung's disease: aetiology, pathogenesis and diagnosis. *Current Topics in Pathology* **59:** 131–179.

Merlob P & Reisner SH (1988) Determination of the normal position of the anus (with reference to idiopathic constipation) (letter). *Journal of Pediatric Gastroenterology and Nutrition* **7:** 630.

Molnar D, Taitz LS, Urwin OM & Wales JKH (1983) Anorectal manometry results in defecation disorders. *Archives of Disease in Childhood* **58:** 257–261.

Neilson IR & Yazbeck S (1990) Ultrashort Hirschsprung's disease: myth or reality. *Journal of Pediatric Surgery* **25:** 1135–1138.

Okamoto E & Ueda T (1967) Embryogenesis of intramural ganglia of the gut and its relation to Hirschsprung's disease. *Journal of Pediatric Surgery* **2:** 437–443.

O'Kelly TJ, Davies JR, Tam P et al (1993) Abnormalities of nitric oxide producing neurones in Hirschsprung's disease, morphology and implications (in press).

O'Regan S, Yazbeck S & Schick E (1985) Constipation, bladder instability, urinary tract infection syndrome. *Clinical Nephrology* **23:** 152–154.

Pilapil VR (1990) A horrifying television commercial which led to constipation. *Pediatrics* **85:** 592–593.

Pinkerton P (1958) Psychogenic megacolon in children: the implications of bowel negativism. *Archives of Disease in Childhood* **33:** 371–380.

Richmond JB, Eddy EJ & Garrard SD (1954) The syndrome of fecal soiling and megacolon. *American Journal of Orthopsychiatry* **24:** 391–401.

Reisner SH, Sivan Y, Nitzan M & Merlob P (1984) Determination of anterior displacement of the anus in newborn infants and children. *Pediatrics* **73:** 216–217.

Rintala R, Rapola J & Lonhimo I (1989) Neuronal intestinal dysplasia. *Progress in Pediatric Surgery* **24:** 186–192.

Rutter R & Maxwell D (1976) Diseases of the alimentary system. Constipation and laxative abuses. *British Medical Journal* **ii:** 997–1000.

Scharli AF & Meier-Ruge W (1981) Localised and disseminated forms of neuronal intestinal dysplasia mimicking Hirschsprung's disease. *Journal of Pediatric Surgery* **16:** 164–170.

Simpser E, Kahn E, Kenigsberg K et al (1991) Neuronal intestinal dysplasia: quantitative diagnostic criteria and clinical management. *Journal of Pediatric Gastroenterology and Nutrition* **12:** 61–64.

Smith B (1968) Effect of irritant purgatives on the myenteric plexus in man and mouse. *Gut* **9:** 139–143.

Soranus (1965) (translated by O. Temkin) *Gynaecology*, Book 2, chap. 13, pp 83–84. Baltimore: John Hopkin Press.

Tolia V, Fleming S & Dubois RS (1984) Use of 'Golytely' in children and adolescents. *Journal of Pediatric Gastroenterology and Nutrition* **3:** 468–470.

Weaver LT & Steiner H (1984) The bowel habit of young children. *Archives of Disease in Childhood* **59:** 649–652.

Whiting BB (ed.) (1963) *Six Cultures. Studies in Child Rearing. Laboratory of Human Development*. New York: John Wiley & Sons.

Yokoyama J, Kuroda T, Matsufugi H et al (1989) *Progress in Pediatric Surgery* **24:** 49–58.

3

Role of small bowel biopsy in diagnosis

A. D. PHILLIPS
J. A. WALKER-SMITH

Proximal small intestinal biopsy in childhood enables an accurate diagnosis to be made of the state of the mucosa in diffuse and patchy lesions. From a practical point of view it has two specific roles: (1) to establish whether an enteropathy is present (i.e. an abnormality seen by light microscopy); and (2) to provide tissue for other diagnostic purposes, e.g. for disaccharidase assay or electron microscopy.

It must be emphasized at the outset that in paediatric practice there are many disorders other than coeliac disease which can cause an enteropathy.

INDICATIONS FOR SMALL BOWEL BIOPSY

In infancy and early childhood the most usual indication is chronic diarrhoea and failure to thrive. When an infant has had diarrhoea for more than 2 weeks with accompanying poor weight gain or weight loss then biopsy is mandatory. Without an associated failure to thrive then a small intestinal biopsy must be considered but the indications are less clear.

A very common cause of chronic diarrhoea without failure to thrive is the syndrome variously known as toddler's diarrhoea or irritable bowel syndrome of infancy (Davidson and Wasserman, 1966), where the mucosa appears normal. A biopsy would not usually be required unless circumstances (such as a family history of coeliac disease, or the presence of circulating anti-endomysial, IgA anti-gliadin or anti-reticulin antibodies) indicate that other disorders may be present. Considerable parental anxiety about the child's condition is a factor which should also be taken into consideration.

Serial small intestinal biopsies in relation to food elimination and challenge are indicated where the diagnosis of coeliac disease is being considered. Children under the age of 2 years who present with coeliac disease should undergo a gluten challenge to confirm the diagnosis before a life-long gluten-free diet is prescribed (Meeuwisse, 1970; Walker-Smith et al, 1990). The observations of Guandalini et al (1989) that coeliac disease was invariably diagnosed when a flat mucosa with crypt hyperplasia was found in children aged over 2 years, indicated that gluten provocation was not necessary in older patients. However, the diagnosis of coeliac disease must be based on the observation of an appropriately abnormal mucosa, either on gluten challenge or on presentation, and should not be made on clinical grounds alone.

Dietary challenges with cows' milk, soy formulae, or other foods associated with a transient intolerance provoking mucosal damage (and carrying the risk of an anaphylactic reaction), are no longer necessary for practical clinical diagnosis. However, such challenges were necessary to establish that these diagnoses exist (Walker-Smith et al, 1978; Vitoria et al, 1982), and may be necessary in communities where the relative importance of temporary food intolerances is debated. Depending on the local conditions and the range of diagnoses considered, a decision should be made regarding the diagnostic approach. Our experience indicates that an initial biopsy is required on presentation as it facilitates diagnosis and expedites clinical action. If it shows the characteristic features of cows' milk-sensitive enteropathy (see later) a presumptive diagnosis of food intolerance is made, and a therapeutic trial of an appropriate elimination diet is instigated which should produce a rapid clinical improvement.

Infants with intractable diarrhoea, particularly if diarrhoea begins in the first week of life, should undergo a biopsy. This can give the specific diagnosis of microvillous atrophy (Phillips et al, 1985; Phillips and Schmitz, 1992), or indicate an autoimmune (Unsworth and Walker-Smith, 1985; Mirakian et al, 1986), or idiopathic, enteropathy.

A proximal small intestinal biopsy is also important to exclude certain diagnoses. Coeliac disease is a frequently considered diagnosis in children with failure to thrive and a biopsy can confidently establish or reject the diagnosis. However, the child should be followed up (by clinical observation and antibody screening tests) in view of the report of latent coeliac disease (Mäki et al, 1990), particularly if no other cause for failure to thrive is found and the problem does not resolve spontaneously.

Although biopsy is not indicated in acute diarrhoeal disease, it is now apparent that some infections can be associated with chronic diarrhoea, e.g. giardiasis (Hjelt et al, 1992), cryptosporidiosis (Phillips et al, 1992), and enteropathogenic *E. coli* (EPEC) infections (Ulshen and Rollo, 1980; Rothbaum et al, 1982). In such circumstances biopsy and stool microbiology may provide valuable information and indicate treatment avenues, i.e. metronidazole in giardiasis; no treatment (apart from relevant management) in cryptosporidiosis unless associated with immune deficiency when passive immunization with hyperimmunized bovine colostrum may be useful (Plettenberg et al, 1993); antibiotics in EPEC infections (Hill et al, 1991).

ADJUNCTS TO SMALL INTESTINAL MUCOSAL BIOPSY

Clinical and/or laboratory data in conjunction with small intestinal biopsy help to indicate diagnoses. Examples include the presence of anti-epithelial cell antibodies in autoimmune enteropathy (Unsworth and Walker-Smith, 1985; Mirakian et al, 1986), hypoproteinaemia and lymphopenia (diagnosis of lymphangiectasia if dilated lacteals are identified; (Waldman, 1966), deficient sucrase and isomaltase activity with a normal lactase level and a normal mucosa in sucrase isomaltase deficiency (Weijers et al, 1960).

Antibody screening

Serum antibody tests (antigliadin, antireticulin, antiendomysial antibodies) provide a useful means of screening certain populations for a possible diagnosis of coeliac disease (family relatives; Corazza et al, 1992, diabetics; Barera et al, 1991, children with Down's syndrome; Castro et al, 1993, atypical Sturge–Weber syndrome; Gobbi et al, 1992). Indeed, the presence of such antibodies is an indication that a small intestinal biopsy should be carried out (Chorzelski et al, 1984; Kapuscinska et al, 1987). They are not sufficient in themselves to make the diagnosis of coeliac disease, despite their high sensitivity, as false positive results (usually in the presence of a normal mucosa (McMillan et al, 1991; Chan et al, 1994a) but also in association with an enteropathy (McMillan et al, 1991; Rossi et al, 1988)) have been reported. They may also assist in assessing whether a patient with coeliac disease is keeping to a strict gluten exclusion diet (thereby avoiding a repeat biopsy) (Valletta and Mastella, 1990) and in monitoring certain patients who have not relapsed histologically after 3 months gluten provocation (thereby predicting when a biopsy might be considered).

Gut epithelial cell antibodies are associated with the diagnosis of autoimmune enteropathy, but are not necessarily consistently positive in such cases (Phillips and Walker-Smith, 1989), and may not be identified at the onset of the illness (Unsworth et al, 1982). Thus, it is of paramount importance to establish the presence or absence of an enteropathy in cases of intractable diarrhoea where the diagnosis of autoimmune enteropathy is considered, and to repeat the gut autoantibody test at regular intervals (particularly if other autoimmune phenomena are identified). Such a finding may indicate that a trial treatment with cyclosporin A is appropriate (Bernstein and Whitington, 1988; Sanderson et al, 1991).

Breath tests

Breath tests are based on the finding that gases released from the digestion of substances in the bowel lumen can diffuse into the blood stream and be released in the breath. The timing at which the gas is detected in the breath can indicate the site of digestion, and nonmetabolized sugars which are fermented in the colon can be used to indicate mouth to caecum transit times (Rumessen, 1992). Thus lactulose, which is a nonmetabolized sugar, can be used to demonstrate small bowel overgrowth when it is rapidly fermented by luminal bacteria to give an early positive hydrogen breath test (Kerlin and Wong, 1988). Malabsorption of sugars which are normally digested and absorbed in the small intestine can be demonstrated by their fermentation in the large bowel to produce hydrogen, e.g. fructose malabsorption (Hoekstra et al, 1993) and sucrose malabsorption in sucrase isomaltase deficiency

(Perman et al, 1978). Likewise a lactose breath test can be used to demonstrate lactose malabsorption in a variety of clinical settings (Davidson et al, 1984; Pettoello et al, 1989; Miller et al, 1991).

Intestinal permeability tests

Permeability tests are based upon the appearance of various sugars in the urine following their oral ingestion as a test of small bowel integrity. Usually two sugars, of small and large relative molecular weight, are given and the result is expressed as a ratio, thereby avoiding errors arising from dilution, variable gastric emptying/transit time, etc. (Ford et al, 1985; van Elburg et al, 1992). The underlying basis of the test remains theoretical, but it is considered that the small molecular weight sugar follows an intracellular route across the epithelium, whereas the larger molecular weight sugar follows the paracellular route, between epithelial cells. Thus, when villous surface area is reduced and the epithelium is damaged, the change in the permeability ratio is thought to be due to less transcellular and greater paracellular traffic of the sugars, respectively.

Although there is a correlation between small bowel morphology and sugar permeability (Ford et al, 1985; Akinbami et al, 1989), the latter is a nonspecific assessment of the general state of the proximal intestine whereas the former gives a view of a small sample and allows specific diagnoses to be recognized. Sugar permeability has been suggested as a screening test for coeliac disease (Troncone et al, 1992) and to monitor changes in the mucosa (van Elburg et al, 1993), but there are reservations concerning its widespread use (Lifschitz and Shulman, 1990). Generally, it is agreed that such tests serve to indicate that a biopsy is required, rather than to act as its replacement (Lifschitz and Shulman, 1990; van Elburg et al, 1993), i.e. sugar permeability is a screen for enteropathy and is not specific for coeliac disease.

Stool microbiology

In all biopsy situations it is important to exclude intercurrent causes of enteropathy, e.g. acute gastrointestinal infection, particularly when there is an exacerbation of clinical symptoms (Phillips and Walker-Smith, 1986). Thus, stool microbiology forms an essential adjunct to the biopsy procedure and the presence of a bacterial or viral pathogen may indicate that a biopsy should be postponed, rather than persevered with.

Stool microbiology is certainly essential in the postenteritis syndrome (postinfectious diarrhoea), as infection may be directly responsible for the illness, either as a single infection or as repeated self-limiting illnesses which appear clinically to be one chronic episode (Phillips and Walker-Smith, 1991; Lanata et al, 1992). Thus, although bacterial and parasitic agents have been directly implicated in chronic diarrhoea (Uhnoo et al, 1986), viruses may be indirectly involved (Phillips and Walker-Smith, 1986, 1991; Lanata et al, 1986), and microbiological screening should include tests for all three classes of pathogens.

Biochemistry

Biopsy samples can be taken and snap-frozen in liquid nitrogen for disaccharidase estimation (Phillips et al, 1980). Such samples can show a generalized depression of enzyme activity which is typically secondary to gut damage (Lee, 1984) or can give the definitive diagnosis of primary sucrase-isomaltase deficiency (Weijers et al, 1960). Isolated lactase deficiency can also be shown; this can be the rare congenital form (Savilahti et al, 1983) or the more common late onset racial lactase deficiency (Simoons, 1978). However, lactase activity is more readily depressed than sucrase or maltase in enteropathies and care should be taken to exclude secondary causes.

TECHNIQUE

This chapter is concerned with the diagnostic value of small intestinal mucosal biopsy. The practicalities of clinical procedures, which will vary between centres, will not be discussed here.

Suction biopsy versus endoscopic avulsion biopsy

There has been some debate recently about the relative merits of endoscopic and suction biopsy (Kirberg et al, 1989; Granot et al, 1993). Combining the techniques has also been suggested (Sullivan et al, 1988).

In our experience suction biopsy has consistently given better preserved and larger samples. However, there are positive, and negative, attributes to each procedure and it is up to each centre to balance these out. These differences are shown in Table 1 and are discussed below.

Younger children can undergo endoscopy and biopsy if a narrow bore endoscope is used. This may allow an earlier diagnosis to be made in children with intractable diarrhoea from birth, e.g. in microvillous atrophy, although caution needs to be exercised in severely marasmic children. Endoscopy provides a macroscopic view of the oesophagus, stomach and duodenum, with the ability to biopsy each of these sites during the one procedure, usually under a general anaesthetic. Suction biopsy does not afford any view of the mucosal surface and provides one or two (Kilby, 1976) biopsy samples, from a sedated patient. The quality of the sample is superior

Table 1. Comparison of suction and endoscopic biopsy techniques.

	Suction biopsy	Endoscopic biopsy
Patient size	Weight > 3 kg (UK)	Weight > 1.8 kg (small bore)
Anaesthesia	Sedation	General anaesthetic
X-ray?	Screening	No screening
Sampling	4th part duodenum	2nd part duodenum
Biopsy technique	Suction	Avulsion
Type of biopsy	Quality	Quantity
Macroscopy	No macroscopic view	Includes gastroscopy
Cost	Low cost	High cost

by suction biopsy but taking multiple biopsies from one site via endoscopy gives sufficient quantity of tissue to overcome this drawback. Orientation of the sample(s) is still a requirement whichever procedure is used. The cost of an endoscope is at least ten-fold higher than a suction biopsy capsule. Thus, while a unit may have several biopsy capsules and there is no wait in between patients, unless two endoscopes are available there must be an enforced pause between cases while the endoscope is sterilized before reuse.

Orientation

It is important that biopsy samples, however obtained, are orientated prior to fixation so that sections are cut perpendicularly to the muscularis mucosae. Without this step a complete analysis of the tissue may not be possible. Similarly, it is prudent to cut a series of sections which will allow patchy abnormalities to be more easily appreciated and afford a view of a greater area of the mucosa so that there is a better chance of detecting the presence of organisms.

INTERPRETATION

Biopsy format and sample handling

A biopsy may form an initial investigative procedure when several diagnoses are under consideration. Alternatively a particular set of circumstances may be organized so that a limited range of diagnoses are possible, e.g. gluten challenge for coeliac disease, fat load for abetalipoproteinaemia or lymphangiectasia. It is important to consider the different diagnosis for each patient prior to the biopsy so that technical requirements for the tissue specimens can be identified and prioritized if necessary. Normally, light microscopy following formalin fixation will be performed on every occasion. Electron microscopy of glutaraldehyde fixed samples should be arranged if infection is a possibility (Kotler et al, 1990; Hill et al, 1991; Phillips and Walker-Smith, 1991; Phillips et al, 1992) and in intractable diarrhoea, particularly if microvillous atrophy is under consideration (Phillips et al, 1985; Phillips and Schmitz, 1992). Disaccharidase estimations should be performed in cases of suspected sucrase-isomaltase deficiency when unfixed, rapidly frozen samples are required (Weijers et al, 1960). Tissue samples can be handled as required following orientation, so long as the tissue is not fixed but is placed in cold, normal saline. In this way the tissue can be viewed under the dissecting microscope for a short period of time and a preliminary interpretation can be performed as well as removal of small fragments for individual tests.

Dissecting microscopy

Dissecting microscopy allows an immediate examination of the biopsy sample to be made following removal from the capsule. Orientation, gross preservation (areas of haemorrhage, trauma, autolysis, etc) and the degree of abnormality, including patchy lesions, can be assessed; dilated lacteals and lymphoid follicles also can be recognized. In addition parents can view the sample and be involved in the diagnostic procedure—this can be particularly helpful in positive gluten challenges when the need for a life-long gluten-free diet can be reinforced. However, it is important to stress to the parents that dissecting microscopy is the first stage of interpretation of the sample as there is a tendency to underestimate minor abnormalities which can be better recognized on light microscopy of stained sections of the mucosa.

The assessment of normality resides mainly in an appreciation of the height of the villi. In childhood the villi are not uniform and can appear ridge-, tongue-, leaf- and/or finger-like [Figure 1(a)]. Older children tend to have less ridge-like and more finger- and leaf-like villi.

An abnormal mucosa shows a reduction in villous height and, where lamina propria cellularity is increased, a thickening of villous width. Minor abnormalities are not readily distinguished from a normal villous pattern; mild to moderate abnormalities exhibit from short ridges (which may appear thin [Figure 1(b)] or thickened) to a low mounded surface; severe abnormalities show a loss of villous pattern, i.e. a flat mucosa [Figure 1(c)], and crypt openings are clearly visible on the mucosal surface. Intra-sample and/or inter-sample patchy abnormalities may be recognized (Manuel et al, 1979).

Light microscopy

Generally haematoxylin and eosin stained 5 μm thick sections of paraffin wax embedded tissue give sufficient detail for most diagnostic situations. Periodic acid–Schiff-stained sections are essential in intractable diarrhoea for the diagnosis of microvillous atrophy, and also give a view of goblet cell numbers and brush border staining.

The various parts of the mucosa should be studied in turn, the main aspects being: villous height, crypt depth, epithelial cell appearance, density and identity of intraepithelial cells, degree of lamina propria cellular infiltration and the cells involved, and the presence of micro-organisms.

The two-dimensional observation of villous height and crypt depth is essentially an indirect assessment of the relative size of the mature and immature cell populations, respectively. Villous height is therefore a measure of the absorptive capacity of the small intestine. Such measurements are obviously approximate, and do not take account of the third dimension which, particularly in paediatric samples (see Figure 1), is complex and variable. However, light microscopy remains an essential means of assessing the mucosal appearance.

Electron microscopy

Ideally, in the transmission electron microscope, the three regions of the mucosa are studied in turn (i.e. the epithelium, the basement membrane,

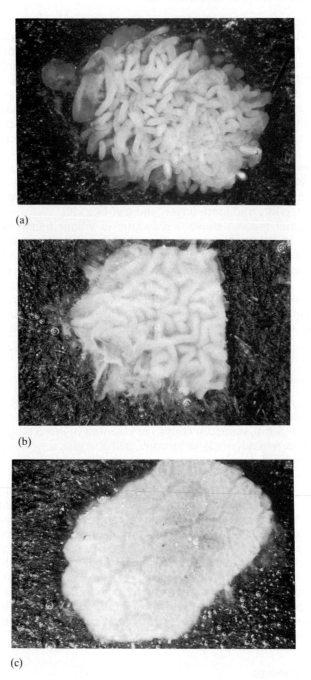

(a)

(b)

(c)

Figure 1. Dissecting microscopy. (a) Normal mucosa showing mixed appearance of ridge-like, tongue-like and finger-like villi. (b) Moderate abnormality demonstrating thin ridges. (c) Flat mucosa (all × 10).

and the lamina propria) and at all levels of the mucosa to ensure a full assessment of the sample. It is particularly important to be aware of the region of the epithelium being examined as organelle appearances can change with cell differentiation; for example, microvillous height varies over the villus and can appear short near the villous tip (Phillips et al, 1979). Scanning electron microscopy is eminently suited to the study of the mucosal surface due to its resolving capacity and to the area of sample that can be analysed. Such studies are very relevant to EPEC infections and cryptosporidiosis.

SPECIFIC DIAGNOSES

Food-related disorders

Coeliac disease

The diagnosis of coeliac disease should be a definitive diagnosis as the patient is required to accept a life-long gluten-exclusion diet. The original European Society of Paediatric Gastroenterology and Nutrition (ESPGN) criteria required three biopsies; however, more recently, the need for three biopsies in all cases has been revised by ESPGN (see earlier). In either case the diagnosis of coeliac disease is indicated in a child on a gluten-containing diet by a small intestinal biopsy showing severe crypt hyperplastic villous atrophy and an increased density of intraepithelial lymphocytes (Figure 2). The density of gamma–delta receptor positive intraepithelial lymphocytes is increased in coeliac disease (Halstensen et al, 1989). This has been suggested to be diagnostic and to remain high when the patient is on a gluten-free diet (Savilahti et al, 1990), although others have shown a fall in numbers with gluten exclusion (Spencer et al, 1991). Also, these cells can be increased in patients without coeliac disease (Chan et al, 1993), so, in common with other markers of coeliac disease such as endomysial antibodies (Chan et al, 1994a), this finding may be sensitive but it is not specific.

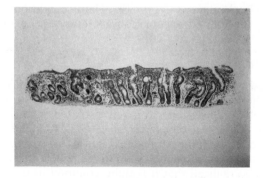

Figure 2. Severe crypt hyperplastic villous atrophy in a child with untreated coeliac disease (×20).

Cow's milk sensitive enteropathy (CMSE)

In the 1970s the enteropathy of CMSE could be as severe as that seen in coeliac disease (Kuitunen et al, 1973). More recently, with the advent of hypoallergenic adapted formulae and a greater awareness of the diagnosis, a milder lesion has been described (Verkasalo et al, 1981). It is our experience that, in the majority of cases, coeliac disease and CMSE can be discriminated on the morphological appearance of the proximal small intestinal mucosa. In CMSE the mucosa appears thinner than in coeliac disease, villous atrophy is mild to moderate, crypts appear normal or show mild hyperplasia, and intraepithelial lymphocytes are in the upper normal to mildly abnormal range (Phillips et al, 1979; Maluenda et al, 1984) (Figure 3). This appearance is similar to that seen in the postenteritis syndrome (Walker-Smith, 1982).

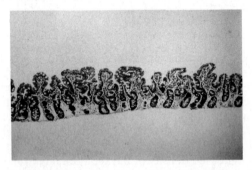

Figure 3. Mild enteropathy seen in cow's milk sensitive enteropathy (× 30).

Lipoprotein disorders (abetalipoproteinaemia, hypobetalipoproteinaemia, Anderson's disease, hypertriglyceridaemia)

In these disorders the biopsy shows an extensive vacuolation of the villous epithelium in an otherwise normal mucosa (Herbert et al, 1984; Roy et al, 1987; Bouma et al, 1988) [Figure 4(a)]. Electron microscopy may help differentiate between some of these disorders on the basis of vacuole size (Roy et al 1987; Bouma et al, 1988). These conditions should not be confused with the limited vacuolation sometimes seen in enteropathies (Variend et al, 1984) [Figure 4(b)].

Lymphangiectasia

Small intestinal biopsy is only one part of the diagnosis as it is necessary to show lymphopenia and protein loss in addition to dilated lacteals (Waldmann, 1966). The lesion may involve isolated regions of the bowel and may be easily missed on biopsy (Hart et al, 1987). For this reason the findings may be missed if the patient has been on a low fat diet and it may be necessary to stress the lymphatic system with a high fat meal prior to biopsy. It should also be realized that it is quite common to observe one or two discrete dilated lacteals on dissecting microscopy in the absence of the other diagnostic criteria, i.e. in patients without lymphangiectasia (Figure 5).

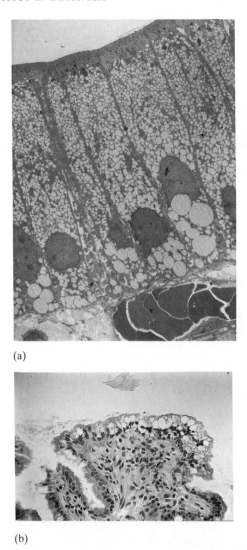

(a)

(b)

Figure 4. (a) Extensive epithelial cell vacuolation seen in abetalipoproteinaemia (×2000). Reproduced with permission from Strich et al (1993, *Journal of Pediatric Gastroenterology and Nutrition*). (b) Limited vacuolation at the villous tip as seen in CMSE and other enteropathies (×400).

Chronic diarrhoea and infection

Enteropathogenic E. coli *(EPEC)*

EPEC have been detected in association with an abnormal proximal small intestinal mucosal biopsy from children with protracted diarrhoea (Ulshen and Rollo, 1980; Rothbaum et al, 1982; Hill et al, 1991). Characteristically

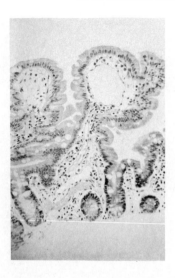

Figure 5. Dilated lacteal in a child *without* lymphangiectasia (× 85).

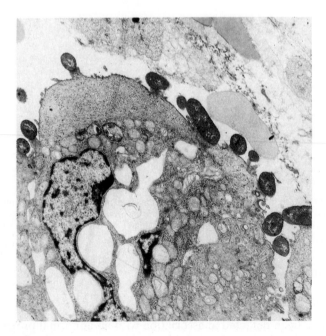

Figure 6. Attaching effacing lesion of EPEC in a child with chronic diarrhoea and failure to thrive (× 6500).

the mucosa shows moderate to severe crypt hyperplastic villous atrophy with neutrophil infiltration of the lamina propria and epithelium (Lewis et al, 1987). Surface adherent bacteria can be identified on light microscopy, but the characteristic lesion of microvillous attachment and effacement at sites of bacterial attachment is seen on transmission electron microscopy (Figure 6). This lesion is also produced by enterohaemorrhagic *E. coli* (differentiated from EPEC by verotoxin production and serotype; Tzipori et al, 1986) and *Hafnia alvei* (Albert et al, 1991). Thus stool microbiology is an important adjunct to biopsy, although non-classic *E. coli*, which would not be recognized in the stool on routine examination, are also capable of causing attachment and effacement (Knutton et al, 1991), underlining the necessity of morphological examination and of in vitro virulence tests.

Enteroaggregative E. coli *(EAggEC) and* Salmonella

Other bacterial organisms have been associated with chronic diarrhoea and failure to thrive (Nataro et al, 1987; Bhan et al, 1989; Khoshoo and Bhan, 1990) raising the possibility that they may be detected on proximal biopsy. There are no reports of the detection of *Salmonella* on small intestinal mucosal samples and a single report of a mild jejunal abnormality enteropathy in association with the presence of EAggEC in the stool (Chan et al, 1994b).

Whipple's disease

Paediatric cases of Whipple's disease are uncommon but the diagnosis can be made on proximal small intestinal biopsy by light and electron microscopy (Maizel et al, 1970).

Cryptosporidiosis

In most immunocompetent individuals *Cryptosporidium* is associated with a self-limiting illness. However, it has also been identified in the stools and mucosa of children with chronic diarrhoea in the absence of overt immunodeficiency, and should form part of the differential diagnosis of chronic diarrhoea with failure to thrive in early childhood (McFarlane and Horner-Bryce, 1987; Sallon et al, 1988; Phillips et al, 1992). In such cases there is no effective treatment although the parasite eventually clears spontaneously. The mucosa shows a mild to moderate crypt hyperplastic villous atrophy [Figure 7(a)], disaccharidase depression, and a variable increase in intraepithelial lymphocyte density (Phillips et al, 1992). Cryptosporidium can be identified on the surface of upper villous epithelium as small basophilic bodies, or more readily by scanning [Figure 7(b)] or transmission electron microscopy (Booth et al, 1980; Kocoshis et al, 1984; Phillips et al, 1992). Cryptosporidiosis has a poor prognosis in immunodeficient patients (Booth et al, 1980; Kocoshis et al, 1984).

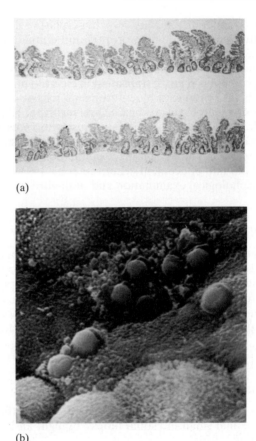

(a)

(b)

Figure 7. (a) Enteropathy seen in a child with cryptosporidiosis ($\times 20$). (b) SEM of adhering *Cryptosporidium* ($\times 2000$).

Giardiasis

It is important to be aware of the diagnosis of giardiasis as it is a treatable infection. Although the clinical picture in giardiasis is variable, ranging from no symptoms to frank malabsorption, the organism has satisfied Koch's postulates as a cause of diarrhoea (Nash et al, 1987), and is associated with failure to thrive and chronic diarrhoea in Europe (Hjelt el al, 1992). *Giardia lamblia* trophozoites are also associated with a variable appearance of the mucosa, minimally by an increase in lamina propria plasma cell infiltration, more often accompanied by mild villous atrophy, and unusually with a moderate to severe crypt hyperplastic villous atrophy which can suggest the diagnosis of coeliac disease. In such a situation antigiardial treatment should be administered first and if the clinical and/or morphological response is not satisfactory then a trial of a gluten exclusion diet should be instigated. The organism can be identified between villi on light and transmission electron microscopy or on the surface and in mucus in the scanning electron microscope.

Cyclospora species

Recent reports have implicated Cyclospora species as a cause of chronic diarrhoea, particularly amongst travellers. It has been found in stools and in proximal small intestinal biopsies implicating the small intestine as a site of infection (Bendall et al, 1993). It is another infective diagnosis to be aware of when interpreting biopsy appearances.

Intractable diarrhoea

Intractable diarrhoea comprises cases of chronic diarrhoea with failure to thrive which persist, and there is no effective treatment. Proximal small intestinal biopsy is useful in this area because it can divide cases into those associated with an enteropathy and those which are not. Intractable diarrhoea from the neonatal period and a normal mucosa would indicate such problems as glucose–galactose malabsorption, chloride diarrhoea, VIP (vasoactive intestinal peptide)-oma, sucrase–isomaltase deficiency, etc. Some of these diagnoses can be established before a biopsy is performed.

If an enteropathy is found then a diagnosis may be made, e.g. auto-immune enteropathy and microvillous atrophy, or cases may remain idiopathic. Total or partial parenteral nutrition is usually required for nutritional support. A recent approach has been to divide patients with an enteropathy and intractable diarrhoea into those in which the immune system appears to be involved and those which appear to have a disorder of epithelial cell differentiation and/or maturation (Cuenod et al, 1990). Thus small intestinal biopsy is affording some means of subdividing this syndrome which may prove fruitful in understanding the pathogenesis of these rare and exceedingly difficult cases.

Microvillous atrophy

The first case of microvillous atrophy was described by Davidson et al (1978) under the general term of familial enteropathy. Characteristic features of the diagnosis were described (Phillips et al, 1985) and two series have been reported (Cutz et al, 1989; Phillips and Schmitz, 1992), with clinical and morphological variants being recognized (Carruthers et al, 1986; Phillips and Schmitz, 1992).

Moderate to severe villous atrophy is seen, usually without severe crypt hyperplastic villous atrophy, producing a thin mucosa (Phillips and Schmitz, 1992). Periodic acid–Schiff (PAS) staining shows an abnormal accumulation of stain in the apical cytoplasm of upper crypt and low villous epithelium, and transmission electron microscopy demonstrates an increased presence of 'secretory granules' and the finding of microvillous inclusions within the cytoplasm of upper villous epithelium (Phillips et al, 1985; Phillips and Schmitz, 1992) (Figure 8). It must be emphasized that the PAS staining

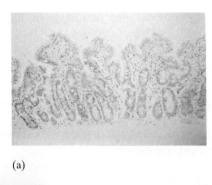

(a)

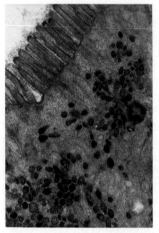

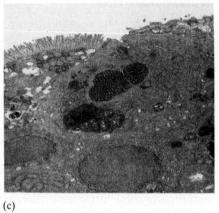

(c)

(b)

Figure 8. Microvillous atrophy. (a) Enteropathy typical of this disorder (×55). (b) Increased presence of secretory granules in upper crypt epithelium (×15 000). (c) Microvillous inclusion (×5000).

abnormality and the microvillous inclusions are different phenomena. The former corresponding in position to the increase in 'secretory granules' (Phillips and Schmitz, 1992), and representing the first abnormality which is seen in the life cycle of the epithelial cell. The PAS staining abnormality affords the possibility of a retrospective diagnosis (Phillips and Schmitz, 1992).

Most patients present in the first week of life, whereas a minority present as 'late onset' cases and may appear clinically as the postenteritis syndrome (Carruthers et al, 1986; Phillips and Schmitz, 1992).

Autoimmune enteropathy

Patients with autoimmune enteropathy tend to present later than other cases of intractable diarrhoea with an enteropathy. The appearance of the mucosa is variable but in cases with extra-gastrointestinal symptoms of autoimmunity it generally shows moderate to severe crypt hyperplastic villous atrophy, with an obviously increased lamina propria cellularity. Some patients have shown a similar lesion to patients with untreated coeliac disease (Unsworth et al, 1982; Mitton et al, 1989) and the diagnosis may be made when no response is shown to a gluten-free diet and gut autoantibodies are detected. The role of the epithelial cell autoantibody in the pathogenesis of the disorder is unclear. Activated T cells have been identified in the lamina propria (Cuenod et al, 1990; Sanderson et al, 1991) and some patients have responded to cyclosporin A therapy (Sanderson et al, 1991). Other patients have resolved spontaneously (Savage et al, 1985).

Idiopathic enteropathy

Small intestinal biopsy serves to demonstrate an enteropathy in these patients but, as yet, does not allow any definitive diagnoses to be made. More research is needed to help unravel the pathogenetic mechanisms involved.

Immune deficiency

Patients with agammaglobulinaemia show an absence of plasma cells in the lamina propria, those with hypogammaglobulinaemia a marked reduction (Lee and Toner, 1980).

Acquired immunodeficiency syndrome (AIDS)

Reports of small intestinal mucosal appearance in AIDS have largely concerned adult patients. The main role of small intestinal biopsy has centred on the diagnosis of opportunistic and/or occult infections (Ullrich et al, 1989; Greenson et al, 1991) and the investigation of HIV-associated enteropathy (Anonymous, 1989; Cummins et al, 1990; Heise et al, 1991). Several studies have suggested the importance of microsporidiosis (Orenstein et al, 1990; Peacock et al, 1991), and in particular the microsporidian, *Enterocytozoon bieneusi* as a cause of diarrhoea (Canning and Hollister, 1990; Orenstein et al, 1992). Electron microscopy of jejunal biopsies may be necessary for the definitive diagnosis of microsporidiosis (Orenstein et al, 1990), although experienced observers can make the diagnosis on light microscopy (Peacock et al, 1991). The site of infection is considered to be the duodeno–jejunal region of the intestine (Orenstein et al, 1992).

It appears most likely that these observations are relevant to paediatric cases of AIDS.

REFERENCES

Akinbami FO, Brown GA & McNeish AS (1989) Intestinal permeability as a measure of small intestinal mucosal integrity: correlation with jejunal biopsy. *African Journal of Medical Science* **18:** 187–192.

Albert MJ, Alam K, Islam M et al (1991) *Hafnia alvei*, a probable cause of diarrhea in humans. *Infection and Immunity* **59:** 1507–1513.

Anonymous (1989) HIV-associated enteropathy. *Lancet* **ii:** 777–778.

Barera G, Bianchi C, Calisti L et al (1991) Screening of diabetic children for coeliac disease with antigliadin antibodies and HLA typing. *Archives of Disease in Childhood* **66:** 491–494.

Bendall RP, Lucas S, Moody A et al (1993) Diarrhoea associated with cyanobacterium-like bodies: a new coccidian enteritis of man. *Lancet* **341:** 590–592.

Bernstein EF & Whitington PF (1988) Successful treatment of atypical sprue in an infant with cyclosporine. *Gastroenterology* **95:** 199–204.

Bhan MK, Raj P, Levine MM et al (1989) Enteroaggregative *E coli* associated with persistent diarrhoea in a cohort of rural children in India. *Journal of Infectious Disease* **159:** 1061–1064.

Booth CC, Slavin G, Dourmashkin R et al (1980) Immunodeficiency and cryptosporidiosis. *British Medical Journal* **281:** 1123–1127.

Bouma ME, Infante R, Jos J & Schmitz J (1988) Chylomicron retention disease. *Gastroenterology* **94:** 554–556.

Canning EU & Hollister WS (1990) Enterocytozoon bieneusi (Microspora): prevalence and pathogenicity in AIDS patients. *Transactions of the Royal Society of Tropical Medicine and Hygiene* **84:** 181–186.

Carruthers L, Dourmashkin R & Phillips AD (1986) Disorders of the cytoskeleton of the enterocyte. *Clinics in Gastroenterology* **15:** 105–120.

Castro M, Crino A, Papadatou B et al (1993) Down's syndrome and celiac disease: the prevalence of high IgA-antigliadin antibodies and HLA-DR and DQ antigens in trisomy 21. *Journal of Pediatric Gastroenterology and Nutrition* **16:** 265–268.

Chan KN, Phillips AD, Walker-Smith JA et al (1993) Density of γ/δ T cells in small bowel mucosa related to HLA-DQ status without coeliac disease. *Lancet* **342:** 492–493.

Chan KN, Phillips AD, Mirakian R & Walker-Smith JA (1994a) Endomysial antibody screening in children. *Journal of Pediatric Gastroenterology and Nutrition* **18:** 316–320.

Chan KN, Phillips AD, Knutton S et al (1994b) Enteroaggregative *E coli*: another cause of acute and chronic diarrhoea in England. *Journal of Pediatric Gastroenterology and Nutrition* **18:** 87–92.

Chorzelski TP, Beutner EH, Sulej J et al (1984) IgA antiendomysial antibody. A new immunological marker for dermatitis herpetiformis and coeliac disease. *British Journal of Dermatology* **111:** 395–402.

Corazza G, Valentini RA, Frisoni M et al (1992) Gliadin immune reactivity is associated with overt and latent enteropathy in relatives of celiac patients. *Gastroenterology* **103:** 1517–1522.

Cuenod B, Brousse N, Goulet O et al (1990) Classification of intractable diarrhoea in infancy using clinical and immunohistological criteria. *Gastroenterology* **99:** 1037–1043.

Cummins AG, LaBrooy JT, Stanley DP et al (1990) Quantitative histological study of enteropathy associated with HIV infection. *Gut* **31:** 317–321.

Cutz E, Rhoads JM, Drumm B et al (1989) Microvillous inclusion disease. *New England Journal of Medicine* **320:** 646–651.

Davidson M & Wasserman R (1966) The irritable colon of childhood (chronic non-specific diarrhoea syndrome). *Journal of Pediatrics* **69:** 1027–1038.

Davidson GP, Cutz E, Hamilton JR & Gall DG (1978) Familial enteropathy: a syndrome of protracted diarrhoea from birth, failure to thrive, and hypoplastic villous atrophy. *Gastroenterology* **75:** 783–790.

Davidson GP, Goodwin D & Robb TA (1984) Incidence and duration of lactose malabsorption in children hospitalized with acute enteritis: Study in a well nourished urban population. *Journal of Pediatrics* **105:** 587–590.

Ford RPK, Menzies IS, Phillips AD et al (1985) Intestinal sugar permeability: relationship to diarrhoeal disease and small bowel morphology. *Journal of Pediatric Gastroenterology and Nutrition* **4:** 568–574.

Gobbi G, Bouquet F, Greco L et al (1992) Coeliac disease, epilepsy, and cerebral calcifications. The Italian Working Group on Coeliac Disease and Epilepsy. *Lancet* **340:** 439–443.

Granot E, Goodman-Weill M, Pizov G & Sherman Y (1993) Histological comparison of suction capsule and endoscopic small intestinal mucosal biopsies in children. *Journal of Paediatric Gastroenterology and Nutrition* **16:** 397–401.

Greenson JK, Belitsos PC, Yardley JH & Bartlett JG (1991) AIDS enteropathy: occult enteric infections and duodenal mucosal alterations in chronic diarrhea. *Annals of International Medicine* 114: 366–372.

Guandalini S, Ventura A, Ansald N et al (1989) Diagnosis of coeliac disease: time for a change? *Archives of Disease in Childhood* 64: 1320–1325.

Halstensen TS, Scott H & Brandtzaeg P (1989) Intraepithelial T cells of the Tcr γδ+, CD8−, Vδ/Jδ+ phenotypes are increased in coeliac disease. *Scandinavian Journal of Immunology* 30: 665–672.

Hart MH, Vanderhoof JA & Antonson DL (1987) Failure of blind small bowel biopsy in the diagnosis of intestinal lymphangiectasia. *Journal of Pediatric Gastroenterology and Nutrition* 6: 803–805.

Heise C, Dandekar S, Kumar P et al (1991) Human immunodeficiency virus infection of enterocytes and mononuclear cells in human jejunal mucosa. *Gastroenterology* 100: 1521–1527.

Herbert PN, Assmann G, Gotto AM Jr & Fredrikson DS (1984) Familial lipoprotein deficiency: abetalipoproteinaemia, hypobetalipoproteinaemia, and Tangier disease. In JB Stanbury, JB Wyngaarden, DS Fredrikson et al (eds) *The Metabolic Basis of Inherited Disease* p 589, 5th edn. New York: McGraw-Hill.

Hill SM, Phillips AD & Walker-Smith JA (1991) Enteropathogenic *Escherichia coli* and life threatening chronic diarrhoea. *Gut* 32: 154–158.

Hjelt K, Paerregaard A & Krasilnikoff PA (1992) Giardiasis causing chronic diarrhoea in suburban Copenhagen: incidence, physical growth, clinical symptoms and small intestinal abnormality. *Acta Paediatrica* 81: 881–886.

Hoekstra JH, van Kempen AA & Kneepkens CM (1993) Apple juice malabsorption: fructose or sorbitol? *Journal of Pediatric Gastroenterology and Nutrition* 16: 39–42.

Kapuscinska A, Zalewski T, Chorzelski TP et al (1987) Disease specificity and dynamics of changes in IgA class anti-endomysial antibodies in celiac disease. *Journal of Pediatric Gastroenterology and Nutrition* 6: 529–534.

Kerlin P & Wong L (1988) Breath hydrogen testing in bacterial overgrowth of the small intestine. *Gastroenterology* 95: 982–988.

Khoshoo V & Bhan AK (1990) Associated factors of protracted diarrhoea. *Indian Paediatrics* 27: 559–569.

Kilby A (1976) Paediatric small intestinal biopsy capsule with two ports. *Gut* 17: 158–159.

Kirberg A, Lattore JJ & Hattard ME (1989) Endoscopic small intestinal biopsy in infants and children: its usefulness in the diagnosis of coeliac disease and other enteropathies. *Journal of Paediatric Gastroenterology and Nutrition* 9: 178–181.

Knutton S, Phillips AD, Smith HR et al (1991) Screening for enteropathogenic *E coli* in infants with diarrhoea. *Infection and Immunity* 59: 365–371.

Kocoshis SA, Cibull ML, Davis TE et al (1984) Intestinal and pulmonary cryptosporidiosis in an infant with severe combined immunodeficiency. *Journal of Pediatric Gastroenterology and Nutrition* 3: 149–157.

Kotler DP, Francisco A, Clayton F et al (1990) Small intestinal injury and parasitic diseases in AIDS. *Annals of International Medicine* 113: 444–449.

Kuitunen P, Rapola J, Savilahti E & Visakorpi JKV (1973) Response of the jejunal mucosa to cow's milk in the malabsorption syndrome with cow's milk intolerance. *Acta Paediatrica Scandinavica* 62: 585–595.

Lanata CF, Black RE, Maurtua D et al (1992) Aetiologic agents in acute vs persistent diarrhoea in children under three years of age in peri-urban Lima, Peru. *Acta Paediatrica* 81 (supplement): 32–38.

Lee PC (1984) Transient carbohydrate malabsorption and intolerance in diarrhoeal diseases in infancy. In Lebenthal E (ed.) *Chronic Diarrhoea in Children*, pp 149–162, Nestle Nutrition Workshop Series vol. 6. New York: Raven Press.

Lee FD & Toner PG (1980) Biopsy pathology of the small intestine. *Biopsy Pathology Series* 111–112.

Lewis DC, Walker-Smith JA & Phillips AD (1987) Polymorphonuclear neutrophil leucocytes in childhood Crohn's disease: a morphological study. *Journal of Pediatric Gastroenterology and Nutrition* 6: 430–438.

Lifschitz CH & Shulman RJ (1990) Intestinal permeability tests: are they clinically useful? *Journal of Pediatric Gastroenterology and Nutrition* 10: 283–287.

McFarlane DE & Horner-Bryce J (1987) Cryptosporidiosis in well nourished and malnourished children. *Acta Paediatrica Scandinavica* **76**: 474–477.

McMillan S, Haughton DJ, Biggart JD et al (1991) Predictive value for coeliac disease of antibodies to gliadin, endomysium, and jejunum in patients attending for jejunal biopsy. *British Medical Journal* **303**: 1163–1165.

Maizel H, Ruffin JM & Dobbins WO (1970) Whipple's disease: a review of 19 patients from one hospital and a review of the literature since 1950. *Medicine (Balt)* **49**: 175–205.

Mäki M, Holm K, Koskimies S et al (1990) Normal small bowel biopsy followed by coeliac disease. *Archives of Disease in Childhood* **65**: 1137–1141.

Maluenda C, Phillips AD, Briddon A & Walker-Smith JA (1984) Quantitative analysis of small intestinal mucosa in cow's milk sensitive enteropathy. *Journal of Pediatric Gastroenterology and Nutrition* **3**: 349–356.

Manuel PD, Walker-Smith JA & France NE (1979) Patchy enteropathy. *Gut* **20**: 211–215.

Meeuwisse GW (1970) Diagnostic criteria in coeliac disease. *Acta Paediatrica Scandinavica* **59**: 461–463.

Miller TL, Orav EJ, Martin SR et al (1991) Malnutrition and carbohydrate malabsorption in children with vertically transmitted human immunodeficiency virus 1 infection. *Gastroenterology* **100**: 1296–1302.

Mirakian R, Richardson A, Milla PJ et al (1986) Protracted diarrhoea of infancy: evidence of an autoimmune variant. *British Medical Journal* **293**: 1132–1136.

Mitton SG, Mirakian R, Larcher VF et al (1989) Enteropathy and renal involvement in an infant with evidence of widespread autoimmune disturbance. *Journal of Pediatric Gastroenterology and Nutrition* **8**: 397–400.

Nash TE, Herrington DA, Losonsky GA & Levine MM (1987) Experimental human infections with *Giadia lamblia*. *Journal of Infectious Disease* **156**: 974–984.

Nataro JP, Kaper JB, Robins-Browne R et al (1987) Patterns of adherence of diarrheagenic Escherichia coli to HEp-2 cells. *Pediatric Infectious Disease* **6**: 829–831.

Orenstein JM, Chiang J, Steinberg W et al (1990) Intestinal microsporidiosis as a cause of diarrhoea in human immunodeficiency virus-infected patients: a report of 20 cases. *Human Pathology* **21**: 475–481.

Orenstein JM, Tenner M & Kotler DP (1992) Localization of infection by the microsporidian Enterocytozoon bieneusi in the gastrointestinal tract of AIDS patients with diarrhea. *AIDS* **6**: 195–197.

Peacock CS, Blanshard C, Tovey DG et al (1991) Histological diagnosis of intestinal microsporidiosis in patients with AIDS. *Journal of Clinical Pathology* **44**: 558–563.

Perman JA, Barr RG & Watkins JB (1978) Sucrose malabsorption in children: non-invasive diagnosis by interval breath hydrogen determination. *Pediatrics* **93**: 17–22.

Pettoello Mantovani M, Guandalini S, Ecuba P et al (1989) Lactose malabsorption in children with symptomatic *Giardia lamblia* infection: feasibility of yogurt supplementation. *Journal of Pediatric Gastroenterology and Nutrition* **9**: 295–300.

Phillips AD & Schmitz J (1992) Microvillous atrophy: a clinico-pathological survey of twenty-three cases. *Journal of Pediatric Gastroenterology and Nutrition* **14**: 380–396.

Phillips AD & Walker-Smith JA (1986) Delayed Recovery in Childhood. In: Walker-Smith JA, McNeish AS (eds) pp 107–112. London: Butterworths.

Phillips AD & Walker-Smith JA (1989) *Proximal small intestinal mucosal morphology in relation to gut epithelial autoantibodies in children with 'autoimmune enteropathy'*. Proceedings of 1st Joint Meeting of British and Italian Paediatric Gastroenterology Societies 19–20.

Phillips AD & Walker-Smith JA (1991) The postenteritis syndrome: opening the box. *Journal of Paediatric Gastroenterology and Nutrition* **13**: 328.

Phillips AD, France NE & Walker-Smith JA (1979) The structure of the enterocyte in relation to its position on the villus: an electron microscopical study. *Histopathology* **3**: 117–130.

Phillips AD, Rice SJ, France NE & Walker-Smith JA (1979) Small intestinal intraepithelial lymphocytes in cow's milk protein intolerance. *Gut* **20**: 509–512.

Phillips AD, Avigad S, Sacks J et al (1980) Microvillous surface area in secondary disacchari-dase deficiency. *Gut* **21**: 44–48.

Phillips AD, Jenkins P, Raafat F & Walker-Smith JA (1985) Congenital microvillous atrophy: specific diagnostic features. *Archives of Disease in Childhood* **60**: 135–140.

Phillips AD, Thomas AG & Walker-Smith JA (1992) Cryptosporidiosis, chronic diarrhoea and the proximal small intestinal mucosa. *Gut* **33**: 1057–1061.

Plettenberg A, Stoehr A, Stellbrink HJ et al (1993) A preparation from bovine colostrum in the treatment of HIV-positive patients with chronic diarrhoea. *Clinical Investigation* **71:** 42–45.

Rossi TM, Kumar V, Lerner A et al (1988) Relationship of endomysial antibodies to jejunal mucosal pathology: specificity towards both symptomatic and asymptomatic celiacs. *Journal of Pediatric Gastroenterology and Nutrition* **7:** 858–863.

Rothbaum R, McAdams AJ, Gianella RA & Partin JC (1982) A clinicopathologic study of enterocyte adherent *Escherichia coli:* a cause of protracted diarrhoea in infants. *Gastroenterology* **83:** 441–454.

Roy CC, Levy EL, Green PHR et al (1987) Malabsorption, hypocholesterolemia, and fat-filled enterocytes with increase intestinal apoprotein B. Chylomicron retention disease. *Gastroenterology* **92:** 390–399.

Rumessen JJ (1992) Hydrogen and methane breath tests for evaluation of resistant carbohydrates. *European Journal of Clinical Nutrition* **46 (supplement 2):** S77–90.

Sallon S, Deckelbaum RJ, Schmid II et al (1988) *Cryptosporidium*, malnutrition, and chronic diarrhoea in children. *American Journal of Diseases of Children* **142:** 312–315.

Sanderson IR, Phillips AD, Spencer J & Walker-Smith JA (1991) Response of autoimmune enteropathy to Cyclosporin A therapy. *Gut* **32:** 1421–1425.

Savage M, Mirakian R, Wozniac ER et al (1985) Specific autoantibodies to gut epithelium in two infants with severe protracted diarrhoea. *Journal of Pediatric Gastroenterology and Nutrition* **4:** 187–195.

Savilahti E, Launiala K & Kuitunen P (1983) Congenital lactase deficiency. A clinical study on 16 infants. *Archives of Disease in Childhood* **58:** 246–252.

Savilahti E, Arato A & Verkasalo M (1990) Intestinal γ/δ receptor bearing T lymphocytes in coeliac disease and inflammatory bowel diseases in children. Constant increase in coeliac disease. *Pediatric Research* **28:** 579–582.

Simoons FJ (1978) The geographic hypothesis and lactose malabsorption. A weighing of the evidence. *Digestive Disease.* **23:** 963–980.

Spencer J, Isaacson PG, MacDonald TT et al (1991) Gamma/delta T cells and the diagnosis of coeliac disease. *Clinical and Experimental Immunology* **85:** 109–113.

Strich D, Goldstein R, Phillips A et al (1993) Anderson's disease: no linkage to the apo B locus. *Journal of Pediatric Gastroenterology and Nutrition* **16:** 257–264.

Sullivan PB, Phillips MB & Neale G (1988) Endoscopic capsule biopsy of the small intestine. *Journal of Paediatric Gastroenterology and Nutrition* **8:** 276–277.

Troncone R, Starita A, Coletta S et al (1992) Antigliadin antibody, D-xylose, and cellobiose/mannitol permeability tests as indicators of mucosal damage in children with coeliac disease. *Scandinavian Journal of Gastroenterology* **27:** 703–706.

Tzipori S, Wachsmuth IK, Chapman C et al (1986) The pathogenesis of haemorrhagic colitis caused by Escherichia coli O157:H7 in gnotobiotic piglets. *Journal of Infectious Disease* **154:** 712–716.

Uhnoo I, Olding-Stenkvist E & Kreuger A (1986) Clinical features of acute gastroenteritis associated with rotavirus, enteric adenoviruses, and bacteria. *Archives of Disease in Childhood* **61:** 732–738.

Ullrich R, Zeitz M, Heise W et al (1989) Small intestinal structure and function in patients infected with human immunodeficiency virus (HIV): evidence for HIV-induced enteropathy. *Annals of International Medicine* **111:** 15–21.

Ulshen MH & Rollo JL (1980) Pathogenesis of *Escherichia coli* gastroenteritis in man: another mechanism. *New England Journal of Medicine* **302:** 99–101.

Unsworth DJ & Walker-Smith JA (1985) Autoimmunity in diarrhoeal disease. *Journal of Pediatric Gastroenterology and Nutrition* **4:** 375–380.

Unsworth J, Hutchins P, Mitchell J et al (1982) Flat small intestinal mucosa and autoantibodies against gut epithelium. *Journal of Pediatric Gastroenterology and Nutrition* **1:** 503–513.

Valletta EA & Mastella G (1990) Adherence to gluten-free diet and serum antigliadin antibodies in celiac disease. *Digestion* **47:** 20–31.

van Elburg RM, Uil JJ, de Monchy JG & Heymans HS (1992) Intestinal permeability in pediatric gastroenterology. *Scandinavian Journal of Gastroenterology* **194 (supplement):** 19–24.

van Elburg RM, Uil JJ, Mulder CJ & Heymans HS (1993) Intestinal permeability in patients with coeliac disease and relatives of patients with coeliac disease. *Gut* **34:** 354–357.

Variend S, Placzek M, Raafat F & Walker-Smith JA (1984) Small intestinal mucosal fat in childhood enteropathies. *Journal of Clinical Pathology* **37:** 373–377.

Verkasalo M, Kuitunen P, Savilahti E & Tillikainen A (1981) Changing pattern of cow's milk intolerance. *Acta Paediatrica Scandinavica* **70:** 289–295.

Vitoria JC, Camarero C, Sojo A et al (1982) Enteropathy related to fish, rice and chicken. *Archives of Disease in Childhood* **57:** 44–48.

Waldmann TA (1966) Protein losing enteropathy. *Gastroenterology* **50:** 422–443.

Walker-Smith JA (1982) Cow's milk intolerance as a cause of postenteritis diarrhoea. *Journal of Pediatric Gastroenterology and Nutrition* **1:** 163–173.

Walker-Smith JA, Harrison M, Kilby A et al (1978) Cow's milk sensitive enteropathy. *Archives of Disease in Childhood* **53:** 375–380.

Walker-Smith JA, Gaundalini S, Schmitz J et al (1990) Revised criteria for diagnosis of coeliac disease. *Archives of Disease in Childhood* **65:** 909–911.

Weijers HA, van de Kramer JH, Mossel DAA & Dicke WK (1960) Diarrhoea caused by deficiency of sugar splitting enzymes. *Lancet* **ii:** 296–297.

4

When to transplant the liver in children

DEIRDRE A. KELLY

The rapid development of paediatric liver transplantation in the 1980s has radically changed the prognosis for many babies and children dying of end-stage liver failure and is now accepted therapy for this condition (Table 1).

Liver transplantation was first attempted in the USA and Europe in 1963 but the first successful transplant was not performed until 1967 in a young girl with a hepatic tumour. Although there were rapid advances in adult transplantation throughout the 1970s, particularly after the introduction of cyclosporin A in 1978 (Starzl et al, 1982), paediatric liver transplantation remained hazardous due to technical difficulties and donor shortages. By 1986, most adult units reported 80% 1-year survival rates, while average 1-year survival in children was only 60% (Shaw et al, 1989). Since that time, there have been considerable advances in both medical and surgical management and international 1-year survival rates for paediatric liver transplantation are now between 85 and 90% (Broelsch et al, 1990; Salt et al, 1992). Of particular relevance to successful paediatric transplantation is the development of reduction hepatectomy (Bismuth and Houssin, 1984; Badger et al, 1992). This innovative surgical technique has not only increased the number of donor grafts suitable for children, especially young babies, but has dramatically reduced the deaths on the waiting list (Langnas et al, 1992). In some centres, living related donor grafts are replacing reduction hepatectomies (Heffron et al, 1993; Rogiers et al, 1993; Katz et al, 1993) in order to overcome the donor shortages.

As the numbers of children receiving transplants has increased so has experience in the perioperative management. By 1990 over 1000 children had receiver liver grafts in the USA (Alexandria, 1990) with a similar number transplanted in Europe by the end of 1991 (European Liver Transplant Registry, 1992). In Europe, 40% of transplants were performed in children under 2 years; 50% in children 2–12 years and 10% in children 12–15 years.

The consequent improvement in survival rates has extended the range of indications for liver transplantation in children from terminally ill, high risk patients, to include semi-elective liver replacement and transplantation for metabolic liver disease.

Despite the recent success of liver transplantation, it remains an expensive procedure with enormous resource implications and an appreciable mortality, thus, careful consideration should be given to the selection of potential recipients.

Table 1. Indications for liver transplantation in children.

I   Chronic liver failure
Neonatal liver disease
  Biliary atresia
  Idiopathic neonatal hepatitis
Inherited metabolic liver disease
  α_1-antitrypsin deficiency
  Cystic fibrosis
  Glycogen storage type I
  Tyrosinaemia type I
  Wilson's disease
Cholestatic liver disease
  Alagille syndrome
  Byler's disease
  Non-syndromic biliary hypoplasia
Chronic hepatitis
  Autoimmune
  Idiopathic
  Post viral (hepatitis B, C, other)
Other
  Cryptogenic cirrhosis
  Fibropolycystic liver disease +/- Caroli syndrome

II   Acute liver failure
Fulminant hepatitis
  Autoimmune
  Halothane exposure
  Paracetamol poisoning
  Viral hepatitis (A, B, C, other)
Metabolic liver disease
  Fatty acid oxidation defects (e.g. Reye's syndrome)
  Galactosaemia
  Neonatal haemochromatosis
  Tyrosinaemia type I
  Wilson's disease

III   Inborn errors of metabolism
  Crigler–Najjar type I
  Familial hypercholesterolaemia
  Primary oxalosis
  Propionic acidaemia
  Urea cycle defects

IV   Liver tumours
  Benign tumours
  Hepatic tumours secondary to
    tyrosinaemia
    α_1-antitrypsin
    glycogen storage type I
    hepatitis B
  Unresectable malignant tumours

INDICATIONS FOR LIVER TRANSPLANTATION

Liver transplantation is now accepted therapy for acute or chronic liver failure. Transplantation for hepatic enzyme deficiency without liver failure is more controversial as is transplantation for hepatic malignancy.

In making the decision to recommend transplantation, the mortality and morbidity of the underlying disease should be compared to the risk of the operation and its complications including life-long immunosuppression.

Chronic liver disease

Chronic liver failure is the commonest indication for transplantation in children (Figure 1) and may arise from neonatal liver disease, including biliary atresia; inherited metabolic liver disease, of which α_1-antitrypsin deficiency is the commonest indication; familial cholestatic syndromes, e.g. Alagille syndrome and Byler's disease; chronic hepatitis with cirrhosis and less commonly from fibropolycystic liver disease or cystic fibrosis (Table 1).

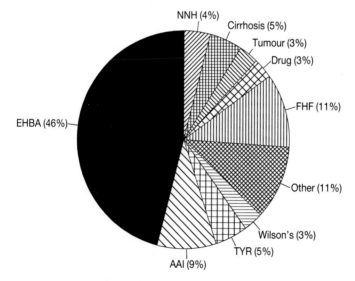

Figure 1. Diagnosis at liver transplantation in 113 children (Paediatric Liver Programme, Birmingham 1982–1992).
Key: AA1—α_1-antitrypsin deficiency; EHBA—extrahepatic biliary atresia; FHF—fulminant hepatic failure; TYR—tyrosinaemia.

Neonatal liver disease

Biliary atresia is the commonest indication for liver transplantation in childhood accounting for 70% of children transplanted under the age of 2 years (European Liver Transplant Registry, 1992). Although palliative surgery (Kasai portoenterostomy) may improve the initial outcome (Ohi et al, 1990), in practice, few children are referred early enough for this surgery to be effective (Hussain et al, 1991a) and urgent transplantation is indicated in those children who do not achieve bile drainage following Kasai porto-enterostomy (Beath et al, 1993a,b).

α_1-antitrypsin deficiency (phenotype protease inhibitor ZZ) is a frequent cause of neonatal cholestasis but although 50–70% of children will develop persistent liver disease progressing to cirrhosis, only 25% will require transplantation in childhood (Hussain et al, 1991b).

The outcome of Alagille syndrome and other cholestatic liver diseases originating in infancy is variable. Liver transplantation may be indicated because of the development of cirrhosis and portal hypertension, but also to alleviate intractable pruritus, unresponsive to maximum medical therapy or biliary diversion, or the development of severe hypercholesterolaemia and xanthomata (Whitington and Balisteri, 1991; Tzakis et al, 1993a).

Liver disease in children over 2 years

The main indications for transplantation in older children include metabolic liver disease (22%) and cirrhosis secondary to biliary atresia (35%) (European Liver Transplant Registry, 1992).

Tyrosinaemia type I. In this autosomal recessive disorder, tyrosine and methionine accumulate secondary to a deficiency of the hepatic enzyme fumaryl acetoacetase. The disease may present acutely in the neonate or with chronic liver failure in the older child. Hepatocellular carcinoma is an inevitable development and until recently transplantation was indicated either to treat hepatic failure or to prevent hepatic malignancy (Esquivel et al, 1989; Sokol et al, 1992). It is difficult to predict when hepatic malignancy may develop, but a rise in serum α-fetoprotein level, or the appearance of hepatic nodularity on ultrasound examination or at CT scan, or the detection of hepatic dysplasia on liver histology may be appropriate indications (Burdelski et al, 1991). However, the recent discovery of a chemical 2-(2-nitro-4-trifluoro-methyl benzoyl)-1,3-cyclo hexanedione (NTBC), which prevents the formation of toxic metabolites in tyrosinaemia and produces rapid clinical improvement may not only alter the natural history of this disease, but the future indications for transplantation (Lindstedt et al, 1992).

Wilson's disease. This autosomal recessive disorder of copper metabolism is rarely diagnosed in children under the age of 3 years but may present with either acute or chronic liver failure. Liver replacement is appropriate if cirrhosis and portal hypertension are present at diagnosis or if liver disease progresses despite adequate penicillamine therapy.

The improved outcome in children with cystic fibrosis has led to the identification of significant liver disease in approximately 20% of patients (Scott-Jupp et al, 1991). Portal hypertension is usually severe but hepatic function remains adequate for many years. It is important to consider liver replacement for only those children with hepatic decompensation and to treat portal hypertension by other therapeutic means, e.g. sclerotherapy

(Revell et al, 1993). If pulmonary disease is severe these children should be considered for heart, lung and liver transplants.

Liver function is usually normal in children with fibropolycystic liver disease even if they develop severe portal hypertension. Thus, liver replacement is only indicated when hepatic decompensation occurs with portal hypertension.

Timing of transplantation

Many children with cirrhosis and portal hypertension remain well compensated for many years, making it difficult to predict accurately their need for liver replacement.

Attempts to predict biochemical decompensation with aminopyrine breath tests or caffeine clearance have been disappointing (Baker et al, 1983, 1990), but recent studies with lidocaine metabolites (MEG X) in both adults and children have shown good correlation with liver function. Some units consider that poor MEG X formation and excretion is an indication for liver transplantation (Oellerich et al, 1990).

Malatack et al (1987) evaluated a combination of clinical and laboratory indices of hepatic decompensation to predict either death or the need for liver transplantation in children. They found that a rise in the proportion of unconjugated bilirubin (indirect bilirubin) $>100\,\mu mol/l$ (6 mg/dl); prothrombin ratio (INR) >1.4; a fall in serum cholesterol $<2.6\,mmol/l$ (100 mg/dl) and albumin $<35\,g/l$ (3.5 mg/dl) were accurate predictors of death. In general, a persistent deterioration of these parameters should alert the clinician to consider transplantation.

As protein energy malnutrition is an inevitable complication of chronic liver disease in the growing child, a decrease in nutritional parameters may be a guide to early hepatic decompensation. Evidence of chronic malnutrition (reduced height for chronological age) is of no value in predicting a potential need for liver transplantation, but evidence of acute malnutrition with reduction in fat stores (triceps skinfold) or protein stores (mid-arm muscle area) are sensitive indicators of hepatic decompensation (Beath et al, 1993b).

Early referral for transplantation should be considered for children with complex hepatic complications, e.g. ascites which is refractory to medical management; variceal haemorrhage which is uncontrolled by endoscopic sclerotherapy, particularly if there are gastric or duodenal varices; and persistent chronic hepatic encephalopathy.

It is now clear that although some aspects of psychosocial development in children with chronic liver disease is well maintained, there is significant reduction in developmental motor skills which may be reversed following liver transplantation if performed early enough (Beath et al, 1993b; Kelly et al, 1993; Wayman et al, 1993). Thus any significant delay in developmental parameters is an indication for early transplantation.

In general, children with chronic liver disease should be referred for transplantation before the complications of their liver disease seriously impairs the quality of their lives and before growth and development are irreversibly retarded.

Acute liver failure

Acute liver failure is a rare but fatal disease with a mortality greater than 70% (Kelly, 1993). The clinical presentation includes the combination of hepatic encephalopathy, coagulopathy, hypoglycaemia and jaundice, but difficulties in appreciating this diagnosis means that many children are referred too late for liver transplantation.

Fulminant hepatitis

The selection of potential recipients for liver transplantation in children with fulminant hepatitis is based on previous experience of mortality in the pretransplant era (Psacharopoulos et al, 1980) and on adult experience (O'Grady et al, 1989). Prognosis is worst in children with non-A, non-B hepatitis; a rapid onset of coma with progression to grade III or IV hepatic coma; a diminishing liver size; falling transaminases; an increasing bilirubin and persistent coagulopathy. Unlike adults, children with a sub-acute illness may have severe coagulopathy, but mild encephalopathy (Kelly, 1993). It is essential that such children should be referred early to a specialist centre for intensive care management and liver transplantation.

In practical terms all children in grade III hepatic coma, who have a persistent coagulopathy (prothrombin ratio INR > 4) and have no evidence of irreversible brain damage from cerebral oedema or hypoglycaemia, should be listed for transplantation. As current management strategies for cerebral oedema are unsatisfactory and methods for determining irreversible brain damage are imprecise, this may be a difficult decision. Careful management of cerebral oedema is critical and best monitored by measurement of intracranial pressure which improves the selection of recipients but not overall survival (Lidofsky et al, 1992). Assessment of cerebral blood flow is not useful as this is reduced in hepatic failure, but assessment of cerebral perfusion pressure is more sensitive. Cerebral CT scans will detect gross cerebral oedema, infarction or intracranial haemorrhage. Serial electroencephalopathy (EEG) may indicate reduction in electrical activity and brain death, although care must be taken in interpreting these results in ventilated patients, as the EEG tracing is affected by sedation and anaesthetic agents.

Paracetamol poisoning. Paracetamol poisoning in children is rare in the USA and Europe, but is becoming increasingly common in Britain. Accidental ingestion is likely in children aged 1–4, while in the adolescent, self-poisoning is usual (Rumack, 1986). The development of liver failure is dose-dependent, and hepatic failure is likely if the ingested dose is greater than 15 g. Children have a lower incidence of liver failure with paracetamol overdose than adults, perhaps because of the effect of age on glutathione production (Lauterberg et al, 1980). Hepatic enlargement and tenderness develop by the second day after ingestion, while jaundice, encephalopathy and renal failure develop between the third and fifth days. Liver transplantation should be considered if there is persistent coagulopathy (INR > 4), metabolic acidosis (pH < 7.3), and rapid progression to hepatic coma grade III.

Metabolic liver disease

Acute liver failure may be the presenting feature of inherited metabolic liver disease such as Wilson's disease and tyrosinaemia type I (Burdelski et al, 1991). The clinical presentation may be subacute and liver failure occurs in the presence of an underlying but undetected cirrhosis. It is unusual to detect a rapid decrease in liver size in these conditions and jaundice may not be present in the early stages.

Babies with infantile haemochromatosis present within the first 6–8 weeks of life with severe coagulopathy and encephalopathy. Although a number of successful transplants in this group of children have now been performed (Lund et al, 1993) liver transplantation may not be feasible, because of their small size, severity of illness and the difficulty in obtaining suitable donor organs in time.

Inborn errors of metabolism

Liver transplantation is also indicated for inherited disorders in which the liver is functionally normal, but where deficiency of a hepatic enzyme may cause severe extrahepatic disease, e.g. Crigler–Najjar type I (Table 1). In considering liver replacement for these disorders it is particularly important to balance the potential mortality and morbidity of the primary disease with that of the complications of liver transplantation and life-long immuno-suppression.

The timing of transplantation in these disorders depends on the rate of progression of the disease, and the quality of life of the affected child. In general, it is important to perform liver transplantation before there is irreversible disease of other organs, e.g. structural brain damage in Crigler–Najjar type I (Kaufman et al, 1986), or coronary artery disease in children with familial hypercholesterolaemia (Sokol et al, 1993). If possible, trans-plantation should be delayed until the child is over 10 kg in order to ensure donor availability and reduce surgical risks. In some cases, liver replacement should be combined with other organ transplantation, e.g. renal trans-plantation for primary oxalosis (Burdelski et al, 1991).

Liver tumours

As primary liver tumours are rare in childhood there is little data on survival following transplantation. Potential indications include: unresectable benign tumours causing hepatic dysfunction; unresectable malignant tumours (hepatoblastoma or hepatocellular carcinoma), which are refractory to chemotherapy and radiation without evidence of extrahepatic metastases; hepatocellular carcinoma secondary to underlying liver disease, e.g. tyrosinaemia type I (Esquivel et al, 1989), α_1-antitrypsin deficiency, glycogen storage type I and hepatitis B, although the latter is associated with a high rate of recurrence of hepatitis B infection (Yandza et al, 1993).

Koneru et al (1991) evaluated liver transplantation for hepatoblastoma in 12 children and reported that there was a worse prognosis in children with extrahepatic metastases, multi-focal tumours, or embryonal/anaplastic tumours. In contrast children who had unifocal tumours with predominantly foetal epithelium had a better prognosis. Thus the transplant evaluation should consider the histological grade of the tumour and perform a bone scan and chest X-ray to exclude extrahepatic metastases.

PRETRANSPLANT EVALUATION

The evaluation process should: assess the need and urgency for transplantation; establish whether the operation is possible or not; establish whether there are any significant contra-indications; establish whether it is appropriate for the child and the family; and prepare the child and family.

Pretransplant assessment

On referral for transplantation the indication for transplantation should be critically evaluated as discussed above. It is particularly important to review the diagnosis, establish the prognosis and consider whether alternative medical or surgical therapy is more appropriate. It is essential to evaluate whether liver transplantation will improve the quality of life for both the child and the family.

The nutritional status and presence of hepatic complications should be determined. Particular attention should be paid to the evaluation of cardiac and respiratory systems, neurological assessment and dental examination.

Cardiac assessment

Some children with liver disease may have congenital cardiac disease, e.g. atrial and ventricular septal defects are associated with biliary atresia, while peripheral pulmonary stenosis is common in Alagille syndrome. Cardiomyopathy may develop secondary to tyrosinaemia type I and propionic acidaemia (Roth et al, 1987). Careful assessment is required to establish whether cardiac function is adequate for transplantation or whether corrective surgery should take place prior to listing. Cardiac catheterization may be necessary in some cases.

Respiratory assessment

A small percentage of children with end-stage liver disease develop intra-pulmonary shunts with or without pulmonary hypertension. Clinical signs of cyanosis and digital clubbing will indicate the need for pulmonary function studies or cardiac catheterization (Laberge et al, 1992).

Neuro-development assessment

In order to evaluate outcome or potential quality of life post-transplantation, it is necessary to determine the nature of any neurological defects and whether they are reversible post-transplantation. This is particularly important in considering transplantation for children with acute liver failure, or those who have developed structural brain damage secondary to severe hypoglycaemia or anoxia. Chronic hepatic encephalopathy is usually reversible and can be diagnosed clinically and confirmed by EEG.

Psychological or developmental assessments using standard tests (Bayley Developmental Scales or Stanford–Binet Intelligence Scales) provide baseline information with which to evaluate progress post-transplantation.

Dental assessment

Chronic liver disease has a devastating effect on the growth and development of young children which includes dentition. Dental problems pre-transplant include hypoplasia and staining of teeth and gingival hyperplasia. It is important to establish good dental hygiene, even in very young children, particularly as gingival hyperplasia will be exacerbated by postoperative medications such as cyclosporin A and the anti-hypertensive drug, nifedipine.

Hepatic function

As discussed above, there are no reliable biochemical tests to evaluate hepatic function and the decision to list for transplantation is based on deterioration in standard liver function tests, with particular reference to prolonged coagulation indices unresponsive to vitamin K. The severity of portal hypertension can be estimated by identifying oesophageal and gastric varices by gastrointestinal endoscopy, which will also detect gastritis or acid peptic disease, which are common complications in these children. If the histological diagnosis is not already apparent, a liver biopsy may be required.

Renal function

Abnormalities of renal function are common in children with end-stage liver disease and include renal tubular acidosis, glomerulonephritis, acute tubular necrosis and hepatorenal syndrome. Careful assessment of renal function is required not only to instigate specific therapy but to provide a base-line, from which to evaluate the potential nephrotoxic effects of post-transplant immunosuppression.

Haematology

Full blood count, platelets, coagulation indices and blood group are obtained.

Serology

Immunity to previous infection is determined (Table 2) with particular reference to cytomegalovirus (CMV), as donor grafts are matched for CMV status where possible.

Table 2. Evaluation for liver transplantation.

1. Nutritional status
   Height, weight, triceps skinfold, mid-arm muscle area

2. Identification of hepatic complications
   Ascites, hepatosplenomegaly, varices on endoscopy

3. Cardiac assessment
   ECG, Echo, Chest X-ray
   (? cardiac catheterization)

4. Neurological and developmental assessment
   EEG
   Bailey developmental scales
   Stanford–Binet intelligence scales

5. Renal function
   Urea, creatinine, electrolytes
   Urinary protein/creatinine ratio

6. Dental assessment

7. Radiology
   Ultrasound of liver and spleen for vascular anatomy
   Wrist X-ray for bone age and rickets

8. Serology
   Cytomegalovirus
   Epstein–Barr virus
   Varicella zoster
   Herpes simplex
   Hepatitis A, B, C
   HIV
   Measles

9. Haematology
   Full blood count, platelets, blood group

Radiology

Doppler ultrasound examination of the liver and spleen is performed to outline the vascular anatomy and identify whether the vessels are patent. It is important to examine the portal vein carefully to assess patency, size and direction of blood flow. Although thrombosis of the portal vein is no longer a contra-indication to transplantation, evidence of retrograde flow indicates severe portal hypertension as does decreasing size of portal vein which is associated with an increase in technical problems perioperatively (Badger et al, 1992). Children with congenital liver disease, such as biliary atresia, have an increased incidence of abnormal vasculature. The hypovascular syndrome consists of an absent inferior vena cava, a preduodenal or absent portal vein, azygous drainage from the liver and polysplenia syndrome. It is often associated with situs inversus, dextrocardia or left atrial isomerism. Pretransplant recognition of these syndromes should reduce technical complications during surgery (Lilly and Starzl, 1974).

X-rays of the wrist or knee will determine bone age, an indication of nutritional status, and detect rickets secondary to vitamin D deficiency.

Contra-indications to transplantation

As surgical skills have improved there are few contra-indications to transplantation. The only contra-indications that remain are as follows.

(a) Severe irreversible disease of another organ system, e.g. severe cardiopulmonary disease not amenable to surgery or severe structural brain damage.

(b) The presence of severe systemic sepsis, particularly fungal sepsis, at the time of operation. These children will not survive the operation and subsequent immunosuppression and such infection should be vigorously treated and the transplant deferred.

(c) Reinfection of the donor graft occurs in over 80% of recipients transplanted for chronic hepatitis B (HBV) (Lucey et al, 1992). Although this is not an absolute contra-indication, a guarded prognosis must be given and reinfection should be prevented using hepatitis B immune globulin although this is not always effective (Gugenheim et al, 1992). Hepatitis B does not recur following transplantation for fulminant HBV.

(d) Transplantation for HIV positive children is currently contra-indicated.

(e) The potential recurrence of malignant tumours post-transplantation may be a relative contra-indication and care should be taken to establish there are no extrahepatic metastases prior to surgery (Koneru et al, 1991).

At one time, babies under 1 year who weighed less than 10 kg were not considered for transplantation because of the technical risks and shortage of available donors (Kahn et al, 1988; Brant de Carvalho et al, 1991). With the development of innovative surgical techniques such as reduction hepatectomy and specialized medical and nursing management, there are now no specific contra-indications related to age and size, although there may be difficulty in obtaining suitable donor livers for very small babies (Beath et al, 1993b).

Preparation for transplantation

Immunization

As live vaccines are contra-indicated in the immunosuppressed child, every effort must be made to ensure that routine immunizations are complete, e.g. diphtheria, pertussis, tetanus and polio, pneumovax for protection against streptococcal pneumonia and HIB for protection against haemophilus influenza. In children older than 9 months, measles, mumps and rubella vaccination should be offered. Varicella vaccine is available but may be limited to named patients only.

Management of hepatic complications

The treatment of specific hepatic complications is an important part of preoperative management. Variceal bleeding may be life threatening and should be managed with sclerotherapy, vasopressin or somatostatin infusions; sepsis, particularly ascending cholangitis and spontaneous bacterial peritonitis requires vigorous treatment. Salt and water retention with ascites is a major problem which is managed with diuretics, fluid and salt restriction. Restriction of fluids may create particular difficulties in providing adequate calories for babies whose enteral intake is dependent on milk feeds.

Haemodialysis or haemofiltration should be instituted if acute renal failure or hepatorenal failure develops, usually secondary to acute liver failure. Haemodialysis is rarely needed in chronic liver failure, unless there is acute decompensation and development of hepatorenal failure (Ellis et al, 1986).

Nutritional support

Rapid advances in the understanding of the pathophysiology of malnutrition in liver disease has led to improved nutritional strategies (Beath et al, 1993c). More than 60% of children referred for transplantation are malnourished and effective therapy has been shown to reduce both morbidity and mortality post-transplantation (Moukarzel et al, 1990; Kelly et al, 1993).

The aim of nutritional therapy is to provide sufficient calories to reverse or prevent malnutrition and to overcome fat malabsorption and ongoing catabolism. A high calorie, protein feed (100–160% RDA) with sufficient medium chain triglycerides (MCT) to reduce fat malabsorption, and long chain triglycerides (LCT) to provide essential fatty acids is utilized (Beath et al, 1993c). It is difficult to provide this high energy intake with standard feeds, particularly in fluid restricted children. Thus a modular feed, in which individual components can be concentrated to maximize energy intake is most appropriate for young babies. As sick babies and children will not take the large volume of concentrated feeds orally, nocturnal nasogastric enteral feeding is usually necessary. A small percentage of children will not tolerate enteral feeds, either because of food intolerance or recurrent complications, and parenteral feeding is mandatory for these children. Generous oral fat soluble vitamin supplementation is essential but occasionally parenteral vitamins may be required.

Psychological preparation

The importance of counselling and preparation of the child and family cannot be sufficiently emphasized. A specialized multidisciplinary team including medical, surgical and nursing staff, a social worker, clinical psychologist, physiotherapist and play therapist is intrinsic to the success of this preparation. Parents and appropriate relatives should be fully informed of the need for liver transplantation in their child, the risks and complications and the long-term implications. Psychological preparation of children over 18 months is essential and can be successfully achieved through innovative play therapy and books suitable for children.

Particularly careful counselling is required for parents of children being considered for transplantation to correct hepatic enzyme deficiencies as they find it more difficult to accept the complications of the operation and the potential mortality. Parents of children who require transplantation for acute liver failure are usually too distressed to understand fully the implications of transplantation and need additional help. Children surviving liver grafting for acute liver failure should have postoperative counselling and play therapy.

THE LIVER GRAFT

The liver graft is matched by ABO blood group, size, and if possible, by CMV status.

Recent advances in organ preservation have been achieved with the development of the Wisconsin solution by the University of Wisconsin. This unique preservation solution allows organs to be preserved for up to 24 h which increases the donor pool as organs can be harvested from long distances and the transplant operation can be planned semi-electively (Kalayoglu et al, 1988).

Operative technique

The traditional form of operation is orthotopic liver transplantation in which the whole diseased organ is removed and replaced with another whole organ. The major shortfall in paediatric donors and the pretransplant mortality of children on the waiting list has led to the development of reduction hepatectomies (Bismuth and Houssin, 1984; Badger et al, 1992). In this procedure, part of a larger liver, usually the left lateral segments, is cut down to fit the child and the cut surface of the liver is sealed with a fibrin glue to prevent leakage (Badger et al, 1992). Graft and patient survival is slightly less with reduction hepatectomy than with whole liver grafts, but this may be because they are normally performed in younger, sicker children (Table 3). Although long-term survival of these grafts are not yet available, this operative innovation has reduced the long wait for donor livers for small babies. Deaths on the waiting list have fallen from 25% (Malatack et al, 1987) to 5% (Cox et al, 1991). Most centres report that reduction hepatectomies make up 60–80% of their total grafts in children and this is particularly true in children under the age of 1 year (Beath et al, 1993a,b; Dunn et al, 1993).

Table 3. Comparison of graft survival in whole and reduced grafts (Paediatric Liver Programme, Birmingham, 1989–1993).

	Whole ($n = 63$)	Reduced ($n = 67$)
*Age (years)	4.9 (5 months–15 years)	1.3 (15 days–10 years)
*Weight (kg)	17 (5.4–55)	8.6 (3.6–36)
Retransplants	10%	27%
1-year graft survival	80%	60%

* Median value.

Although reduction hepatectomies have increased the donor pool for paediatric donors, this innovation has not increased the total donor pool. Historically, split liver grafts, in which a single donor liver graft is offered to two recipients, have 1 year graft survival rates of 30–50% (Langnas et al, 1992). However, more recent results suggest that controlled liver splitting for transplantation may have a future (Houssin et al, 1993), and a prospective study is underway in Europe.

Auxiliary liver grafts, in which the original liver remains in situ, and part of the donor liver is inserted beside or in continuity with the original liver may have a role in transplantation for inborn errors of metabolism when the liver is functionally normal, or in fulminant hepatitis, when the liver might recover. Although progress has been made there are a number of technical problems which have yet to be resolved (Terpstra, 1993).

The most recent operative innovation is that of living related donor grafts. This technique was pioneered by Christoph Broelsch in Chicago and is the only form of transplantation permissible in Japan (Tanaka et al, 1993). Although there are many ethical problems associated with this form of transplantation in which a relative or parent donates part of their liver to the child, it is currently strongly advocated in a number of American centres (Heffron et al, 1993; Katz et al, 1993). It is clear that there is a considerable donor morbidity (Rogiers et al, 1993) and to date a single death in a mother (Burdelski, personal communication). The overall results in the recipient child are equivalent to those obtained with reduction hepatectomies with 80–85% 1-year survival (Rogiers et al, 1993).

Postoperative management

The immediate postoperative management is concerned with monitoring graft function, initiating immunosuppression and the prevention and management of immediate complications. Primary nonfunction of the transplanted liver is most likely to occur within 48 h and graft function is monitored by evaluating acid–base status, blood sugar levels, coagulation times, hepatic amino transferases, bilirubin, alkaline phosphatase. Primary graft failure is most likely to be due from nonfunction, or thrombosis of hepatic artery or portal vein (Brant de Carvalho et al, 1991). Hepatic artery thrombosis is more common in children (10–20%) than adults (5–8%) but is less common with reduction hepatectomies because of larger donor blood vessels (Langnas et al, 1991). It may be prevented by prophylactic administration of aspirin (3 mg/kg/day) and dipyridamole (25–50 mg t.d.s.).

Immunosuppression regimes vary between centres, but the majority of centres currently use triple immunosuppression with prednisolone (2 mg/kg), cyclosporin A (2 mg/kg) and azathioprine (2 mg/kg). Immunosuppression is maximal for the first 2 weeks post-transplant and most centres reduce immunosuppression with time (Beath et al, 1993b; Andrews et al, 1993).

Monoclonal antibodies, OKT3 and anti-lymphocytic globulin are not routine medications but are reserved for resistant rejection (Cosimi et al, 1987).

The novel immunosuppressive drug FK506 has not yet been adequately evaluated in children, but preliminary experience suggests that it is very much more effective than cyclosporin A in preventing rejection, but there is a higher risk of lymphoproliferative disorder (Tzakis et al, 1993).

Early postoperative complications

Hepatic or portal vein thrombosis is a life-threatening event which may require retransplantation (Brant de Carvalho et al, 1991). The diagnosis is suggested by evidence of graft dysfunction (hypoglycaemia, metabolic acidosis, rising hepatic amino transferases) and confirmed by Doppler ultrasound and/or hepatic angiography.

Oliguria may develop with poor graft function, hypovolaemia or cyclosporin therapy and strict fluid balance is mandatory. Less than 10% of children require dialysis for renal failure (Ellis et al, 1986).

Hypertension secondary to cyclosporin or prednisolone is common (Lawless et al, 1989) and responds to fluid restriction and anti-hypertensive therapy with nifedipine (5–10 mg sublingually), sodium nitroprusside (0.5–8 mg/kg/min) and atenolol (25–50 mg/day).

Fluid balance is particularly difficult in young babies because of the pre-existing salt and water retention associated with chronic liver disease. It is important to restrict fluid to these children to half their maintenance fluids and to treat vigorously with diuretics (Poulson et al, 1987).

Although most children are mechanically ventilated for 24–48 h postoperatively, prolonged ventilation leads to respiratory complications, including collapse and consolidation of the lung, recurrent infection and pulmonary oedema. A right pleural effusion secondary to operative trauma is common. These complications increase initial morbidity but usually respond to standard therapy.

Acute cellular rejection occurs between 7 and 10 days postoperatively. The incidence of acute rejection varies from 60 to 80% (Emond et al, 1987; Brant de Carvalho et al, 1991) and there is some evidence to suggest that infants under the age of 1 year are immunologically tolerant of the liver graft, as the rate of rejection in these infants is 20–30% (Murphy et al, 1993). In over 80% of instances, acute rejection responds to increased immunosuppression with methyl prednisolone or an increase in cyclosporin A dosage. Chronic rejection occurs in approximately 16% of children (Murphy et al, 1993). It is characterized by irreversible loss of bile ducts and leads to retransplantation (Ludwig et al, 1987).

Gastrointestinal complications may develop in the first 14 days. Intestinal perforation occurs in 21% of children with previous abdominal surgery (Kelly et al, 1988). Gastrointestinal bleeding (Kelly et al, 1988) is also common and is effectively prevented by infusion of ranitidine (Dimand et al, 1989).

Biliary complications due to technical problems or vascular thrombosis remain a challenge in 15–20% of children. Reduction hepatectomies are associated with an increased incidence of biliary leaks and anastomotic strictures, while hepatic artery thrombosis leads to ischaemic biliary strictures, sepsis and sometimes retransplantation (Yandza et al, 1994).

Modern techniques for treatment of biliary complications include the use of biliary dilatation and biliary stents (Yandza et al, 1994), although surgical biliary reconstruction may be required.

The most common complication post-transplantation is sepsis related to immunosuppression which is a lifelong problem and a major cause of death (Zitelli et al, 1987). In the immediate postoperative stage, bacterial infections (e.g. *Streptococcus faecalis* and *viridans*, *Pseudomonas* and *Staphylococcus aureus*) are likely and may be associated with central line infections (Beath et al, 1993b).

Fungal infections with *Candida albicans*, or aspergillosis are documented in 23% of patients, particularly if acute hepatic necrosis is present (Castaldo et al, 1991).

CMV infections occur 5–6 weeks later and are more common in children than in adults as children are more likely to be CMV-negative at the time of transplantation. The risk of CMV disease is indirectly related to receiving a CMV-positive donor (Davison et al, 1993) and may be treated effectively with high dose DHPG (ganciclovir) and hyperimmune CMV globulin. Effective prophylaxis with ganciclovir is currently being evaluated.

Retransplantation

In the initial post-transplant phase, 20–25% of children will require retransplantation for primary nonfunction, hepatic artery thrombosis or severe acute rejection. Retransplantation for chronic rejection occurs in 10–15% of children (Brant de Carvalho et al, 1991).

Late complications post-transplantation

Late complications of transplantation are related to cyclosporin nephrotoxicity (Ellis et al, 1986), or growth retardation due to excess steroid dosage, although this can be reduced by discontinuation of steroids (Beath et al, 1993b; Andrews et al, 1993).

Long-term prophylaxis against *Pneumocystis carinii* is mandatory with low dose co-trimoxazole and systemic fungal infections should be prevented with prophylactic oral anti-fungals (nystatin and amphotericin).

The development of primary Epstein–Barr virus (EBV) is a serious long-term problem. As the majority of children are nonimmune to EBV at the time of transplantation, the majority seroconvert to EBV within 18 months (Davison et al, 1993), but only approximately 10% develop lympho-proliferative syndrome (LPS) which is reversible with discontinuation of immunosuppression (Renard et al, 1991). The incidence of LPS has increased with the use of FK506 (Tzakis et al, 1993b).

Survival post-liver transplantation

The increased international experience with liver transplantation in children has led to a welcome improvement in survival rates. One- and 2-year actuarial survival in world centres is now in excess of 85% (Otte et al, 1988; Salt et al, 1992; Beath et al, 1993b). Five-year survival figures are less impressive ranging from 56 to 70% and represent earlier results (Shaw et al, 1988; Chin et al, 1991). The main causes of death remain primary non-function of graft, hepatic infarction and sepsis.

The long-term management of this group of children requires monitoring of hepatic function, growth, development and maintaining immunosuppression at a level to prevent rejection. Continued family support is a vital part of postoperative management as some parents and children need encouragement to resume a normal life.

Quality of life post-transplantation

Children who survive the initial 3 month post-transplantation without major sequelae should achieve a normal life-style, despite the need for continuous medical monitoring of immunosuppressive therapy (Zitelli et al, 1987; Chin et al, 1991; Beath et al, 1993b).

Recent evidence suggests that there is remarkable improvement in catch-up growth. Beath et al (1993b) prospectively evaluated 25 children transplanted under the age of 1 year and noted that weight, muscle and fat scores returned to normal within 1 year, although height catch-up growth was initially delayed. Rodeck et al (1993) evaluated growth in survivors over a 5-year period and noted that there was complete rehabilitation by the second and third year post-transplant, although the extent of linear growth was related to the degree of stunting preoperatively.

There are few studies on prospective evaluation of psychosocial development. Beath et al (1993b) reviewed the psychosocial development of infants under 1 year and noted that pretransplant, there was a disproportionate reduction in motor skills, compared to other developmental parameters, such as eye–hand co-ordination, social and language skills. One year post-transplant, there was a dramatic improvement in motor skills with some regression of eye–hand and language skills, although the values remained within the normal range. Another recent study (Wayman et al, 1993) evaluated children under the age of 3 years before, and 1 year after liver transplantation and found very similar findings, although 57% of children continued to have motor deficits while 62% of children had language deficits. The difference between these findings may have been related to the severe degree of developmental delay in the older group compared to the babies under 1 year. A 5-year follow-up in older children post-transplant indicated that the majority of children attended normal school with excellent quality of life (Chin et al, 1991).

SUMMARY

Remarkable advances in paediatric liver transplantation have been achieved in the last decade with improvement in both medical and surgical expertise. Current indications for liver transplantation include acute or chronic liver failure, unresectable hepatic tumours and replacement of hepatic enzyme deficiencies. The majority of children are transplanted for liver failure, secondary to biliary atresia following a failed Kasai portoenterostomy.

The timing of transplantation depends on the aetiology of the liver failure. Children with chronic liver disease should be grafted before nutritional parameters deteriorate, growth and development become significantly impaired, and quality of life is unacceptable.

Children with acute liver failure should be transplanted before there is irreversible brain damage from hypoglycaemia or cerebral oedema and should be referred early to a specialist centre for management.

The evaluation process should establish the urgency for transplantation, exclude alternative management, assess technical feasibility and confirm the medical and nutritional status of the child. Preoperative management includes treatment of hepatic complications, intensive nutritional support, and psychological preparation of the child and family.

The majority of paediatric recipients receive a reduced liver graft which has reduced the deaths on the waiting list and achieves similar mortality (10–15%), but increased morbidity compared to whole graft transplantation.

Current 1-year survival figures are 85%, the main causes of death being primary graft function, hepatic infarction and sepsis. Postoperative morbidity remains high with many complications including sepsis, rejection, vascular thrombosis and biliary problems. The majority of survivors achieve a normal life-style within 3 months of the operation with dramatic improvement in catch-up growth and maintenance of normal psychosocial development. The long-term outcome for these children will be determined by the effects of immunosuppression and the development of viral illnesses, such as Epstein–Barr virus and the subsequent development of lymphoproliferative disease.

REFERENCES

Alexandria BA (1990) *National Association in Children's Hospitals and Related Institutions Inc*.
Andrews WS, Shimaoka S, Sommerauer J et al (1993) Steroid withdrawal after paediatric liver transplantation. *Transplantation Proceedings*, June 25, 1990.

Badger IL, Czerbiak A, Beath S et al (1992) Hepatic transplantation in children using reduced size allografts. *British Journal of Surgery* **79**: 47–49.

Baker A, Kitak EA & Schoeller D (1983) Clinical utility of breath tests for the assessment of hepatic function. *Seminar in Liver Disease* **3**: 318–329.

Baker AJ, Ballentine N & Kelly DA (1990) Does sequential caffeine half-life predict deteriorating liver function in children. *Gut* **30**: A1473.

Beath S, Pearmain G, Kelly D et al (1993a) Liver transplantation in babies and children with extra-hepatic biliary atresia. *Journal of Pediatric Surgery* **28**: 1044–1047.

Beath SV, Brooks GD, Kelly DA et al (1993b) Successful liver transplantation in babies under 1 year. *British Medical Journal* **307**: 825–828.

Beath S, Kelly D & Booth I (1993c) Nutritional support in children with liver disease. *Archives of Disease in Childhood* **69**: 545–547.

Bismuth H & Houssin D (1984) Reduced size orthotopic liver grafts in hepatic transplantation in children. *Surgery* **95**: 367–370.

Brant de Carvalho F, Reding R, Falchetti D et al (1991) Analysis of liver graft loss in infants and children below 4 years. *Transplantation Proceedings* **23**: 1454–1455.

Broelsch CE, Whitington PF & Emond JC (1990) Evolution and future perspective for reduced-size hepatic transplantation. *Surgery, Gynaecology, Obstetrics* **171**: 353–360.

Burdelski M, Rodeck B, Latta A et al (1991) Treatment of inherited metabolic disorders by liver transplantation. *Journal of Inherited Metabolic Disease* **14**: 604–618.

Castaldo P, Stratta RJ, Wood RP et al (1991) Clinical spectrum of fungal infections after orthotopic liver transplantation. *Archives of Surgery* **126**: 149–156.

Chin SE, Shepherd RW, Kleghorn GJ et al (1991) *Journal of Pediatrics & Child Health* **27**: 380–385.

Cosimi AB, Cho SI, Delmonico SL et al (1987) A randomised clinical trial comparing OKT3 and steroids for treatment of hepatic allograft rejection. *Transplantation* **43**: 91–95.

Cox K, Nakazato P, Berquist W et al (1991) Liver transplantation in infants weighing less than 10 kgs. *Transplantation Proceedings* **23**: 1579–1580.

Davison SM, Murphy MS, Adeodu OO & Kelly DA (1993) Impact of cytomegalovirus and Epstein Barr virus infection in children following liver transplantation. *Gut* **34**: S32.

Dimand RJ, Burckart G, Concepcion W et al (1989) The prevention of gastrointestinal bleeding and metabolic alkalosis by control of gastric pH using continuous infusion Ranitidine in post-operative paediatric liver transplant patients. *Hepatology* **10**: 569A.

Dunn S, Weintraub W, Winocur C et al (1993) Is age less than 1 year a high risk category for orthotopic liver transplantation? *Journal of Paediatric Surgery* **28**: 1048–1049.

Eckhoff D, D'Alessandro AM & Knechtle SJ (1993) Management of biliary complications following liver transplantation in children. *Transplantation Proceedings* (in press).

Ellis D, Avner E & Starzl TE (1986) Renal failure in children with hepatic failure undergoing liver transplantation. *Journal of Pediatrics* **108**: 393–398.

Emond JC, Thistlethwaite JR, Baker AL et al (1987) Rejection in liver allograft recipients, clinical characterisation and management. *Clinical Transplantation* **1**: 143–150.

Esquivel CO, Mieles L, Marino IR et al (1989) Liver transplantation for hereditary tyrosin-aemia in the presence of hepatocellular carcinoma. *Transplantation Proceedings* **21**: 2445–2446.

European Liver Transplant Registry (1992) Hopital Paul Brousse, Villejuif, France.

Gugenheim J, Crafa F, Fabiani P et al (1992) Recurrence of virus B hepatitis after liver transplantation. *Gastroenterologie Clinique et Biologique* **16**: 430–433.

Heffron TG, Langnas AN, Fox IJ et al (1994) Paediatric living related transplantation affords optimal donor utilisation. *Transplantation Proceedings* **26**: 135–137.

Houssin D, Boillot O, Soubrane O et al (1993) Controlled liver splitting for transplantation in two recipients; technique, results and perspectives. *British Journal of Surgery* **80**: 75–80.

Hussain M, Howard ER, Mieli-Vergani G & Mowat AP (1991a) Jaundice at 14 days of age—exclude biliary atresia. *Archives of Disease in Childhood* **66**: 1177–1179.

Hussain M, Mielie-Vergani G & Mowat AP (1991b) Alpha-1-antitrypsin deficiency in liver disease; Clinical presentation, diagnosis and treatment. *Journal of Inherited Metabolic Disease* **14**: 497–511.

Kahn D, Esquivel CO, Mandrigal-Torres M et al (1988) An analysis of the causes of death after paediatric liver transplantation. *Transplantation Proceedings* **20**: 613–615.

Kalayoglu M, Stratta RJ, Hoffmann RN et al (1988) Extended preservation of the liver for clinical transplantation. *Lancet* **1:** 617–619.

Katz SM, Ozaki CF, Fonteno TD et al (1994) Living related donation is equally as successful as cadaveric donation in paediatric liver transplantation. *Transplantation Proceedings* **26:** 145–146.

Kaufman S, Wood R, Shaw B et al (1986) Orthotopic liver transplantation for type I Crigler Najjar Syndrome. *Hepatology* **6:** 1259–1262.

Kelly D (1993) Fulminant hepatitis and acute liver failure. In Buts JP & Sokol EM (eds) *Management of Digestive & Liver Disorders in Infants and Children*, pp 551–568. Elsevier Science Publishers.

Kelly D, Kaufman S, Wood RP et al (1988) Gastrointestinal complications in children post orthotopic liver transplantation. *Gut* **29:** A1476–A1477.

Kelly DA, Beath SV, Brook GD et al (1994) Improving outcome of liver transplantation in babies less than 1 year. *Transplantation Proceedings* **26:** 180–182.

Koneru B, Wayneflye M, Busuttil RW et al (1991) Liver transplantation for hepatoblastoma. *Annals of Surgery* **213:** 118–121.

Laberge JM, Brandt M, Lebecque P et al (1992) Reversal of cirrhosis related pulmonary shunting in two children by orthotopic liver transplantation. *Transplantation* **53:** 1135–1165.

Langnas A, Marujo W, Stratta RJ et al (1991) Vascular complications after orthotopic liver transplantation. *American Journal of Surgery* **161:** 76–83.

Langnas A, Wagner C, Marujo W et al (1992) The results of reduced-size liver transplantation including split livers in patients with end-stage liver disease. *Transplantation* **53:** 387–391.

Lauterberg BH, Vaishnar Y, Stillwell WB & Mitchell JR (1980) The effects of age in glutathione depletion on hepatic Glutothione turnover in vivo determined by acetaminophen probe analysis. *Journal of Pharmacology and Experimental Therapeutics* **213:** 54–58.

Lawless S, Ellis D, Thompson A et al (1989) Mechanisms of hypertension during and after orthotopic liver transplantation in children. *Journal of Pediatrics* **115:** 372–379.

Lidofsky SD, Bass NM, Prager MC et al (1992) Intracranial pressure monitoring and liver transplantation for fulminant hepatic failure. *Hepatology* **16:** 1–7.

Lilly JR & Starzl TE (1974) Liver transplantation in children with biliary atresia and vascular anomalies. *Journal of Pediatric Surgery* **9:** 707–714.

Lindstedt S, Holme E, Lock E et al (1992) Treatment of hereditary Tyrosinaemia Type I by inhibition of 4-hydroxyphenyl pyruvate dioxygenase. *Lancet* **340:** 813–817.

Lucey MR, Graham DM, Martin P et al (1992) Recurrence of hepatitis B and delta hepatitis after orthotopic liver transplantation. *Gut* **33:** 1390–1396.

Ludwig J, Wiesner RH, Batts KP et al (1987) The acute vanishing bile duct syndrome (acute irreversible rejection) after orthotopic liver transplantation. *Hepatology* **7:** 476–483.

Lund DP, Lillehei CW, Kevy F et al (1993) Liver transplantation in new born liver failure; treatment for neonatal haemochromatosis. *Transplantation Proceedings* **25:** 1068–1071.

Malatack JJ, Schald DJ, Urbach AH et al (1987) Choosing a paediatric recipient of orthotopic liver transplantation. *Journal of Pediatrics* **112:** 479–489.

Moukarzel AA, Najm I, Vargas J et al (1990) Effective nutritional status on outcome of orthotopic liver transplantation in paediatric patients. *Transplantation Proceedings* **22:** 1560–1562.

Murphy MS, Harrison RF, Hubscher S et al (1994) Liver allograft rejection is less common in children transplanted in the first year of life. *Transplantation Proceedings* **26:** 157–158.

O'Grady J, Alexander G, Hayllar KM & Williams R (1989) Early indicators of prognosis in fulminant hepatic failure. *Gastroenterology* **97:** 439–445.

Oellerich M, Burdelski M, Lautz HU et al (1990) Lidocaine metabolite formation as a measure of liver function in patients with cirrhosis. *Therapeutics and Drug Monitoring* **12:** 219–226.

Ohi R, Nio M, Chiba T et al (1990) Long-term follow-up after surgery for patients with biliary atresia. *Journal of Pediatric Surgery* **25:** 442–445.

Otte JB, Yandza T, De Ville DE et al (1988) Paediatric liver transplantation report on 52 patients with a two year survival of 86%. *Journal of Pediatric Surgery* **23:** 250–253.

Poulson RJ, Park GR & Lindop MJ (1987) The prevention of renal impairment in patients undergoing orthotopic liver grafting by infusion of low dose Dopamine. *Anaesthesia* **42:** 15–19.

Psacharopoulos HT, Mowat AP, Davies M et al (1980) Fulminant hepatic failure in childhood. *Archives of Disease in Childhood* **55:** 252–258.

Renard DH, Andrews WS & Foster ME (1991) Relationship between OKT3 administration, EBV sero-conversion, and the lymphoproliferative syndrome in paediatric liver transplant recipients. *Transplantation Proceedings* **23:** 1473–1476.

Revell SP, Noble-Jamieson G, Robertson NR & Barnes ND (1993) Liver transplantation in cystic fibrosis. *Journal of the Royal Society of Medicine* **86:** 111–112.

Rodeck B, Melter M, Hoyer PF et al (1994) Growth in long-term survivors after orthotopic liver transplantation (OLT). *Transplantation Proceedings* **26:** 165–166.

Rogiers X, Burdelski M, Gundlach N et al (1994) Living related liver transplantation; the Hamburg experience. *Transplantation Proceedings* **26:** 192–194.

Roth B, Younossi-Hartenstein A, Skopnik H et al (1987) Haemodialysis for metabolic decompensation in propionic acidaemia. *Journal of Inherited Metabolic Disease* **10:** 147–151.

Rumack BH (1986) Acetoaminophen overdose in children and adolescents. *Pediatrics Clinics of North America* **33:** 691–701.

Salt A, Noble-Jamieson G, Barnes ND et al (1992) Liver transplantation in 100 children: Cambridge & King's College Hospital Series. *British Medical Journal* **304:** 416–421.

Scott-Jupp R, Lama M & Tanner MS (1991) Prevalence of liver disease in cystic fibrosis. *Archives of Disease in Childhood* **66:** 698–701.

Shaw BW, Wood RP, Kaufmann SS et al (1988) Liver transplantation therapy for children part II. *Journal of Pediatric Gastroenterology and Nutrition* **7:** 797–815.

Shaw BW, Wood PR, Kelly DA et al (1989) Liver transplantation in children. In Lebenthal E (ed.) *Textbook of Gastroenterology and Nutrition in Infancy*, pp 1045–1070. Raven Press.

Sokol EM, Bustos R, Van Hoof F & Otte JB (1992) Liver transplantation for hereditary tyrosinaemia. *Transplantation* **54:** 937–939.

Sokol EM, Ulla L, Harveng TC & Otte JB (1993) Liver transplantation for familial hyper-cholesterolaemia before the onset of cardiovascular complications. *Transplantation* **55:** 432–433.

Starzl TE, Iwatsuki S, Van Thiel DH et al (1982) Evolution of liver transplantation. *Hepatology* **2:** 614–636.

Tanaka K, Uemoto S, Tokunaga Y et al (1993) Liver transplantation in children from living related donors. *Transplantation Proceedings* **25:** 1084–1086.

Terpstra O (1993) Auxiliary liver grafting: a new concept in liver transplantation. *Lancet* **342:** 758.

Tzakis AG, Reyes J, Tepetes K et al (1993a) Liver transplantation for Alagille's Syndrome. *Archives of Surgery* **128:** 337–339.

Tzakis AG, Reyes J, Todo S et al (1993b) Two year experience with FK506 in paediatric patients. *Transplantation Proceedings* **25:** 619–621.

Wayman KI, Cox K, Berquis TW & Esquivel C (1994) Developmental status of children with end-stage liver disease secondary to biliary atresia—one year post transplant. *Transplantation Proceedings* (in press).

Whitington PE & Balisteri WF (1991) Liver transplantation in paediatrics; indications, contra-indications and pre-transplant management. *Journal of Pediatrics* **118:** 169–177.

Yandza T, Alvarez F & Laurent J (1993) Paediatric liver transplantation for primary hepato-cellular carcinoma associated with hepatitis virus infection. *Transplant International* **6:** 95–98.

Yandza T, Hiromi H & Gauthier F (1994) Biliary complications associated with choledocho-jejunostomy without biliary stent in paediatric liver transplantation. *Transplantation Proceedings* **26:** 169–170.

Zitelli BJ, Gartner JC, Maltack JJ et al (1987) Paediatric liver transplantation, patient evaluation and selection, infectious complications and life-style after transplantation. *Transplantation Proceedings* **19:** 3309–3316.

5

The role of gastrointestinal motility studies

P. J. MILLA

For years a relationship has been assumed to exist between abnormal gastrointestinal motility and abdominal symptoms. Until the last 15 years the evidence for this statement from systematic investigation was sparse and understanding of the physiology of motor activity of the gut was rudimentary. Latterly there has, however, been an increase of knowledge regarding both basic aspects of enteric nerve and muscle, of disease processes affecting the neuromusculature of the gut and of its function in a variety of gastrointestinal disease processes affecting both the mucosa and other abdominal organs. The practical applications of this knowledge are now influencing clinical paediatrics and, in this chapter, the role of studies of gastrointestinal motor activity will be discussed and those tests that the author finds helpful in clinical practice, highlighted.

Knowledge of the ways in which food can move in the gut may clarify symptoms, provide insights into the origin and control of abnormal movements and may indicate novel and effective treatments of the patients' symptoms. It is, however, only in the last 5 years or so that sufficient information has been available for this to become a reality. There are probably no more than 20 gastroenterology units, both paediatric and adult, throughout the world that are using motility tests routinely to investigate patients. As a consequence each of these units does its own thing and it takes time to gain sufficient experience to make confident predictions and to devise effective treatments. At the present time it is probable that this situation will continue and it is premature, other than in a few well-defined circumstances such as intra-oesophageal pH monitoring and anorectal manometry, to lay down rules for the conditions under which such tests should be performed. In some areas it is clearer than in others what the current use of tests of gastrointestinal motility should be and I hope that this chapter will clarify some of these areas.

Detailed observations are being carried out in children with gastrointestinal motor disorders that have identified new phenomena which challenge our concept of disease and pose important questions. Do these phenomena represent a primary disturbance in the control of gastrointestinal motility? For example, patterns of fasting motor activity have been described in association with neuropathic disease of the bowel, yet it is now becoming apparent that very similar changes may occur as a consequence of enteropathic disorder of the mucosa (Cucchiara et al, 1993). So,

Baillière's Clinical Paediatrics—
Vol. 2, No. 4, November 1994
ISBN 0–7020–1866–X

are these so called primary phenomena also secondary to the presence of inflammation of the mucosa in the bowel or toxins for infection in the bowel lumen? Thus the observation of characteristic motor phenomena may not be as helpful in identifying particular diseases as was once thought.

Clinically, the identification of specific abnormalities is only useful if it allows us to arrive at a precise diagnosis and/or institute treatment which is associated with resolution of the patient's symptoms. Unfortunately, treatment options are often limited; surgery is only feasible if the defect is confined to a particular region of gut and that section of gut can either be removed, bypassed or, in the case of disturbed sphincter activity, modified. Pharmacotherapy of gastrointestinal motility disorders seems restricted at the present time, to agents that will relax smooth muscle and a few gastro-intestinal prokinetic agents that improve peristalsis. The pharmaceutical industry has, however, risen to the challenge of producing new gut selective drugs by producing specific antagonists to particular receptors in the gut, for example 5HT3 receptor antagonists, which are beginning to prove useful for the treatment of specific disorders. The continued investigation of disorders of gut motility are necessary to reveal the range of specific disorders of the enteric neuromusculature that must exist in order to provide the impetus for the investment to develop specific and effective drugs.

TESTS OF GASTROINTESTINAL MOTILITY

Clinical tests should be simple to perform, tolerable and safe for the patient and provide information that discriminates accurately between different disorders and treatment options. Which test is used depends upon the questions that are being asked; different tests may be used in different situations. However, in investigating patients with suspected motility disorders of the gastrointestinal tract two types of investigations are mandatory. These are radiology and scintigraphy, and manometry. Other methods are useful in certain circumstances, for example intra-oesophageal pH monitoring in suspected gastro-oesophageal reflux.

Radiology

Radiology is the oldest and probably most widely available test of gastrointestinal motor function that there is (Smith et al, 1957). It provides the clearest indication of disturbances in contractile activity and movement of luminal contents. It provides us, however, with very little insight into the cause of such changes. A video fluoroscopy with barium is the most appropriate investigation in patients with disorders of swallowing or dysphagia. A plain abdominal X-ray followed by a barium meal and follow-through examination is the initial work-up for any patient with recurrent vomiting or who is suspected of having chronic intestinal pseudo-obstruction. In the former patients the follow-through examination need only be as far as the duodeno-jejunal flexure whereas, in those with chronic intestinal pseudo-obstruction, effort must be made to follow the barium through to the terminal ileum. A radiological study of the distribution of the radio-opaque pellets is the simplest and most useful test in the investigation of constipation.

Especially in childhood the dose of radiation limits the length and number of studies that can be performed and thus radiology can only demonstrate gross and persistent disturbances in motor activity. Unfortunately many motility disorders are intermittent and may only occur under certain conditions. As is clear in the investigation of gastro-oesophageal reflux, radiology often fails to detect conditions which only occur intermittently.

The effective use of radiology in investigating disorders of gastrointestinal motility takes time and commitment. The radiologist must be experienced, highly motivated and prepared to make a considerable effort in obtaining the appropriate conditions for demonstrating disturbed motor function. Many disorders are subtle and difficult to identify and interpret. Therefore, dynamic studies such as barium swallow and barium meal and follow-through should be recorded on video tape and several examinations of the tape may be required to exact all the information available.

Scintiscanning

Gamma scintigraphy can also be used to image gastrointestinal contents and observations can be made over a much longer period of time than with conventional radiology. The radiation exposure is the same irrespective of the duration of the study. Scintigraphy, however, lacks the resolution of radiology and individual contractions can only be seen providing images are collected at very frequent intervals and, even then, the detail is quite blurred. Consequently scintiscanning is mostly used for the measurement of transit of material through different regions of gastrointestinal tract. Food, especially infant milk feeds, can be labelled with small amounts of gamma-emitting radio-isotopes which allow studies to be conducted under normal digestive conditions. Scintiscanning has been used for the detection of gastro-oesophageal reflux, it is probably the most accurate method for studying gastric emptying and it is the only method capable of measuring both solid and liquid components of a meal, simultaneously. In paediatric practice it has been little used to measure whole bowel transit or colonic transit.

Like radiology, scintiscanning requires expensive and sophisticated equipment and trained technicians. In most nuclear medicine departments in Children's Hospitals, gamma cameras are often in demand for the investigation of life-threatening conditions involving other organs. Access to the equipment is, therefore, often restricted and in few institutions is there sufficient work to justify the purchase of a gamma camera to be devoted entirely to gastrointestinal investigation.

Manometry

Gastrointestinal manometry is clinically useful when multilumen probes are used to measure intraluminal pressure at closely spaced sites. Today multiport manometric probes can be constructed so that they are sufficiently narrow and flexible for it to be introduced through the nose and tolerated for long periods of time by patients as small as 26–28 week pre-term infants (Bisset et al, 1988) to adolescents. A variety of devices are available including water-perfused catheter systems, catheter-mounted sub-miniature strain gauges, and pressure sensitive radio pills. These systems permit the examination of patterns of contractile activity and to determine their possible function that is propulsive, retropulsive or mixing. If many ports closely sited together are arrayed across a sphincter, a dynamic impression of the function of the whole sphincter region can be gained which is much more useful than pulling a single manometric sensor back through the sphincter. If a continuous record of sphincter activity is required then the incorporation of a sleeve sensor can accommodate the axial mobility of the sphincter. In addition to measuring intraluminal pressure, electrodes for the measurement of other parameters can be included, for example the measurement of pH in oesophageal and gastroduodenal manometric probes may provide greater insight into the function of contractile activity around the lower oesophageal sphincter or pylorus. Similarly, silver–silver chloride electrodes may be incorporated to measure electromyographic activity or to measure transmural potential difference.

Whilst manometry is inexpensive, when compared with radiography and scintigraphy, and can be used to investigate patients over long periods of time, and during provocative tests, it should not be regarded as a simple technique. Manometry requires skilled technicians and obsessional attention to methodological detail if high fidelity reproducible recordings are to be made. The rapid development of multiport techniques and the gathering of data over long periods of time requires sophisticated and complex computer analysis if all the information contained within the records is to be obtained.

Ambulatory or provocative studies

It is clear that even though stationary records of motor activity can be made over long periods of time, intermittent abnormalities may still be missed or abnormalities may only occur under certain specific conditions. In the field of intra-oesophageal pH monitoring, which provides an overall test of the lower body of the oesophagus and lower oesophageal sphincter function, ambulatory monitoring has become the gold standard. Ambulatory monitoring is also now available for prolonged intraluminal pressure recordings and signals from pressure-sensitive radio pills or from intra-luminal strain-gauge transducers can be recorded onto solid-state data loggers and then played back into a personal computer for analysis or a chart recorder to provide a permanent record. With solid-state systems it is now possible to store data from eight channels or more over a 12 h period or from three or four channels for up to 72 h at a time (Kellow et al, 1990).

Provocative tests may be particularly useful if they can simulate a situation which the patient or the relevant part of their gut may encounter. Perhaps the earliest of these studies was the infusion of acid into the lower oesophagus or balloon distension to provoke pain and abnormal contractile activity in patients with a disturbed oesophageal motility. Similarly acid perfusion studies used to examine duodenal motor activity, and rectal distension to provoke relaxation of the internal anal sphincter, as a test for Hirschsprung's disease, are but a few examples. These manoeuvres provide important insights into patient's disabilities and should, wherever possible, be incorporated into tests of gastrointestinal motility.

In these days of cost-effective investigation and treatment, is prolonged ambulatory recording more or less likely to detect an intermittent disorder than specific manoeuvres designed to provoke abnormalities? At the present time the role of ambulatory pressure recording is being defined and clear guidelines as to the circumstances under which it should be used are not yet available and thus the utility of prolonged ambulatory studies is not clear.

THE OESOPHAGUS

Most children are referred for tests of oesophageal motility, either because they have a disorder of swallowing or because they have symptoms suggestive of gastro-oesophageal reflux. Unlike adult practice it is unusual for a child to be referred for investigation of chest pain of uncertain origin. There is no single investigation that is suitable for all purposes and the choice of investigation depends upon the nature of the patient's symptoms and the question that is being asked.

Disorders of swallowing

The single most useful investigation into disorders of swallowing is the video fluoroscopy or the video recording of a barium swallow (Ekberg and Nylander, 1982). In this technique all phases of swallowing from ingestion of the test meal, be it liquid or solid, are carefully observed from the time that the food is placed in the patient's mouth to it entering the stomach. The technique does, however, require a radiologist who is skilled in the perform-ance of the investigation and its interpretation. In our practice it is usual for a speech therapist and radiologist to carry out the investigation together. Not only is this a good technique for observing the initial oral and pharyngeal phases of swallowing to determine whether aspiration occurs or not, or whether laryngeal movement is co-ordinated with pharyngeal movement, it is also very useful in detecting abnormal oesophageal motility. However, abnormal contractile activity may be missed or misinterpreted unless the radiologist records the procedure on video tape and is prepared to spend time reviewing it later with other members of the diagnostic team. It is important that the test meals that are used are appropriate for the infant's age, e.g. it is inadequate in a toddler for a study to be done with liquid barium alone and the patient should also be asked to swallow barium labelled foods of different textures, such as bread or barium labelled marshmallow.

Oesophageal manometry

If radiology fails to establish a definitive diagnosis then it should be followed by manometric recording of oesophageal motor activity, which must include defining the activity of the lower and upper oesophageal sphincters. Under these conditions oesophageal manometry is useful in identifying both achalasia of the lower oesophageal sphincter and cricopharyngeal spasm, since both of these can be missed or mis-diagnosed on radiological examination. Oesophageal manometry is also the most sensitive way of diagnosing diffuse oesophageal spasm. Finally developmental anomalies of the enteric neuromusculature, particularly at the junctions of the striated and smooth muscle are often best detected manometrically, as are disorders of peristalsis of the lower oesophagus associated with pseudo-obstructive disorders.

In the author's practice, a multiport manometric system is used with a perfused sleeve sensor to record lower oesophageal sphincter activity (Arndorfer et al, 1977; Mahony et al, 1988). In our laboratory, assemblies made up of water-perfused catheters are less expensive, more robust, more reliable and more comfortable for the patient than probes using intraluminal strain-gauge transducers.

Gastro-oesophageal reflux

In many children a carefully taken history will suffice to make a diagnosis of gastro-oesophageal reflux and, where there is no indication of associated disease, treatment can be initiated without the need for an investigation. Investigation is, however, indicated when either symptoms are severe and are associated with failure to thrive, disordered feeding, haematemesis or respiratory symptoms, or where they persist despite treatment and recur as soon as treatment is finished. Investigation has three functions: to define the presence and severity of reflux; to detect the presence of associated complicating disorders such as oesophagitis, stricture or respiratory condition; and to elucidate the nature of the underlying disorder causing the reflux. It is clear, therefore, that for patients with complicated gastro-oesophageal reflux disease a whole variety of investigations are required (Milla, 1990). These will range through tests of oesophageal motor function and upper gastrointestinal endoscopy to magnetic resonance imaging of the brain stem and tests of immunological function. In this section only tests of motor function of the oesophagus or stomach will be considered.

24 Hour pH monitoring

The majority of gastro-oesophageal reflux is acid in nature and can be reliably detected by interoesophageal pH monitoring. At the present time there is no doubt that ambulatory 24 h intra-oesophageal pH monitoring provides a gold standard for identifying gastro-oesophageal reflux. The normal ranges for reflux under postprandial and supine conditions during wakefulness and sleep have been carefully documented so that patients can be given a score which indicates the degree of exposure of the lower oesophagus to acid (Johnson and Demeester, 1986; Vandenplas and Sacre-Smits, 1987). It is, however, dependent upon the degree of gastric acidity and some controversy exists regarding the cut-off levels for threshold pHs. Recently, attempts have been made to negate these problems by using double pH probe recordings in which one probe is placed in the conventional position in the lower oesophagus and the other in the stomach. The other area which causes difficulty, in practice, is where respiratory symptoms occur as a consequence of gastro-oesophageal reflux. The symptoms may be as diverse as recurrent episodes of apnoea, bronchospasm and aspiration causing chest infection. In the predisposed patient, the symptoms do not appear to be related to prolonged exposure of the lower oesophagus to acid, but may occur following relatively short lived episodes of reflux both during the day, in small infants, and in association with changes of sleep state when asleep. In order to define the association of respiratory symptoms with reflux it has become the practice, in our laboratory, to combine pH studies with recordings of oxygen saturation. Dips in oxygen saturation being associated with clinically significant episodes of bronchospasm or episodes of apnoea. For those patients who have repeated chest aspiration, examination of specimens of sputum for fat-laden macrophages is of use.

Oesophageal manometry

Measurement of lower oesophageal sphincter pressure is of little value in assessing the individual patient. The major advantage of the technique is that it can identify different mechanisms that lead to abnormal exposure of the lower oesophageal mucosa to acid. These include transient, inappropriate lower oesophageal sphincter relaxation, lower oesophageal sphincter pressure, abnormal clearance of acid due to impaired secondary peristalsis and a displaced lower oesophageal sphincter (Mahony et al, 1988). Currently manometry does not appear to be very useful in evaluating patients with gastro-oesophageal reflux.

Hiatus hernia and gastro-oesophageal reflux

Sliding hiatus hernia and episodes of reflux are common in patients who have recurrent regurgitation. Surgical treatment of gastro-oesophageal reflux involves much time and effort being spent in ensuring that a proportion of the oesophagus remains in the abdomen and in recreating normal anatomical abnormalities. It does, however, seem likely that the sliding hiatus hernia is a function of the length of the oesophagus which tends to be relatively shorter in the first 2 years of life and motor activity of the oesophagus. It seems likely that shortening of the oesophagus still further occurs during contraction of the longitudinal muscle of the oesophagus and that this may occur in relationship to impaired acid clearance (Dodds et al, 1974). Hence the most likely explanation of the sliding hiatus hernia is that this is a radiological appearance induced by the function of the oesophagus rather than solely an anatomic abnormality.

Gastric emptying and gastro-oesophageal reflux

Studies of gastric emptying in children with gastro-oesophageal reflux have shown that those who have complicated gastro-oesophageal reflux are more likely to have delays in gastric emptying (Hillemeier et al, 1981). In the experimental animal, one documented mechanism for the initiation of transient relaxation of the lower oesophageal sphincter is that of gastric distention. Consequently, if gastric emptying is impaired, gastric distention is more likely to occur and hence there may indeed be a relationship between gastric emptying and severe gastro-oesophageal reflux. Unfortunately whilst surgical procedures to control gastro-oesophageal reflux are reasonably successful, surgical procedures to improve gastric emptying are often far from successful.

THE STOMACH

In the stomach the first stage of digestion is initiated and gastric emptying is one of the most important motor functions in the gastrointestinal tract. It limits the rate of absorption of nutrients and drugs by controlling delivery into the small intestine. The rate of delivery is modulated by feedback from nutrient and other receptors in the small intestine, by the central nervous system via the vagus and sympathetic nerves, and by the release of a variety of hormones.

Many patients complain of upper gastrointestinal symptoms for which no obvious cause can be found. Such symptoms may include nausea, reflex vomiting, epigastric pain and a sense of bloating and early satiety. Both excessively rapid and excessively slow gastric emptying are known to be associated with the above symptoms, yet in spite of this, tests of gastric motor function are rarely carried out on such patients. It is possible to rectify abnormal rates of gastric emptying with prokinetic drugs, smooth muscle relaxants or, in some instances, diet. Thus the knowledge that a disorder of gastric emptying exists in a patient may influence not only drug treatment but also a choice of diet or formula for the infant.

Despite the very obvious indications for tests of gastric motor function, these are only routinely conducted in a very few research centres. One of the reasons for this is that apart from measuring mouth to caecal transit time by breath hydrogen or observation of the emptying of barium from the stomach, most tests of gastric motor function are not easily available. They either require a detailed understanding of complex analytical techniques or sophisticated and expensive gamma camera facilities.

In addition to these difficulties, the symptoms related to disturbances in gastric motor function are often intermittent. Unless the patient is willing to undergo several examinations, a disorder of emptying or motor function may be missed and if present its relevance may be questionable. There is thus an argument for carrying out tests under conditions that provoke the symptoms. Certainly provocative test meals can be designed but it is often difficult to reproduce other stressful conditions under laboratory conditions or to carry out sufficient control studies to be able to interpret the results.

Gamma scintigraphy or scintiscanning is almost certainly the most accurate test of gastric emptying and is the only test that allows the emptying of solids and liquids to be carried out simultaneously. Its disadvantages are, however, that it is inconvenient, expensive and radio isotopes are required which preclude multiple studies in the same patient and, at the present moment, would be unethical in children. There are, however, a number of alternatives.

Ultrasound

Ultrasound is safe and comfortable for the patient and can be repeated on multiple occasions but can only be used with meals of specific composition (Bolondi et al, 1985). The images are not always very clear and require great skill in both the acquisition and interpretation. Nevertheless, there are indications that it may be useful as a means of measuring gastric emptying.

Radiology

A barium meal is of little value in assessing many gastric motor disorders as it determines gastric emptying under fasting conditions. The majority of motor disorders of the stomach, which result in abnormality of gastric emptying, appear to be most prominent in the postprandial phase when there is a very high degree of gastroduodenal co-ordination. A barium meal is, of course, essential in determining an anatomical obstructing lesion to the gastric outlet.

Electrical impedance tomography

Of the alternative methods to scintiscanning electrical impedance tomography (EIT) or applied potential tomography is probably the most useful. The equipment is cheap, portable and easy to operate so that tests can be conducted at the bedside. The technique is non-invasive, it does not employ radio-isotopes and the results compare favourably with results of syntigraphy or dye dilution tests (Avill et al, 1987). There are, however, a number of problems with EIT, the major one being the necessity to use drugs to block acid secretion. EIT measures the conductance of gastric contents which can be altered by the ionic composition as well as the volume. Therefore, changes in gastric acid secretion that take place during the digestion of a meal may distort gastric emptying profiles as measured by EIT. In addition to this EIT has not been validated to monitor the emptying of solid meals, although it appears to be perfectly capable of measuring the emptying of semi-solids such as porridge or sausages and mash. Despite its obvious advantages and its few drawbacks, EIT has not, at the present time, enjoyed widespread favour as a means of measuring gastric emptying. It should, perhaps also be said that it is perfectly possible, using EIT, to measure contractile activity of the antral wall and gastro-oesophageal and duodenal gastric reflux (Ravelli and Milla, 1993).

Electrogastrography

Electrogastrography is another very old methodology first used by Alvarez (1992) which latterly has seen a resurgence of interest. In this case the interest has been due to improved methods of analysis made possible by the advent of personal computers and the development of analytical techniques (Van der Schee and Grashuis, 1987). We have found the technique useful in the case of children with intractable vomiting and have found a high correlation especially with nausea and the presence of antral dysrhythmias (Devane et al, 1989). Advances in understanding the neurophysiology of the emetic reflex have shown that dysrhythmia of the gastric antrum is one of a number of autonomic consequences of activation of the emetic reflex and that these occur during the pre-ejection phase when nausea is common. Studying patients with neuromuscular disease, we have been able to show particular patterns of disturbance of gastric antral electrical control activity which are persistent when measured in the fasting phase. It would thus seem that electrogastrography would be an excellent screening test for patients with idiopathic pseudo-obstruction (Devane et al, 1992).

Barostat and gastroduodenal manometry

The two major motor functions of the stomach are receptive relaxation to receive a meal and antral motor activity to break up food particles and to deliver the ingested meal in a controlled fashion to the small intestine. Methods to measure these motor functions of the stomach are, at present, research tools only and are helping us to understand the motor events that control gastric emptying. These tools will probably only be useful as clinical procedures if it can be established that there are specific disturbances of the individual components of gastroduodenal motor activity and if treatment of these disturbances rectifies gastric emptying and improves symptoms. At the present time this is not the case.

SMALL INTESTINE

Motor activity of the small intestine is closely related to its physiological function of digestion and absorption. In the postprandial state, contractile activity results in segmentation, mixing and exposure of the intestinal contents to the mucosa in as efficient a way as possible. Once the nutrients have largely been absorbed from the intraluminal contents a fasting, or interdigestive, pattern of activity is returned to and this results in sweeping the intraluminal contents out of the small intestine and into the colon. Identification of abnormal patterns of activity in the small intestine is relatively simple compared with the colon or stomach since our knowledge of normal patterns of small intestinal motor activity is much greater. Whilst this knowledge applies almost entirely to the fasting state, greater insight is being gained into the organization of postprandial activity and this is beginning to be applied to patients who have disturbance of small bowel motility who complain of symptoms after meals. The two tests for small intestinal motor function that are routinely employed are those of small bowel manometry and of small bowel transit by breath hydrogen analysis of a lactulose test meal.

Manometry

Like oesophageal manometry small bowel manometry may be undertaken using either small bore multilumen water perfused catheter systems or intraluminal strain-gauge transducers mounted on a catheter at fixed points apart. The former have the advantage of being robust, small enough to be passed through the nose of a small infant but the disadvantage that it must be a stationary technique, and very long term or ambulatory recordings are not possible. Intraluminal strain-gauge transducers at the present time have the disadvantage of being relatively bulky, are fragile and extremely expensive. They do, however, have the advantage of it being possible to make ambulatory and very long-term recordings.

Manometry is employed in one of two ways. Either the fasting or inter-digestive pattern of motor activity is recorded and used as a probe of the integrity of the enteric nervous system or the ability of the smooth muscle coat to contract. A number of studies have suggested that small bowel manometry may be a useful investigation in investigating patients with suspected intestinal pseudo-obstruction. A normal pattern of contractile activity with abnormally low pressures might suggest an intestinal myopathy while an abnormal configuration or migration of the interdigestive migrating motor complex (MMC), or loss of the cyclical pattern of the fasting activity, suggests an enteric or intrinsic neuropathy (Stanghellini et al, 1987). Other abnormalities such as the failure of a meal to convert the fasting motor pattern to a fed motor pattern or a prolonged burst of phasic activity superimposed on a tonic elevation in the base line have also been suggested as indicative of neuropathy. However, very recent studies of patients with coeliac disease have shown similar patterns of activity suggesting that these abnormalities may not be as specific as once thought (Cucchiara et al, 1993). The problem appears to be that patterns of motor activity that occur in normal subjects under fasting conditions are relatively well understood and known. We have very inadequate insight, however, into the range of normality and in particular the influence of changes in luminal contents or the effect of physical discomfort, psychic stress or disease processes affecting other areas of the gut such as the mucosa. Disorder of extrinsic nerves may well affect the fasting motor pattern and, for example, post-vagotomy diarrhoea is associated with a rapid postprandial return to the fasting motor pattern (Thompson et al, 1982). These abnormalities are also seen in neonates, in some dysmorphic syndromes such as Noonan's syndrome and Turner's syndrome, and in toddler diarrhoea (Fenton et al, 1983).

Other features may be observed in normal subjects, e.g. contraction clusters, giant migrating clusters, but if they occur frequently in regions of the small intestine where they are not usually seen they may then be abnormal. The presence of giant migrating contractions in the upper small intestine is abnormal and may be secondary to drugs, toxins or infection.

Similarly frequent clusters of contraction are unusual in normal man but may occur where there is sub-acute intestinal obstruction or in the irritable bowel syndrome.

As more experience is gained in recording small intestinal motility many abnormal features are being detected and described. However, whether these relate more to primary disturbances of the enteric or extrinsic nerves or whether they are secondary to other factors is often unclear. When more of these questions have been answered, small intestinal manometry may become a useful clinical procedure. It certainly shows great promise but, at the moment, is probably not used other than in a unit that has great experience in performing it.

Mouth to caecal transit by breath hydrogen analysis

Breath hydrogen analysis using a nonabsorbable sugar as a test meal is a simple, safe, noninvasive method of measuring mouth to caecal transit time (Corbett et al, 1981). This test is probably of very limited value and is a composite of gastric emptying and small bowel transit. It has the disadvantage that the relationship between the transit time at the head of the meal and the transit time at the bulk of the meal varies considerably between patients. The results may also be distorted where there is bacterial overgrowth of the small intestine. Furthermore, a very early postprandial rise in breath hydrogen concentration may occur leading the unwary investigator to conclude that the patient has a very rapid transit. At present, this measurement does not appear to be very useful clinically.

COLONIC AND ANORECTAL FUNCTION TESTS

The colon is the least accessible region of the gastrointestinal tract and its normal functions of salvage of nutrients and concentration of salt and water are poorly understood. In recent years patterns of colonic motility have been detected and a little is known regarding it.

Whilst the whole panoply of motility tests of manometry, myoelectric recordings, scintigraphy have all been employed in clinical practice only two investigations are clearly of value and a third may be. At present the most useful test of colonic motor activity is the simple measurement of colonic transit time using radio-opaque markers. This study may be carried out in one of two ways. A number of small radio-opaque markers—we use 25–50 small rings of 2.5 mm diameter radio-opaque tubing cut into 1 mm lengths—are fed at time 0 either in ice-cream or mashed potato and X-rays are taken at 48 and 72 h after ingestion. The distribution of markers on the abdominal X-rays is then measured and useful information can be gained from the distribution of the markers around the colon or in the rectum (Martelli et al, 1978). A variation on this method is to use different shaped markers on three successive days and for one single plain abdominal X-ray to be taken on the fourth day (Metcalfe et al, 1987). This, however, requires specially shaped pellets in order to be able to distinguish each days marker.

In our experience in patients with constipation related to disturbance in colonic propulsion, marker studies may reveal either slow transit through all regions or through the proximal colon or the distal colon. These patients appear to behave differently from those that have rectal holding which appears to be the commonest form of constipation seen in preschool children.

Anorectal manometry

The other investigation that clearly is of value in childhood in the diagnosis of Hirschsprung's disease is that of anorectal manometry (Aaronson and Nixon, 1972). Whilst in adult practice anorectal manometry is used extensively for the investigation of patients with constipation it has only found lasting favour in childhood for the diagnosis of Hirschsprung's disease. Attempts to investigate other forms of constipating disorder by anorectal manometry have shown it to have a relatively low sensitivity and specificity. A good example of this is the investigation of intestinal neuronal dysplasia (Koletzko et al, 1992).

In our laboratory, however, anorectal manometry is now very rarely undertaken as the sensitivity and specificity for the diagnosis of Hirschsprung's disease of suction rectal biopsy with acetylcholinesterase staining is so much greater.

Provocative manometry

In patients with slow transit constipation, some form of provocative recto-sigmoid motility may have a place. In the author's laboratory in patients with slow transit constipation two forms of provocative study are used. Firstly, the so-called gastrocolonic response in which sigmoid motility is measured in response to a standardized test meal, usually of milk in toddlers of 30 ml per kilo to a maximum of 300 ml. It is suggested that the increased motor activity in response to food is an index of the integrity of the neurohumoral control of colonic motility. The second provocative test which is used, tests local enteroenteric reflexes and a few ml of bisacodyl syrup is injected into the lumen of the sigmoid colon above the perfused catheter system used and the motility record observed for an increase in activity induced by the bisacodyl. These investigations should be regarded as screening tests and the results of them may indicate more definitive procedures such as full-thickness rectal biopsy. It is beyond the scope of this chapter to discuss the various histological findings that might occur in slow transit constipation and interested readers are referred to a recent excellent review (Milla and Smith, 1994).

CONCLUSION

Only 8 years ago, in a review of intestinal motility disorders in childhood, it was remarked that the increased understanding of the basic science of the enteric neuromusculature had, as yet, hardly influenced the clinical practice of paediatric gastroenterology. It is today, quite clear that studies of gastrointestinal motility are beginning to have clinical relevance to the diagnosis and treatment of disorders of the enteric neuromusculature. At the present time progress is restricted more by the lack of a base of knowledge regarding pathological changes of intestinal motor activity than by the techniques necessary to obtain that data. It is hoped that the above discussion will indicate the usefulness of gastrointestinal motor activity and inspire others to undertake such studies to add to the growing base of information regarding the pathophysiology of gastrointestinal motility disorders.

REFERENCES

Aaronson I & Nixon HH (1972) A clinical evaluation of ano-rectal pressure studies in the diagnosis of Hirschsprung's Disease. *Gut* **13**: 138–146.

Alvarez WC (1922) The electrogastrogram and what it shows. *Journal of the American Medical Association* **78**: 1116–1119.

Arndorfer RC, Stef JJ, Dodds WJ et al (1977) Improved infusion system for intra-luminal oesophageal manometry. *Gastroenterology* **73**: 23–27.

Avill R, Mangnall YF, Bird NC et al (1987) Applied potential tomography a new non-invasive technique for measuring gastric emptying. *Gastroenterology* **92**: 1019–1026.

Bisset WM, Watt JB, Rivers RPA & Milla PJ (1988) Measurement of small intestinal motor activity in the premature infant. *Journal of Biomedical Engineering* **10**: 155–158.

Bolondi L, Bartolotti M, Santi V et al (1985) Measurement of gastric emptying time by real time ultra-sinography. *Gastroenterology* **89**: 752–759.

Corbett CL, Thomas S, Reid NW et al (1981) Electro-chemical detector for breath hydrogen determination: measurement of small bowel transit time in normal subject and patients with the irritable bowel syndrome. *Gut* **22**: 836–840.

Cucchiara S, Bassatti G, Bastellycci G et al (1993) Abnormalities of small intestinal motility in children with active coeliac disease. *Journal of Paediatric Gastroenterology and Nutrition* **17**: 469.

Devane SP, Bisset WM & Milla PJ (1989) Persistent tachygastria in severe nausea and vomiting. *Paediatric Research* **26**: 275.

Devane SP, Ravelli AM, Bisset WM et al (1992) Gastric antral dysrhythmia in children with chronic idiopathic intestinal pseudo-obstruction. *Gut* **33**: 1477–1481.

Dodds WJ, Stewart ET, Hogan WJ et al (1974) Effect of oesophageal movement on intra-luminal oesophageal pressure recording. *Gastroenterology* **67**: 592–600.

Ekberg O & Nylander G (1982) Scintiradiography of the pharyngeal stage of deglutition in 250 dysphageal patients. *British Journal of Radiology* **55**: 258–262.

Fenton TR, Harries JT & Milla PJ (1983) Abnormalities of post-prandial small intestinal motor activity in childhood: their role in the pathogenesis of the irritable bowel syndrome. In Labo G & Bortolotti M (eds) *Gastrointestinal Motility*, pp 207–213. Verona: Cortina International.

Hillemeier C, Lange R, McCallum R et al (1981) Delayed gastric emptying in infants with gastro-oesophageal reflux. *Journal of Paediatrics* **98**: 190–193.

Johnson LF & Demeester TR (1986) Development of the 24 hour intra-oesophageal pH monitoring computer scoring system. *Journal of Clinical Gastroenterology* **8**: 52–58.

Kellow JE, Gill RC & Wingate DL (1990) Prolonged ambulant recordings of small bowel motility demonstrated abnormalities in the irritable bowel syndrome. *Gastroenterology* **98**: 1208–1218.

Koletzko S, Ballauff A, Hadziselimovic C & Enck P (1992) Ano-rectal manometry in Hirschsprung's Disease and neuronal intestinal dysplasia. In Hadziselimovic F & Herzog B (eds) *Fauk's Symposium 65. Paediatric Gastroenterology: Inflammatory Bowel Diseases and Morbus Hirschsprung*, pp 263–282. Dordrecht: Clear Academic Publishers.

Mahony MJ, Migliavacca M, Spitz L & Milla PJ (1988) Motor disorders of the oesophagus in gastro-oesophageal reflux. *Archives of Disease in Childhood* **63**: 1333–1338.

Martelli H, Devroede GH, Arhan P & Duguay C (1978) Mechanisms for idiopathic constipation: outlet obstruction. *Gastroenterology* **75**: 623–631.

Metcalfe AM, Phillips SF, Zinsmeister AR et al (1987) Simplified assessment of segmental colonic transit. *Gastroenterology* **924**: 40–47.

Milla PJ (1990) Reflux vomiting. *Archives of Disease in Childhood* **65**: 996–999.

Milla PJ & Smith VV (1994) Aganglionosis hypoganglionosis and hyperganglionosis: clinical presentation and histopathology. In Kamm MA & Lennard Jones JE (eds) *Constipation*, pp 183–192. Petersfield: Wrightson Biomedical Publishing.

Ravelli AM & Milla PJ (1993) Detection of gastro-oesophageal reflux by electrical impedance tomography. In Holder DA (ed.) *Electrical Impedance Tomography*, pp 159–164. London: University College Press.

Smith AWM, Code CF & Schlegel JF (1957) Simultaneous scintiradiographic and kimographic studies of human gastric antral motility. *Journal of Applied Physiology* **11**: 12–16.

Stanghellini V, Camilleri M & Malagelada J-R (1987) Chronic idiopathic intestinal pseudo-obstruction: clinical and intestinal manometric findings. *Gut* **28**: 5–12.

Thompson DG, Ritchie HD & Wingate DL (1982) Patterns of small intestinal motility in duodenal ulcer patients before and after vagotomy. *Gut* **23**: 517–523.

Vandenplas Y & Sacre-Smits L (1987) Continuous 24 hour oesophageal pH monitoring in 285 asymptomatic infants 0–15 months old. *Journal of Paediatric Gastroenterology and Nutrition* **6**: 220–224.

Van der Schee EJ & Grashuis JL (1987) Running spectrum analysis as an aid in the representation and interpretation of electrogastrographic signals. *Medical and Biological Engineering and Computer* **25**: 57–62.

6

Home parenteral nutrition in children

W. M. BISSET
N. J. MEADOWS

The rapid rates of growth and development seen in young children are dependent on a steady supply of nutrients which are assimilated through the digestive and absorptive processes of the gastrointestinal tract. Where gastrointestinal function is severely compromised by disease, this supply of nutrients is reduced and intravenous nutrition may be the only means by which the normal growth and development of the child can be maintained (Amarnath et al, 1987). As a result of improvements in the compounding and formulation of parenteral feeding regimes and in the insertion technique and nursing care of central venous catheters, it is now possible to maintain children on total parenteral nutrition for many years. Previously, many of these children spent prolonged periods in hospital receiving their parenteral nutrition, where many died from the complications of treatment, but now with the realization that treatment out of hospital has many advantages, there has been an understandable move towards the provision of parenteral nutrition in the family home (Scribner et al, 1970; Revesz and Wesley, 1991).

Home parenteral nutrition (HPN) was first described in the early 1970s and shortly afterwards its use was reported in children with severe intestinal disease (Cannon et al, 1980). Although this treatment has been most widely used in North America (Ament et al, 1986) and France (De Potter et al, 1992), there have subsequently been reports of home parental nutrition in children from most developed countries. Until the techniques of gut transplantation are perfected, the use of HPN as a supportive therapy for children with severe intestinal failure is likely to continue to increase (Hiyama, 1993).

INDICATIONS FOR HOME PARENTERAL NUTRITION

Any patient who is dependent on parenteral nutrition and who does not require complex nursing support should be considered as a candidate for home parenteral nutrition. Many health professionals underestimate the ability of parents to care for their own children and it is likely that where the parents are motivated, their expertise in the delivery of HPN to their child, will be at least equal to, if not better than that of the carers in hospital.

Baillière's Clinical Paediatrics—
Vol. 2, No. 4, November 1994
ISBN 0–7020–1866–X

The major indications for home parenteral nutrition in children are outlined in Table 1. In the majority of reported cases, the underlying problems are primarily gastrointestinal. Gastrointestinal functions can be seriously compromised as a consequence of: (i) reduction of absorptive surface area as occurs in the short bowel syndrome (Goulet et al, 1991); (ii) motility disturbances of the gastrointestinal tract (Pitt et al, 1985) where there is a failure of the normal propagation of nutrients along the gut; and (iii) a range of intractable diarrhoeal processes which result in serious structural or functional abnormalities of the small intestinal mucosa. In addition, home parenteral nutrition has been used to support children with neoplastic disease and the acquired immune deficiency syndrome.

Table 1. Common indications for home parenteral nutrition.

(a)	Gastrointestinal disease
	Reduced length of gut
	Intestinal resection
	Necrotising enterocolitis
	Volvulus
	Multiple intestinal atresia
	Crohn's disease
	Congenital short intestine
	Motility disturbance
	Myopathic pseudo-obstruction
	Neuropathic pseudo-obstruction
	Hirschsprung's disease involving small intestine
	Intractable diarrhoea of infancy
	Congenital enteropathy
	Autoimmune enteropathy
	Congenital secretory diarrhoea
(b)	Systemic disease
	Malignant disease
	Acquired immune deficiency syndrome

While it may be technically possible to support any child, irrespective of their underlying disease, this may not always be desirable and the success of home parenteral nutrition, in a well organized centre, is largely down to the ability of the family to cope with the management of their child. If parents are highly motivated and are able to learn the techniques required, their child is likely to do well at home. However, if neither of the parents or a family member is dedicated to providing the treatment required, home parenteral nutrition will almost certainly fail.

If the child is suffering from a condition which is potentially reversible or where adaptation with time may compensate for the defect (i.e. short gut syndrome) the decision to send a child home on parenteral nutrition will be determined by the likely length of time adaptation will take, compared to the time required to train the parents and set up the provision of parenteral nutrition at home. Where the provision of HPN is well organized it should be possible to make all the necessary arrangements within a few weeks and thus many young babies with the short gut syndrome will complete their adaptation at home. Where this is not the case, many of these children will remain in hospital and are more likely to succumb from the complications of their treatment.

ADMINISTRATION OF HOME PARENTERAL NUTRITION

In order to administer reliably home parenteral nutrition to a child, one requires a reliable form of venous access, a means of regulating the delivery of the nutrient solutions and finally one has to provide a solution which is bacteriologically safe and meets the nutrient requirements of the child.

Venous access

In most reported series venous access has been provided through the insertion of a surgically implanted silastic Hickman–Broviac (Bard Inc., C.R. Murray Hill, NJ) type of catheter (Broviac et al, 1973; Broviac and Scribner, 1974). The line is inserted with full aseptic precautions, via the internal jugular or subclavian vein, with the tip of the line placed either at the junction of the superior vena cava and the right atrium or high in the right atrium. There is some debate about the ideal position for the tip of central venous catheters in HPN patients, although it is clear that when the tip is lying high in the superior vena cava the risk of venous thrombosis is greatly increased, and alternatively, if the tip either touches or passes through the tricuspic valve, damage or infection of the valve leaflets may occur. The cuffed venous catheter should be inserted through a sub-cutaneous tunnel as this not only improves the anchorage of the line but also acts as a microbiological barrier to prevent the migration of micro-organisms along the line (Pokorny et al, 1987). The best results are likely to be obtained with a single lumen, as opposed to a multilumen catheter, as the risk of sepsis is reduced and the larger internal diameter makes the risk of occlusion less likely.

An alternative to the traditional silastic catheter is the use of an infusion port. Devices such as the Port-A-Cath (Pharmacia Deltec, Inc., St Pauls, MN) have the advantage that external dressings are not required, making swimming or showering a simple procedure (Pomp et al, 1989). They do, however, require a needle stick with each use and this may eventually lead to skin ulceration with fenestration and contamination of the infusion port membrane. With the increasing use of these devices in children on HPN it is clear that they can be used very successfully in some patients although it is not yet clear whether they are superior to traditional catheters (Howard et al, 1989). A more recent development has been the introduction of the Cuff Cath (Viggo-Spectramen, Swindon, UK) which is made of polyurethane and has the advantage of a reduced external diameter for a given lumen size, compared to traditional silastic catheters.

Irrespective of the type of catheter or infusion port used, it is most important that it is only handled by a person fully trained in the care of central lines. It is most people's experience that when untrained staff handle central lines or when they are used for multiple sampling of venous blood the risk of line sepsis increases dramatically.

Delivery system

A reliable paediatric infusion pump which will deliver the correct volumes of nutrient solutions at the correct rate is required for safe HPN. Such a pump should alarm at the end of the infusion or when the line becomes occluded and should be both safe and reliable so that it can be left unattended while the child is sleeping. If problems do arise during an infusion, the parents should be fully trained to cope with the situation and it is recommended that the pump should be supported by a 24 hour service contract which allows for immediate repair or replacement if a fault develops.

Intravenous infusion pumps are almost exclusively powered from the mains and require a drip stand which ties the child to a single room or severely limits their mobility. This problem can be overcome by the use of portable, battery-powered infusion pumps which allows the patient to be mobile during their infusion (Anonymous, 1991a,b). This is particularly valuable in children with large fluid requirements, where it may be necessary to continue their i.v. infusion for more than 12 h of the day or during holiday periods where greater flexibility is required.

In hospital it is usual for patients to receive their parenteral nutrition continuously over 24 h. This is clearly not acceptable for patients at home as it would greatly restrict their mobility and in children would prevent them going to school and from playing normally. For this reason most groups give the daily nutrient intakes over a period of 10–12 h overnight, allowing the child complete independence during the day. In children with residual intestinal function it may be possible to restrict the infusion of HPN to 5 or 6 days a week, allowing the child and family even greater freedom. The higher infusion rates of nutrients that this inevitably requires are well tolerated by children and lead to very few problems. It must, however, be remembered that when the infusion is being stopped in the morning it is best to reduce the infusion rate in stages over a period of approximately 1 h in order to prevent the development of reflex hypoglycaemia.

Nutrients

Without adequate nutrition, growth and development will be compromised. While guidelines exist for nutritional requirements in healthy children, the requirements for children with severe gastrointestinal disease may be difficult to predict and are likely to vary greatly from one child to the next. Estimates can be made of the parenteral nutrient requirements for a child on HPN by making allowances for nutrient and electrolyte losses in stool or vomit and by assessing the degree of residual enteral food tolerance (Just et al, 1991) (see Table 2). However, it is only once the HPN regime has been used and the growth and nutritional response of the child has been monitored, that the adequacy of the formulation can be properly assessed.

Table 2. Average daily nutrient requirements in health. Values for energy requirement are higher for boys than girls above 1 year of age. Details of trace metal and vitamin requirements are given in Ament (1991).

Age (years)	Volume (ml/kg)	Energy kJ (kcal/kg)	Protein (g/kg)
Newborn	150	483 (115)	2.2
1	110	399 (95)	2.0
3	100	399 (95)	1.8
5	90	357 (85)	1.5
7	80	310 (74)	1.4
9	70	273 (65)	1.2
12	60	252 (60)	1.0
Adult	40	189 (45)	0.8

Although this chapter primarily concerns the use of parenteral nutrition, it must be emphasized that in patients on HPN, enteral nutrition should be maintained up to the level of tolerance. The only group of patients where this might not apply are the minority of children who are unfortunate enough to have such severe gastrointestinal disease that the addition of any enteral intake will stimulate the increased loss of salt and electrolytes.

Enteral nutrition is of importance for a number of reasons. Firstly, in children with the short gut syndrome, the adaptation of the residual small intestine is dependent to a large extent on the presence of luminal nutrients. Without adequate enteral nutrition, adaptation will be severely compromised and HPN will be more prolonged. Secondly, the hepatic complications of parenteral nutrition, cholestasis and cholelithiasis, are more common in children with no enteral intake. These problems can be largely overcome by the use of bolus enteral feed, which stimulates the normal flow of bile from the liver. Thirdly, it should be remembered that eating is a major social activity and in children who have received prolonged periods of parenteral nutrition without enteral intake, major behavioural feeding problems are likely to develop when attempts are made to introduce oral feeds. Unless these problems are addressed at an early stage, the child's ability to feed normally by mouth may lag far behind the ability of their gut to digest and absorb the ingested food. Finally, if the child has a significant oral intake it may be possible to deliver nutrients enterally, which might otherwise cause instability problems in the formulation of the HPN.

Parenteral nutrient solutions

The standard parenteral nutrition which children receive in hospital is a two infusion system with one bag containing the amino acid, dextrose and minerals, and the other containing the lipid and vitamins (Cochran et al, 1988). Such a system works well in hospital, although the complexity of two infusions and two pumps is likely to compromise the success of treatment at home. With the aim of making things as simple as possible for the parents, the HPN should, where possible, use a single bag infusion. With recent advances in the understanding of the stability of parenteral nutrition solutions, there has been a move towards the formulation of 'all-in-one' bags where all the intravenous nutrients are mixed together (Campos et al, 1990). The main problem with these systems is that the stability of the lipid within the solution is, to a large extent, determined by the concentration of di- and trivalent salts and particular problems develop due to the high calcium and phosphate requirements of young children (Drwal et al, 1990). There are, however, ways to overcome some of these problems. Firstly the 'all-in-one' solution may be given on certain days of the week and then on the other days, when lipid is omitted, larger amounts of calcium and phosphate can be added to the parenteral nutrition. Using this regime the patient requires two different parenteral nutrition bags, but on any one day the parents only have to connect up and run one solution. However, to some extent this problem may be resolved in the future by the use of organic phosphate solutions, such as sodium glycerophosphate. Secondly, in older children in whom the calcium and phosphate requirements are lower than those in young children, it may be possible to formulate all the nutrients in one solution. Finally, in children with good residual intestinal function it may be possible to give enough lipid by the enteral route to overcome the need to give any parenterally. Although traditionally up to 30 or 40% of the energy in enteral and parenteral nutrition is given as lipid, it is our experience that this can be reduced to as little as 10% without deleterious effect on essential fatty acid status or liver function.

Home parenteral nutrition should, in all cases, be formulated in a pharmacy under full aseptic conditions and as such is likely to have a shelf-life of between 1 and 3 months. Particular problems arise, however, with the stability of intravenous vitamin solutions. The stability of some preparations when exposed to light at room temperature can be measured in hours (Billion Rey et al, 1993) and even when refrigerated and kept in the dark there are serious questions about the stability of some solutions (Hariz et al, 1993). This problem can be overcome if the vitamins are added in the pharmacy, but this will inevitably lead to solutions with a short shelf-life. In children with good residual intestinal function, that is up to 30% of their nutrients absorbed orally, it has been our experience that if large doses of oral vitamins are given it is possible to maintain good levels of fat and water soluble vitamins. In many children, however, there may be no alternative to the parents adding intravenous (i.v.) vitamins to the HPN solution.

The methods described above should simplify the administration of home parenteral nutrition while ensuring that the child continues to receive an adequate nutrient intake. The philosophy of making HPN as simple as possible for the parents ensures the high success rate seen with this therapy.

ORGANIZATION OF HOME PARENTERAL NUTRITION

The discharge of a child on home parenteral nutrition is a major undertaking not only for the hospital and community services but particularly for the parents. It is essential therefore that this form of therapy is supervised by a centre with experience of HPN in children. Discharging a child home on HPN without adequate supervision by the hospital and without adequate training of the parents or support in the community is a recipe for disaster (Anonymous, 1992). It is important that before any decision is made on discharge, that the parents are fully aware of what they are undertaking and that the parents and the child's medical and nursing carers are all agreed that this is the most appropriate treatment for this child at the present time. The well-being of the child should be a priority at all times and it should be this that determines the timing of discharge.

Funding

It is generally accepted that it is cheaper to treat a child at home on parenteral nutrition than keep the same child in hospital (Dzierba et al, 1984; Goel, 1990). It is likely that home treatment is between a half and a third of the cost of treatment in hospital (Wateska et al, 1980). One would think therefore that arranging funding to discharge a child home on parenteral nutrition should be relatively straightforward, but in different countries where different funding systems exist this is not always the case. In countries such as the USA, where health care is largely funded by medical insurance, there are major incentives for discharging children home early on parenteral nutrition. These incentives are largely financial and the premature discharge of a child on parenteral nutrition may not necessarily be in that child's best interest. In France, central government funding is available for the provision of home parenteral nutrition through designated centres of excellence, thus removing all financial barriers to the provision of HPN. In the UK (Milewski et al, 1980), there is no special provision for home parenteral nutrition and because of the system of funding, the discharge home of a child on parenteral nutrition is not necessarily perceived as a saving. The first approach for funding should be via the general practitioner, who will have responsibility for the prescription of the nutrient solutions and to the local community paediatric budget holder who will be responsible for the funding of the infusion pump and consumables. For the person taking on this funding, HPN may be seen as a major burden (Bisset et al, 1992). The lack of adequate funding for the community care of children with complex medical problems exists in many countries and may seriously compromise the chances of children on parenteral nutrition being cared for at home. As a consequence many children who would benefit from home parenteral nutrition are never offered the treatment and as a result they either languish in hospital for prolonged periods or die from complications of their treatment.

Training

It is important that the parents or carers of children to be discharged home on parenteral nutrition are well trained in the handling and care of the central venous catheter and have a full understanding of how to cope with any emergencies that may develop, due to equipment failure or disconnection, during treatment (Cady and Yoshioka, 1991; Evans et al, 1993). This training should be undertaken by a nurse specialist in nutrition (Dewar, 1986) and it is important that both parents are resident for at least part of the training period so their aseptic techniques can be adequately supervised and their competence ascertained.

Prior to the discharge of a child home on parenteral nutrition it is important that clear lines of communication are established between the discharging hospital, the parents and the providers of health care within the community. It has therefore been our experience that the organization of a professionals meeting, involving the child's general practitioner, community paediatric nurse, the Social Services Department and Education Department for older children, has been most helpful in ensuring these aims are met. Most parents are very anxious and nervous when they are discharged home with a child on parenteral nutrition and they find it reassuring to know that there is a net of people available to support them.

Formulation and delivery of HPN solutions

Commercial home care companies have a great deal of experience in the provision of HPN and are often in the best position to formulate and deliver parenteral nutrition solutions. It is very important that the parents have regular, reliable deliveries of the HPN solutions and of the giving sets and other consumables which are required. When items are delivered separately or where suppliers are unreliable, this greatly increases the work load and stress level on the parents. In some centres, where large numbers of patients on HPN are supported, well organized hospital pharmacies may be able to compete successfully with the services provided by home care companies.

Monitoring and support

Once a child has been discharged home on parenteral nutrition it is important that the progress of the child is adequately monitored. Immediately following discharge it may be necessary to see the child every 2 or 3 weeks, but thereafter, if the home TPN regime has been correctly formulated and the parents are coping well, review every 2–3 months may be adequate and where patients live a long way from the referral centre, care can be shared with the local hospital. The growth and development of the child should be checked, the biochemical and nutritional state should be monitored and attempts should be made to detect the development of any complications at an early stage. A suggested protocol is shown in Table 3. The needs of the child and their family are best served when the care is supervised by a nutrition team with access to expertise in pharmacy, medical and nursing matters, dietetics (McCrae et al, 1993) and biochemistry. A member of the hospital nutrition team should be on-call 24 hours a day so that when the parents do have problems they know that they can speak to a professional who knows their child.

Support for the family is also essential. When the parents visit the hospital with their child, for review, they should have access to a psychologist who

Table 3. An investigation protocol for the monitoring of HPN (Bisset et al, 1992).

Time (before discharge)	Investigation	
6 weeks	Anthropometry	Weight
		Height
	Haematology	Full blood count
	Biochemistry	Urea and electrolytes
		Calcium
		Magnesium
		Liver function tests
		Urine electrolytes
	Bacteriology (if indicated)	Urine culture
		Line site
3 months	Haematology	Ferritin
		Clotting
	Biochemistry	Copper
		Zinc
		Selenium
6 months	Haematology	Folate
		Vitamin B12
	Biochemistry	Vitamin B1, 2, 6
		Vitamin A, E, D
	If indicated	Aluminium
		Chromium
		Manganese
		Essential fatty acids
	Radiology	Liver ultrasound
		Chest X-ray
	Cardiology	Doppler echo
1 year	Psychology	Developmental assessment

can advise them on the management of their child if behavioural feeding problems develop (Handen et al, 1986) and to a social worker (Johnston, 1981) who can make them aware of all the benefits to which they are entitled. It is helpful if the parents can meet together informally, as they can often learn much from each others experiences (Payne James and Ball, 1991).

OUTCOME

Almost every published report of home parenteral nutrition in childhood has shown that normal growth and development can be maintained while on HPN (Amarnath et al, 1987; Berry and Jorgensen, 1988). Patients who have previously spent prolonged periods in hospital are likely to have grown poorly and very often their developmental milestones lag behind. It is only once these children are discharged home that their growth and development improves (Dahlstrom et al, 1985; O'Connor et al, 1988). Most children at home on parenteral nutrition have a good quality of life and are able to partake in normal schooling and the full activities of their family (Ralston et al, 1984). Although home parenteral nutrition can be quite demanding on time and effort, most parents find this preferable to their child spending prolonged periods in hospital and feel that it is much less disruptive to family life.

The outcome of HPN is dependent on the quality of care that the child receives and on the underlying problem which initiated the need for parenteral nutrition. No two series of patients on HPN are the same and survival figures will be determined by the type of patients treated (Burnes et al, 1992). In a large series of adult patients, the annual survival rate of patients with Crohn's disease was 95%, falling to 25% in those with active cancer, 50% of whom were dead within 6–9 months (Howard, 1992). Although results in childhood cancer seem better than adults, the results remain disappointing as do those obtained in patients with acquired immune deficiency syndrome (AIDS) (Leibowitz and Iberti, 1992).

Complications

With the high quality of care delivered by most parents, problems with HPN are much lower than one might predict (Herfindal et al, 1992). Repeated studies show that the complication rate at home is significantly less than those found in hospital. Most children, however, are likely at some time, to develop a complication of their treatment and most frequent problems arise with the central venous catheter (Schmidt-Sommerfeld et al, 1990).

Central line infection

With meticulous attention to the detail of aseptic technique, the risk of sepsis can be reduced to a minimum and it is likely that most infections are due to some lapse in this technique. The majority of infections will enter the blood through the central venous catheter although in some cases sepsis may track along the external surface of the line, through the skin tunnel and occasionally where other focuses of sepsis exist, the central venous catheter may become chronically colonized (Rammen et al, 1986). The organisms most commonly seen are *Staphylococcus epidermidis* though infection with fungi such as candida and Gram-negative organisms such as pseudomonas and *Escherichia coli* are frequently seen. The rate of line infections is quite markedly reduced when children are discharged home from hospital. The skills of highly motivated parents in caring for their own child's central line may be equal to or even better than those found among hospital nursing staff. It is likely also that there is less opportunity for contamination of the line in the home environment compared to hospital (see Table 4). The central line should be used exclusively for HPN and should never be handled by staff who are not fully familiar with the aseptic handling of central venous devices.

A central line infection should be diagnosed with central and peripheral venous culture and treatment with systemic antibiotics, tailored to the sensitivity of the organism, should be given through the central line. If the sepsis is not life-threatening the line should be left in situ and treatment continued for 10 days. The majority of central lines can be salvaged following

Table 4. Central line survival and infection, at home and in hospital in a consecutive series of 20 children from The Hospital for Sick Children, London. Total follow-up of 47.6 patient years.

	Hospital	Home
Infection rate	1 in 140 days	1 in 566 days
Average line life	175 days	623 days

an infective episode but where sepsis recurs with the same organism, following a course of treatment with an appropriate antibiotic, it should be removed.

Some children have very few problems with sepsis, while others, with identical intestinal disease may have repeated infections. When this occurs one should strongly suspect that the aseptic technique of the parents falls short of that required and it is only by re-education that there is any chance of overcoming this problem.

Line blockage

Blockage of the central venous catheter can occur either due to fibrin deposition at the tip or through precipitation of the parenteral nutrients within the lumen of the line, in particular the lipid component or the calcium and phosphate salts (Breaux et al, 1987). The management of blocked lines depends on the cause of the problem and the site of blockage (ter Borg et al, 1993). Fibrin deposition is best treated with urokinase (5000 units in 2 ml) instilled and left in the line for a period of 3 or 4 h or if this fails with a urokinase infusion (10 000–20 000 units over a 6 h period). Lipid deposition can be treated by the installation of 70% alcohol within the lumen. Many lines block at the hub rather than the tip and this may be detected by inspection of the lumen through the hub, which may be seen to be occluded. Proximal occlusion can be relieved with the use of a catheter repair kit which replaces the hub and a short length of catheter. It is important that suspected blockage is treated early in order to prolong the life of the line.

The central lines may become dislodged and this most frequently occurs within the first month after insertion when the fibrous tissue between the line hub and the skin tunnel has not fully developed. The central line may also become damaged due to trauma or may occasionally split near the hub due to wear and tear. Experience shows that central lines last considerably longer while cared for at home as opposed to hospital for reasons similar to those discussed for line infection (see Table 4).

Thrombosis may also develop at the tip or along the length of the catheter and this is often related to the siting of the line and to the concentration of hyperosmolar solutions given through it. Where high concentrations of dextrose are given into a catheter which is not centrally placed, the risk of thrombosis increases. Patients with an underlying inflammatory problem or repeated line sepsis may also be at increased risk. Catheter thrombosis may present ocultly with symptoms of breathless less or more acutely with a massive pulmonary embolism or superior vena caval obstruction (Graham and Gumbiner, 1984).

Any complication which requires a central line to be removed will inevitably mean that further venous access will be required. If central lines are cared for well, new lines should only be required infrequently and venous access will not become a problem. However, when repeated venous access is required, central veins become thrombosed or damaged following insertion and a lack of venous access can become a very major problem. Lines can if necessary, be inserted into the femoral vein with a tunnel onto the anterior abdominal wall but in small children this almost always causes problems because of the proximity to the napkin area. Occasionally even the azygous vein can be used for venous access but this will inevitably require a thoracotomy for line insertion.

Liver disease

Progressive liver disease is a widely reported complication of long-term parenteral nutrition. The exact reasons why children develop liver disease remains unclear but there are quite definite factors which appear to predispose to its development (Gerard Boncompain et al, 1992). The pathological problem is essentially one of cholestasis associated with progressive biliary cirrhosis which will progress eventually to cirrhosis, liver failure and the death of the child (Cohen and Olsen, 1981). These problems appear to be most common in preterm or very young infants undergoing gastrointestinal surgery, in infants who have repeated episodes of sepsis, and children who have either no or only minimal oral intake. In children with established cholestasis due to parenteral nutrition it may be possible to reverse the jaundice by meticulous attention to aseptic technique which reduces the incidence of sepsis and by the promotion of enteral feeding which will further stimulate biliary flow. The use of oral bile salts such as ursodeoxycholic acid has been suggested in the treatment of cholestasis in patients with total parenteral nutrition (TPN) liver disease (Lindor and Burnes, 1991). In jaundiced children an improvement of liver function frequently occurs after discharge home due to the associated reduced rate of sepsis and with the increased time and attention given by the parents to enteral feeding. Gallstone formation is a well-recognized complication of long-term TPN (Roslyn et al, 1983) and again if an adequate oral intake is introduced the resulting improvement in biliary flow should result in dissolution of the gallstones.

In children in whom cirrhosis has progressed and does not respond to the measures outlined above it is likely that liver transplantation combined with gut transplantation offers the only means of survival.

Nutritional deficiencies

The more the child relies on HPN for their total nutritional requirements the more vulnerable they are to the development of nutritional deficiencies. When the parenteral nutrition regime is being formulated great care and attention should be taken in ensuring that all the essential nutrients are present within the solution. Despite these precautions nutritional deficiencies may develop for a number of reasons. The underlying requirements of the child may change with time, due to the effects of growth and to alteration in losses. When HPN or other nutrient supplements are prescribed it should be remembered that deficiencies may also arise as a result of non-compliance with therapy. By keeping a close eye on the growth of the child it should be possible to ascertain whether the child is receiving adequate energy and protein and from detailed biochemical monitoring it should be possible to detect most deficiency states before major problems have arisen. It must, however, be remembered that a very large number of micro- and macro-nutrients are required for normal health and that the cost of monitoring every single nutrient, at frequent intervals, is likely to be prohibitive. A compromise will therefore have to be reached (see Table 3). While deficiencies of some nutrients may take months to develop, one should be particularly aware that the body stores of water soluble vitamins may be very limited and major deficiency states can develop within 1–2 weeks and should always be suspected when a child shows acute neurological deterioration.

The most commonly reported deficiency states relate to problems with trace metals such as zinc or selenium (Kien and Ganther, 1983) although many other deficiencies have been reported in patients on HPN (Dahlstrom et al, 1986). With most regimes it is difficult to provide an optimal intake of iron and many patients will require blood transfusion periodically to maintain their haemoglobin.

As well as omissions from the HPN it should be remembered that contamination of nutrient solutions can occur. Although aluminium contamination of amino-acid solutions has reduced significantly since the introduction of synthetic solutions, many of the trace metal mixtures on the market are still contaminated with significant amounts of aluminium (Koo et al, 1986). As the body has no efficient way of excreting this metal, the consequences for HPN patients, treated for prolonged periods, remains unclear.

CONCLUSIONS

Home parenteral nutrition is now well established as an effective treatment in children unfortunate enough to suffer from severe disease of their gastrointestinal tract. To many it offers support while the gut is adapting following a major insult, while in others, where recovery is unlikely ever to occur, it offers a vital lifeline. Irrespective of the underlying pathology it is clear that any child requiring long-term parenteral nutrition, is best treated in their own home. This not only offers an improved quality of life (Detsky et al, 1986), compared to prolonged hospital admission but also offers the prospect for normal growth and development (Bisset et al, 1992). Where children on HPN are cared for by centres with experience of this treatment, and the parents are highly motivated, long-term survival, particularly among those without neoplastic disease or AIDS is now the norm (Vargas et

al, 1987). Some unfortunate children, however, develop major complications either from their treatment or their underlying disease and ulti-
mately die.

Over the last 5 years there have been major advances in the area of gut
transplantation and early results would suggest that when combined with
transplantation of the liver, long-term survival may be possible. It must be
remembered, however, that the quality of life and survival of many children
on HPN, at present, greatly exceed that which might be obtainable from
transplantation and it is likely that for many years to come, HPN will remain
the first line treatment for children with intestinal failure (Hiyama, 1993).

SUMMARY

As a result of improvements in the management of intravenous nutrition it is
now possible to maintain children on total parenteral nutrition for many
years. Previously many of these children spent prolonged periods in hospital
receiving their parenteral nutrition, where many died, but now with the
realization that treatment out of hospital has many advantages, there has
been a move towards the provision of intravenous nutrition in the family
home.

Any child with severe gastrointestinal disease who requires parenteral
nutrition for more than 2 or 3 months and who does not need intensive
nursing care should be considered for HPN. While many such patients have
the short gut syndrome or severe motility disturbances of their gut, more
recently children with AIDS and neoplastic disease have been treated in this
manner. Successful HPN is dependent on good venous access, impeccable
aseptic technique, well formulated nutrient solutions and the care and
attention of dedicated parents and support staff. Where treatment is
successful, there are substantial savings in the cost of health care when one
compares home with hospital. In addition, there is less disruption to family
life and normal growth and development is an attainable goal. It is only in
those children with complex multisystem disease or those in whom home
care is suboptimal that the outcome may be poor.

Complications of treatment relate primarily to the central line with
infection and blockage being major problems. Nutrition and hepatic
complications are also widely reported but it seems clear that where
treatment is managed well and the child is able to maintain an enteral intake,
complications can be reduced to a minimum. Most studies also show fewer
complications at home compared to hospital.

Until the outcome of gut transplantation improves significantly HPN is
likely to remain the treatment of choice for children with chronic severe
intestinal disease.

REFERENCES

Anonymous (1991a) Ambulatory infusion pumps. *Health Devices* **20**: 324–358.
Anonymous (1991b) Home infusion therapy. *Health Devices* **20**: 323.

Anonymous (1992) Standards for home nutrition support. American Society for Parenteral and Enteral Nutrition. *Nutritional Clinical Practice* **7**: 65–69.

Amarnath RP, Fleming CR & Perrault J (1987) Home parenteral nutrition in chronic intestinal diseases: Its effect on growth and development. *Journal of Pediatric Gastroenterology and Nutrition* **6**: 89–95.

Ament ME (1991) Home total parenteral nutrition. In Walker WA, Durie PR, Hamilton JR et al (eds) *Pediatric Gastrointestinal Disease*, pp 1676–1688. Philadelphia: BC Decker Inc.

Ament ME, Vargas J & Berquist WE (1986) Home parenteral nutrition in the infant. *Clinics in Perinatology* **13**: 213–226.

Berry RK & Jorgensen S (1988) Growing with home parenteral nutrition: adjusting to family life and child development. *Pediatric Nursing* **14**: 43–45.

Billion Rey F, Guillaumont M, Frederich A & Aulagner G (1993) Stability of fat-soluble vitamins A (retinol palmitate), E (tocopherol acetate), and K1 (phylloquinone) in total parenteral nutrition at home. *Journal of Parenteral and Enteral Nutrition* **17**: 56–60.

Bisset WM, Stapleford P, Long S et al (1992) Home parenteral nutrition in chronic intestinal failure. *Archives of Disease in Childhood* **67**: 109–114.

ter Borg F, Timmer J, de Kam SS & Sauerwein HP (1993) Use of sodium hydroxide solution to clear partially occluded vascular access ports. *Journal of Parenteral and Enteral Nutrition* **17**: 289–291.

Breaux CWJ, Duke D, Georgeson KE & Mestre JR (1987) Calcium phosphate crystal occlusion of central venous catheters used for total parenteral nutrition in infants and children: prevention and treatment. *Journal of Pediatric Surgery* **22**: 829–832.

Broviac JW & Scribner BH (1974) Prolonged parenteral nutrition in the home. *Surgery, Gynecology and Obstetrics* **139**: 24–28.

Broviac JW, Cole JJ & Scribner BH (1973) A silicone rubber catheter for prolonged parenteral nutrition. *Surgery, Gynecology and Obstetrics* **136**: 606.

Burnes JU, O'Keefe SJ, Fleming CR et al (1992) Home parenteral nutrition—a 3-year analysis of clinical and laboratory monitoring. *Journal of Parenteral and Enteral Nutrition* **16**: 327–332.

Cady C & Yoshioka RS (1991) Using a learning contract to successfully discharge an infant on home total parenteral nutrition. *Pediatric Nursing* **17**: 67–71.

Campos AC, Paluzzi M & Meguid MM (1990) Clinical use of total nutritional admixtures. *Nutrition* **6**: 347–356.

Cannon RA, Byrne MJ, Ament ME & Gates B (1980) Home parenteral nutrition in infants. *Journal of Pediatrics* **96**: 1098–1104.

Cochran EB, Phelps SJ & Helms RA (1988) Parenteral nutrition in pediatric patients. *Clinical Pharmacology* **7**: 351–366.

Cohen C & Olsen MM (1981) Pediatric total parenteral nutrition. Liver histopathology. *Archives of Pathological and Laboratory Medicine* **105**: 152–156.

Dahlstrom KA, Ament ME, Medhin MG & Meurling S (1986) Serum trace elements in children receiving long-term parenteral nutrition. *Journal of Pediatrics* **109**: 625–630.

Dahlstrom KA, Strandvik B, Kopple J & Ament ME (1985) Nutritional status in children receiving home parenteral nutrition. *Journal of Pediatrics* **107**: 219–224.

Detsky AS, McLaughlin JR, Abrams HB et al (1986) Quality of life of patients on long-term total parenteral nutrition at home. *Journal of General Internal Medicine* **1**: 26–33.

Dewar BJ (1986) Total parenteral nutrition at home. *Nursing Times* **82**: 35–38.

Drwal LA, Cochran EB & Helms RA (1990) Solubility of calcium and phosphorus in parenteral nutrition solutions. *Journal of Pediatrics* **116**: 319–320.

Dzierba SH, Mirtallo JM, Grauer DW et al (1984) Fiscal and clinical evaluation of home parenteral nutrition. *American Journal of Hospital Pharmacy* **41**: 285–291.

Evans MA, Liffrig TK, Nelson JK & Compher C (1993) Home nutrition support patient education materials. *Nutrition and Clinical Practice* **8**: 43–47.

Gerard Boncompain M, Claudel JP, Gaussorgues P et al (1992) Hepatic cytolytic and cholestatic changes related to a change of lipid emulsions in four long-term parenteral nutrition patients with short bowel. *Journal of Parenteral and Enteral Nutrition* **16**: 78–83.

Goel V (1990) Economics of total parenteral nutrition. *Nutrition* **6**: 332–335.

Goulet OJ, Revillon Y, Jan D et al (1991) Neonatal short bowel syndrome. *Journal of Pediatrics* **119**: 18–23.

Graham L & Gumbiner CH (1984) Right atrial thrombosis and superior vena cava syndrome in children. *Pediatrics* **73**: 225–229.

Handen BL, Mandell F & Russo DC (1986) Feeding induction in children who refuse to eat. *American Journal of Diseases of Children* **140**: 52–54.

Hariz MB, De Potter S, Corriol O et al (1993) Home parenteral nutrition in children: Bioavailability of vitamins in binary mixtures stored for 8 days. *Clinical Nutrition* **12**: 147–152.

Herfindal ET, Bernstein LR, Wong AF et al (1992) Complications of home parenteral nutrition. *Clinical Pharmacology* **11**: 543–548.

Hiyama DT (1993) The current role of small-bowel transplantation in intestinal failure. *Nutrition in Clinical Practice* **8**: 5–11.

Howard L (1992) Home parenteral nutrition in patients with a cancer diagnosis. *Journal of Parenteral and Enteral Nutrition* **16**: 93S–99S.

Howard L, Claunch C, McDowell R & Timchalk M (1989) Five years of experience in patients received home nutrition support with the implanted reservoir: A comparison with the external catheter. *Journal of Parenteral and Enteral Nutrition* **13**: 478–483.

Johnston JE (1981) Home parenteral nutrition: the 'costs' of patient and family participation. *Social Worker and Health Care* **7**: 49–66.

Just B, Messing B & Darmaun D (1991) Oral nutrition in patients receiving home cyclic parenteral nutrition: pattern of substrate utilization. *American Journal of Clinical Nutrition* **54**: 560–564.

Kien CL & Ganther HE (1983) Manifestations of chronic selenium deficiency in a child receiving total parenteral nutrition. *American Journal of Clinical Nutrition* **37**: 319–328.

Koo WW, Kaplan LA, Horn J et al (1986) Aluminium in parenteral nutrition solution—sources and possible alternatives. *Journal of Parenteral and Enteral Nutrition* **10**: 591–595.

Leibowitz AB & Iberti TJ (1992) Home TPN and AIDS patients (letter). *Journal of Parenteral and Enteral Nutrition* **16**: 496–497.

Lindor KD & Burnes J (1991) Ursodeoxycholic acid for the treatment of home parenteral nutrition-associated cholestasis. A case report. *Gastroenterology* **101**: 250–253.

McCrae JD, O'Shea R & Udine LM (1993) Parenteral nutrition: hospital to home. *Journal of the American Dietetic Association* **93**: 664–670.

Milewski PJ, Gross E, Holbrook I et al (1980) Parenteral nutrition at home in management of intestinal failure. *British Medical Journal* **280**: 1356–1357.

O'Connor MJ, Ralston CW & Ament ME (1988) Intellectual and perceptual-motor performance of children receiving prolonged home total parenteral nutrition. *Pediatrics* **81**: 231–236.

Payne James J & Ball P (1991) Support group for patients receiving home nutritional support (letter; comment). *British Journal of Hospital Medicine* **46**: 269.

Pitt HA, Mann LL, Berquist WE et al (1985) Chronic intestinal pseudo-obstruction. Management with total parenteral nutrition and a venting enterostomy. *Archives of Surgery* **120**: 614–618.

Pokorny WJ, Black CT, McGill CW et al (1987) Central venous catheters in older children. *American Surgeon* **53**: 524–527.

Pomp A, Caldwell MD & Albina JE (1989) Subcutaneous infusion ports for administration of parenteral nutrition at home. *Surgery, Gynecology and Obstetrics* **169**: 329–333.

De Potter S, Goulet O, Lamor M et al (1992) 263 patient-years of home parenteral nutrition in children. *Transplant Proceedings* **24**: 1056–1057.

Ralston CW, O'Connor MJ, Ament M et al (1984) Somatic growth and developmental functioning in children receiving prolonged home total parenteral nutrition. *Journal of Pediatrics* **105**: 842–846.

Rammen T, Ladefoged K, Tvede M et al (1986) Catheter related septicaemia in patients receiving home parenteral nutrition. *Scandinavian Journal of Gastroenterology* **21**: 455–460.

Revesz S & Wesley JR (1991) The use of home parenteral nutrition in pediatric patients. *Current Opinion in Pediatrics* **3**: 497–502.

Roslyn JL, Berquist WE & Pitt HA (1983) Increased risk of gallstones in children receiving total parenteral nutrition. *Pediatrics* **71**: 784–789.

Schmidt-Sommerfeld E, Snyder G, Rossi TM & Lebenthal E (1990) Catheter-related complications in 35 children and adolescents with gastrointestinal disease on home parenteral nutrition. *Journal of Parenteral and Enteral Nutrition* **14**: 148–151.

Scribner BH, Cole JJ & Christopher TG (1970) Long-term total parenteral nutrition. *Journal of the American Medical Association* **212:** 457.

Vargas JH, Ament ME & Berquist WE (1987) Long-term home parenteral nutrition in pediatrics: Ten years of experience in 102 patients. *Journal of Pediatric Gastroenterology and Nutrition* **6:** 24–32.

Wateska LP, Sattler LL & Steiger E (1980) Cost of a home parenteral nutrition program. *Journal of the American Medical Association* **244:** 2303–2304.

7

Gastrointestinal food allergy

MARTIN STERN

Gastrointestinal (GI) food allergy has been known since classical ancient times (Goldstein and Heiner, 1970). Since the beginning of this century, with the introduction of cow's milk into child nutrition, public awareness has increased of GI food allergy in children, in particular to cow's milk (Bahna and Heiner, 1980). To overcome misinterpretations, over- as well as under-diagnosis of food allergy, a clear-cut definition has to be used. In this chapter, a rational approach is suggested for diagnosis and management in order to minimize misdiagnosis of food allergy and, as a consequence, of unnecessary elimination diets that may be harmful to infants and children with respect to growth and development.

DEFINITION AND EPIDEMIOLOGY

Many terms have been used almost synonymously in this field such as adverse reactions to foods, food intolerance and idiosyncrasy, hypersensitivity and allergy to food. According to Soothill (Brostoff and Challacombe, 1987) the general term is food intolerance that splits into biochemical forms (e.g. lactose intolerance, favism), and the allergic form, based on a pathological immune reaction to food. Food intolerance appears to be a frequent problem in children (8% according to Bock, 1987), but only a fraction of this is due to food allergy.

The definition of food allergy thus requires two tests: (i) a clinically reproducible intolerance reaction to a given food or food substance; and (ii) proof of a pathological immune reaction towards the same food. This definition rules out biochemical intolerances as well as symptoms wrongly assumed to be food allergic on circumstantial evidence.

Food allergy occurs on different levels of contact with the offending agent, the GI tract (50–80%), the skin (20–40%), and the respiratory system (10–25%). Multi-system involvement is common, and systemic (anaphylactic) reactions occur. There are immediate- and delayed-onset patterns of food allergy, with respect to pathogenetic mechanisms and clinical reaction. Comprehensive data on this subject are given in some excellent recent books and reviews (May, 1986; Bock, 1987; Brostoff and Challacombe, 1987; Bishop et al, 1990; Metcalfe et al, 1991; Sampson and Metcalfe, 1992; Symposium proceedings, 1992; Walker-Smith, 1992). Frequency data for

Baillière's Clinical Paediatrics—
Vol. 2, No. 4, November 1994
ISBN 0–7020–1866–X

food allergy are conflicting. Sound epidemiological data are missing due to selection bias of studies, use of different diagnostic criteria and insufficient follow-up (Kardinaal, 1991; Strobel, 1993).

Prospective Scandinavian studies reported a prevalence close to 2.0% for cow's milk allergy (Jakobsson and Lindberg, 1979; Høst and Halken, 1990). Because of the transient nature of many forms of GI food allergy in infancy and because of the possible shift of symptoms between GI, respiratory and skin reactions, long-term prevalence data are difficult to obtain and a wide range of figures has been reported (0.2–7.5%, Gerrard et al, 1973; Bahna and Heiner, 1980; Metcalfe et al, 1991). There is a strong pathogenetic relation between food allergic reactions, in particular of the immediate type, and atopic disease. In this context, newborn IgE levels can be used as an epidemiological predictor (Croner et al, 1982). However, prevalence of atopy by far exceeds that of food allergy, and there are many cases of GI food allergy not related to atopy.

Risk factors for the development of food allergy have been postulated, such as prematurity and early introduction of cow's milk. Data, however, are conflicting (Lucas et al,1990; Lindfors et al, 1992; Savilahti et al, 1993). Epidemiology of food allergy, while bearing definite potential for preventive programmes still awaits definite analysis.

There is also a psycho-social dimension to GI food allergy. For instance, many parents believe their children to have food allergy, based on very little evidence (Rona and Chinn, 1987; Price et al, 1990; Metcalfe et al, 1991). A feeling of 'environmental hypersensitivity' (Jewett et al, 1990) is also common among adults, and only a small minority of those individuals can be identified to be food allergic by the appropriate challenge test. Self-deception and abnormal psychological reactions by parents (e.g. Münchhausen's syndrome by proxy; compare Webb et al, 1992) have to be considered by any physician dealing with children with symptoms suggestive of food allergy.

BASICS: FOOD ANTIGENS, GALT, AND PATHOGENESIS

Food antigens (Table 1)

Many foods and food substances can act as an antigen in man (Metcalfe et al, 1991). Since cow's milk, in most children, is the first foreign protein introduced into nutrition, cow's milk proteins range first during infancy. From school age on, egg proteins become more important. The molecular basis of food antigen epitopes have been identified in some cases (e.g. allergen M from cod fish with a molecular weight of 12 328 Da, 113 amino-acid residuals, a protein that is stable to heat and proteolysis).

Soy protein is another common food antigen, in particular in infants with primary cow's milk allergy who have been given a soy formula (Perkkiö et al, 1981; Giampietro et al, 1992). Minute amounts of foreign proteins contained in breast milk can act as food antigens in breast-fed infants (Machtinger and Moss, 1986). Antigenic properties might still be retained in hydrolyzed cow's milk protein used for special infant formula (Rosenthal et

Table 1. Important food antigens.

Cow's milk proteins
  Caseins
  Whey proteins
Soy proteins, Egg proteins
Others
  Fish, Crustacea
  Pork
  Peanut, legumes, beans, peas
  Nuts and seeds, cocoa, chocolate
  Citrus fruits, apple, strawberry
  Wheat, cereals
  Spices
  Food additives

al, 1991). Processed food sometimes contains additives causing allergy in children (Wilson and Scott, 1989).

Cross-reactivity exists between allergens from related vegetable families and foods from related animal sources (Bernhisel-Broadbent and Sampson, 1989; Metcalfe et al, 1991). Cross-reactivity might even exist between substances causing GI and respiratory allergy such as apple (fruit) and birch (pollen), cereals and grasses (De Blay et al, 1991; Jones et al, 1993). Sometimes it is extremely difficult to identify the food allergen from the patient's history and symptoms, and extensive reference sources have to be used systematically (Brostoff and Challacombe, 1987).

Macromolecular uptake and gut-associated lymphoid tissue (GALT)

Gastrointestinal uptake of macromolecules, such as food antigens, is basically a physiological process (Sanderson and Walker, 1993). Antigen uptake was found to be increased, however, in children with gastroenteritis, and with cow's milk allergy (Heyman et al, 1988; Husby et al, 1990; Jalonen et al, 1991; Juvonen et al, 1991).

GI food antigen uptake is an endocytosis/exocytosis process involving intracellular lysosomes. Cellular antigen handling and degradation may decrease allergenicity of food proteins, but it can also unfold new antigenic epitopes. It is still incompletely understood why, in most cases, oral tolerance is the consequence of food antigen uptake and why, in a few cases, sensitization occurs (Strobel, 1990). Enterocytes are able to act as antigen-presenting cells at the basal lateral membrane, with the help of linkage to MHC II molecules (major histocompatibility complex class II) that interact with T-cell receptors. Increased antigen uptake and activation of the local immune system are operative in the pathogenesis of GI food allergy.

The gut is a major lymphoid organ and contains a complicated network of macrophages, mast cells, immunoglobulin-producing cells, intraepithelial lymphocytes, helper and suppressor T-cells, at the subepithelial level (elements of GALT). This network is structurally organized (e.g. Peyer's patches) and subject to immunoregulation (Strobel, 1990; Brandtzaeg et al, 1991; Crowe and Perdue, 1992). Physiologically, this system acts as a specific mucosal barrier against the uncontrolled penetration of antigens. Pathologically, it is the site of allergic reactions. These comprise different types according to the Gell–Coombs classification.

Pathogenetic mechanisms (Figure 1)

There are different factors which influence the development of food allergy. One of them is a positive family history of atopic disease. This is particularly true for immediate allergic reactions to food. Another predisposing factor is low colostral IgA in mothers of breast-fed infants (Savilahti et al, 1991). A GI mucosal barrier defect has been postulated to be the cause of post-enteritis cow's milk allergy (Walker-Smith, 1982). However, in only a very few cases has this sequence been proven by short-term challenge studies.

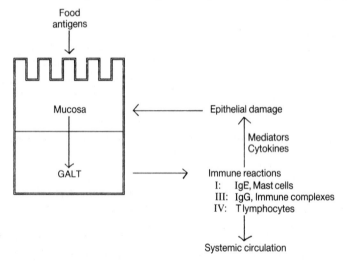

Figure 1. Pathogenesis of gastrointestinal food allergy.

Finally, early antigen exposure during postnatal development of gut mucosal barrier and immune function has been thought to influence food allergy. Small quantities of cow's milk given during the first few days of life at the maternity wards apparently increases the risk of sensitization. However, data on this are contradictory (see Epidemiology section). Finally, food antigen provocation can induce an immune response to unrelated dietary 'bystander' antigens (Suomalainen et al, 1992). Thus, soy protein allergy occurs secondary to initial cow's milk allergy (Perkkiö et al, 1981).

Immediate-onset allergic reaction (type I)

Degranulation of intestinal mast cells with release of mediators that act directly on the epithelium is a basic mechanism for type I food allergic reactions (Sampson et al, 1989; Crowe and Perdue, 1992). Mast cell mediators primarily affect immunoregulatory mechanisms of the GALT network. In type I GI food allergies, mucosal oedema, disruption of enterocytes, alterations of motility and disturbed gut barrier function, are consequences of IgE antibody and mast cell mediator action (Crowe and Perdue, 1992).

Local production and systemic distribution of specific reaginic IgE food antibodies play a significant role in this type of food allergy (Dannaeus and Johansson, 1979; Rosekrans et al, 1980; Björksten et al, 1983; Hattevig et al, 1987; Kemeny et al, 1991; Høst et al, 1992). Specific IgE food protein antibodies are also found in delayed-type reactions and in food-related atopic dermatitis (Sampson and Albergo, 1984). However, IgE antibody titres do not reflect the degree of clinical sensitivity.

Immune complex-mediated allergic reaction (type III)

Direct and antibody-dependent cytotoxic effects (type II) have not been proven in food allergy. There is, however, vast evidence on the occurrence of IgG food protein antibodies. This finding just signifies antigen exposure but not necessarily sensitization (Strobel, 1990). Demonstration of excessive antigen–antibody complex deposition and immune complex formation involving IgG, however, indicate type III reactions in GI food allergy, together with activation of the complement system (Paganelli et al, 1987; Husby et al, 1990). In addition to these IgG antibody and immune complex findings, ultrastructural and immunohistochemical studies (Shiner, 1981) have demonstrated features of type III reactions in the small intestine of children with cow's milk allergy.

Circulating immune complexes with food antigen specificity have also been found in IgA-deficient patients. It is conceivable that a food allergic reaction can spread from the GI tract to distant sites, e.g. kidney and skin via the systemic circulation (Brostoff and Challacombe, 1987).

IgG and IgE food protein antibody findings by some groups appear to differentiate between food allergic reactions of immediate or delayed type (Firer et al, 1987), and between patients retaining allergy or becoming tolerant (Isolauri et al, 1992; James and Sampson, 1992). These data still await corroboration by others. There is, as yet, no immunological test predicting clinical outcome of food allergies (cf. Prognosis section).

Delayed-onset allergic reaction, cell-mediated immunity (type IV)

Morphological studies (Phillips et al, 1979; Kosnai et al, 1980) demonstrated the role of GI T-cells such as intraepithelial lymphocytes for pathogenesis of GI food allergy. Lymphocyte reactions were closely linked to epithelial changes (villus–crypt cell kinetics). An enterotropic lymphokine was postulated to be the connecting link between subepithelial T-cell reactions and epithelial damage. Animal models using GI parasitic infection and graft versus host reaction produced GI reactions very similar to human food allergic enteropathy (Strobel, 1990). Food sensitized T-lymphocytes were found in patients with food-sensitive atopic dermatitis. This combined evidence points to the relative importance of cell-mediated immunity in GI food allergy, but there are still 'missing links' in the chain of pathogenetic events.

CLINICAL FEATURES (Table 2)

Clinical features of GI food allergy are manifold. They depend not so much on specificity of the offending food antigen, but on genetic predisposition and circumstantial factors such as the age of the infant or child and the site of food antigen exposure. The gut is not only the main target organ in GI food allergy, but is also a vehicle for delivery of food antigens to cause reactions at distant sites (cf. Pathogenesis section, Figure 1). Clinical symptoms also vary due to the participation of different pathogenetic mechanisms, e.g. immediate or delayed allergic reactions. Food allergy can cause many symptoms and syndromes (Table 2). General anaphylaxis and shock, GI, respiratory and skin reactions have been widely accepted in this context, whereas others like arthritis and central nervous system dysfunctions have not.

All the symptoms observed are not specific, or pathognomonic, for food allergy and it is only after a careful diagnostic procedure involving elimination and challenge that a symptom can be ascribed to food allergy.

Table 2. Clinical symptoms and syndromes.

Symptoms	Syndromes
General	
Anaphylaxis	Shock
Gastrointestinal	
Nausea, vomiting	
Diarrhoea, malabsorption,	Enteropathy
Failure to thrive	
GI loss: blood, protein	Colitis
Abdominal pain, bloating	
Constipation	
Skin	
Lip swelling, angioedema	
Itching, rash	Urticaria
Eczema	Atopic dermatitis
Respiratory	
Sneezing, rhinorrhoea	Rhinitis, Otitis
Wheezing, cough	Bronchitis
Bronchospasm, dyspnoea	Asthma
Others (?)	
Joint swelling, pain	Arthritis
Headache, apathy	Migraine
Irritability, hyperkinesis	Hyperactivity
Proteinuria	Nephrotic syndrome

Anaphylaxis and shock

Severe systemic reactions including anaphylaxis and shock have been described in food allergic children and adolescents (Sampson et al, 1992). Fatal and near-fatal courses are possible, although rare. The fact points to the relevance of exact diagnosis of food allergy and to the necessity of taking the appropriate precautions (epinephrine kit). This is particularly important in asthmatic patients sensitized to food allergens.

Most fatal reactions occurred after incidental ingestion of the respective food. Any diagnostic challenge is contra-indicated in children with a known anaphylactic reaction to food, since fatal cases on such occasion have been reported.

Shock fragments such as urticarial rashes, lip swelling and angio-oedema, larnyngeal and bronchial spasms may occur in food allergy. All of these symptoms have to be taken seriously in order to prevent fatal outcome of GI food allergy in later life.

Gastrointestinal manifestations

Since the prevailing level of confrontation with food antigens is in the GI tract, clinical reactions of its organs are most common in GI food allergy. Historically, morphological examination of the GI tract in food allergy has provided us with insight into the interrelation between immune reactions on the local level and GI epithelial damage. Diagnostic relevance of these findings is, however, limited (Savilahti, 1992). Gastric, small intestinal, and colonic manifestations of GI food allergy are well known; the two syndromes of food allergic enteropathy and of colitis are the most prominently defined syndromes.

Food allergic enteropathy

The demonstration of an enteropathy caused by specific food proteins (e.g. cow's milk, soy) has become a paediatric classic (Kuitunen et al, 1973; Manuel et al, 1979; Verkasalo et al, 1981; Walker-Smith, 1982). Classical symptoms are vomiting, diarrhoea, malabsorption and failure to thrive. Intestinal protein and blood losses with the consequences of general oedema and anaemia are possible. Acute reactions, such as vomiting and diarrhoea, are accompanied by delayed ones, e.g. malabsorption and failure to thrive.

In infants with these clinical signs, the degree of small intestinal damage varies from slight changes to partial villous atrophy and to subtotal villous atrophy (flat mucosa). Enteropathy tended to become less severe in cases observed after 1974 (Verkasalo et al, 1981). A changing clinical and morphological pattern of cow's milk allergic enteropathy was observed, the severity generally decreasing. The non-homogeneous 'patchy' lesion (Manuel et al, 1979) was found typical. This further limits the interpretation of single blind small intestinal biopsies.

Electron microscopic and immuno-histochemical studies have helped to describe the local immune reaction precisely (Phillips et al, 1979; Perkkiö et al, 1981; Shiner, 1981; Brandtzaeg et al, 1991). Cell kinetic and morphometrical studies have indicated links between immune reactions and epithelial changes (Kosnai et al, 1980; Perkkiö et al, 1981).

Enteropathy in GI food allergy fully subsides after elimination of the offending food. Food allergic enteropathy most often occurs during infancy and tends to disappear after 2–3 years. Thus, it is an example of an allergic reaction with transient character (cf. Prognosis section).

Eosinophilic gastroenteropathy is a related, rare entity to be differentiated from food allergic enteropathy by morphological means. Often, there is a positive family history of atopy, and the symptoms of protein-losing enteropathy are predominant. In gastric and small intestinal biopsies, eosinophilic infiltration of lamina propria is revealed (Waldmann et al, 1967; Katz et al, 1984). The connection of eosinophilic gastroenteropathy with IgE-mediated food allergic reaction has been established. Corticosteroids are often required in this syndrome.

Food allergic colitis

There is no solid evidence that inflammatory bowel disease (e.g. ulcerative colitis, Crohn's disease) is influenced by allergic reactions to foods. The leading symptom of bloody diarrhoea, however, can be caused by the separate clinical entity, namely, food allergic colitis. This typically presents in children with atopic family history before the age of 2 years (Rosekrans et al, 1980; Jenkins et al, 1984; Goldman and Proujansky, 1986; Berezin et al, 1989; Hill and Milla, 1990). Rectosigmoidoscopy shows mucosal erythema, aphthous lesions, ulcerations and eosinophilic infiltration. Immunohistochemistry reveals an increase in IgE-containing cells of lamina propria (Rosekrans et al, 1980). Endoscopy and biopsy are important tools for differential diagnosis in this syndrome. Cow's milk and soy proteins, again, are the most relevant food antigens for this disease which is benign and responds well to dietary elimination.

Other GI manifestations

Many more non-specific GI reactions have been ascribed to food allergy, such as recurrent oral aphthae, bowel oedema and obstruction, constipation, occult GI bleeding and anaemia (Ziegler et al, 1990; Sullivan, 1993) and infantile colic (Lothe et al, 1982; Forsyth, 1989; Iacono et al, 1991). Even if these syndromes are reversible after an elimination diet, it could not be convincingly shown that the underlying mechanism was an immune reaction to food.

Skin manifestations

Extra-gastrointestinal manifestations may occur independently of, or in combination with, GI symptoms (Vandenplas et al, 1992b). Lip swelling, angio-oedema and urticarial rashes immediately after ingestion of the offending food are sometimes indicative of food allergy. The existence of a separate 'oral allergy syndrome' consisting of lip-swelling, stomatitis and oral ulcers is disputed.

Contrary to acute urticaria which is more common in the paediatric age group, chronic urticaria with pruritus more often occurs in adult age. Only in a minority of cases was food allergy found to be the underlying disease (Metcalfe et al, 1991). Food additives were found to be relevant. Some clinical overlap exists between urticarial rashes and atopic eczema.

Atopic dermatitis or eczema is a frequent, multi-factorial disease with a genetic predisposition. It is characterized by an itching, erythematous, papulovesicular rash and occurs at typical sites, (e.g. head, flexural sides of extremities). As many as 12% of pre-school children are involved. Frequently, atopic dermatitis is combined with, and usually precedes, asthma and hay fever. Food allergy can be one of many factors influencing this disease (Pike et al, 1989; Sampson and Scanlon, 1989; Sloper et al, 1991; David, 1992; Guillet and Guillet, 1992).

About 80% of children with atopic dermatitis show positive skin tests and specific serum IgE antibodies to food allergens. In addition to immediate reactions, an IgE-dependent 'late phase' reaction to food has been postulated for this disease (Metcalfe et al, 1991). Egg, peanuts, milk and soy proteins have been identified most frequently to trigger pathological IgE production and to add to the development of atopic dermatitis. Only after unequivocal identification of food allergy is dietary elimination justified for treatment of eczema. This applies to severe cases, refractory to common local and systemic therapy. An uncontrolled trial of multiple dietary elimination lacks scientific basis and bears substantial risk to produce protein calorie malnutrition and multiple deficiencies in growing children.

Respiratory manifestations

Upper respiratory symptoms, such as nasal congestion and serous rhinitis with sneezing and itching, are the most common respiratory signs of food allergy. However, respiratory manifestations are rare compared to GI and skin reactions (King, 1992). Symptoms occur within minutes after exposure. Chronic serous otitis and sinusitis can also be a consequence of food allergy. Direct exposure of the nasal mucosa appears to be more important than ingestion.

Wheezing, bronchial spasm and asthma may be a main symptom in severe cases of food allergy (Onorato et al, 1986; Bousquet et al, 1992). Bronchial asthma due to food allergy is underestimated, although potentially highly dangerous (see anaphylactic course, above). Symptoms may occur with a delay of hours or even days after ingestion of the offending food. Food allergic children with asthma tend to be older than children with predominant GI manifestations of the disease. However, during adulthood, bronchial asthma due to food allergy (2%) is not as frequent as in children (6.8%, according to Onorato et al, 1986). Laboratory results are unreliable. Bronchial response after food ingestion challenge is the only reliable diagnostic criterion, and it is the only acceptable basis for an elimination diet in asthmatic children. The efficacy of oral disodium cromoglycate and of ketotifen in food allergic bronchial asthma is incompletely established. In any case, patients should always be treated for bronchial inflammation and obstruction as well as being treated for food allergy (Metcalfe et al, 1991).

Heiner's syndrome is a rare disease consisting of rhinitis, otitis, wheezing, pulmonary infiltration, and haemosiderosis. It has not yet been proven that this is a chronic pulmonary disease of infants induced by cow's milk proteins. Aspiration and sensitization by respiratory food exposure appear to play a role in some neonates and infants.

Other extra-gastrointestinal manifestations

Arthralgia and arthritis have been linked to food allergy based on blind, placebo-controlled challenge in single patients. Although this could be compatible with an immune complex-mediated allergic reaction (type III), direct evidence of food allergy in arthritis is scanty. The same is true for nephrotic syndrome and immune complex glomerulopathy.

A matter of considerable dispute is the possible involvement of central nervous symptoms in food allergy, such as headaches, apathy, tension–fatigue and hyperactivity (Egger et al, 1983, 1992). Double-blind trials have shown that migraine can be induced by many different foods such as egg, coffee, wheat, milk and cheese. It cannot be ruled out that pharmacologically active food components (e.g. tyramine) are the offending agent in these cases. Even more doubtful than the connection of CNS symptoms with food is the existence of an allergic reaction, since there was never a direct proof of any of the accepted types of immune reactions in these cases. Sleep disturbances and behavioural abnormalities have not convincingly been shown to be food allergic. Dietary elimination in these cases is highly speculative and potentially dangerous.

In summary, clinical symptoms of food allergy vary with respect to time between exposure and reaction from minutes to days. The sites of food allergic reactions imply mainly the GI tract and skin, and, to a lesser extent, the respiratory system, whereas other manifestations, at present, remain doubtful. A combination of symptoms is frequent. The transient character of clinical reactions is not uncommon, and infancy is the predominant age. Transition from GI to respiratory reactions in later childhood is a possibility to be aware of. GI food allergy bears short-term risks (anaphylaxis) as well as long-term risks (failure to thrive). All these characteristics point to the crucial role of a reliable diagnosis when food allergy is suspected.

DIAGNOSIS (Table 3)

Franz Ingelfinger stated in 1949 that 'gastrointestinal allergy is a diagnosis frequently entertained, occasionally evaluated and rarely established' (cited after Crowe and Perdue, 1992). This verdict still holds true today. In view of frequent misdiagnosis and mistreatment, recent cooperation between paediatric allergologists and gastroenterologists has produced major advances towards standardization of diagnostic procedures in GI food

Table 3. Diagnostic tests.

Elimination and challenge
    Open/blind/double-blind   (Gold standard)
Immunological tests
    Skin-prick tests, defined antigens
    IgE food antibodies   (RAST)
    IgG food antibodies
    Circulating immune complexes, C_{1q} binding
    Plasma histamine, basophil histamine release
    Leukocyte migration inhibition
Gastroenterological tests
    Gastric biopsy
    Small intestinal biopsy
    Rectosigmoidoscopy and biopsy
    Sugar absorption studies (e.g. xylose)
    Stool analysis (α_1-antitrypsin, blood)

allergy (Sampson and Albergo, 1984; Leinhaus et al, 1987; Bock and Atkins, 1990; Metcalfe, 1992; Savilahti, 1992; Symposium proceedings, 1992; Walker-Smith, 1992).

The cornerstone of diagnosis in GI food allergy is a complete history and an unequivocal, reproducible reaction to elimination and challenge. History based on parents' observations, however, is sometimes misleading. Diagnosis based solely on history and some laboratory tests, without defined food challenge, is not justified and adds to misconceptions of food allergy on the iatrogenic side.

Physical examination should reveal any of the clinical signs of food allergy listed above, depending on the target organ affected, primarily the GI tract, the skin and respiratory system. Any of these signs has to be reproduced during challenge before the diagnosis can be accepted.

Elimination and challenge (Figure 2)

Typical symptoms of GI food allergy disappear upon elimination of the suspected food within a few days. In malabsorption and enteropathy it may take weeks. If symptoms continue upon elimination, they may be caused by different foods or by non-allergic mechanisms.

Originally, three consecutive elimination and challenge procedures were postulated for GI food allergy diagnosis (Goldman et al, 1963). This was a puristic and non-realistic approach, since challenge in anaphylaxis and multiple challenges in different types of reactions are unethical and impossible to impose on families with a food allergic child. A standard protocol for single open challenge in infants and young children should be followed (modified after Powell, 1978; Savilahti et al, 1993) as given below.

1. Challenges should be done under clinical control on an in-patient basis. A known anaphylactic reaction should preclude any challenge. None of the initial symptoms should persist and infants should be thriving upon elimination prior to challenge.

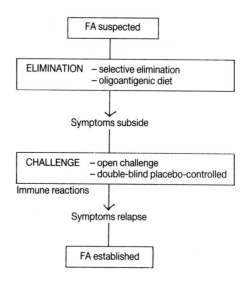

Figure 2. Clinical diagnosis of food allergy (FA).

2. In suspected cow's milk allergy, lactose intolerance should be excluded (for instance, by H_2 breath testing after oral lactose load).
3. Pre-testing liquid food should include subsequent exposure of (a) an unaffected skin area, and (b) the lips to one drop of the liquid (for instance, cow's milk). A heparin lock should be installed and the usual precautions (e.g. i.v. fluids, epinephrine, antihistamines, steroids) should have been prepared.
4. The oral challenge should start with small amounts (e.g. a few drops of milk). The child should be carefully observed under medical control for development of rhinorrhea, respiratory changes, wheezing, lip-swelling, rashes, vomiting and diarrhoea. A written protocol on clinical symptoms should be followed. If there is no obvious reaction, challenge dose should be increased in 5 ml steps at hourly intervals.
5. Four hours after beginning the challenge, oral feeding (e.g. hydrolysate formula) should be resumed. If there is no reaction at this point, challenge dose should be increased to reach 10 ml/kg after 48 h, and full strength after 96 h. The child may now be dismissed. Observation period should be extended to 7 days. Stool samples should be tested for occult blood, pH and carbohydrate.

Natural, unprocessed food is used for open challenge. Single food proteins or standardized food extracts are currently not widely available and cannot be recommended for general patient testing.

In doubtful cases, particularly in older children with an unreliable history of multiple allergies, double-blind placebo–controlled food challenge (DBPCFC) is the therapeutic gold standard (Bock and Atkins, 1990; Jewett et al, 1990; Sloper et al, 1991; Metcalfe, 1992). The suspected food is eliminated 7–14 days before challenge, and medical treatment is discontinued. The suspected food is hidden in some neutral, tolerated food or in capsules. Placebo and verum are administered in a randomized way. The dose is increased from 125 mg to 10 g. Time and character of reactions vary. IgE-mediated acute reactions are never missed. The duration of observation depends on the type of reaction to be expected (Metcalfe et al, 1991; Symposium proceedings, 1992). Delayed reactions are still a problem in DBPCFC. In any case, the endpoint of a positive challenge has to be an objective observation of one or more of the typical symptoms by professional staff. The endpoint of challenge has to be defined beforehand, considering acute and delayed reactions.

If there is no direct suspicion of a single food in clearly allergic reactions in older children, oligoantigenic diets (Brostoff and Challacombe, 1987); e.g. lamb, rice, potato, carrots and lettuce, can be used. After the disappearance of symptoms, definitive challenge is carried out using single foods. The use of 'rotary diets' without definite challenge has to be disfavoured since psychogenic factors, e.g. a placebo effect of strong dietary rules, are enforced by such practice beyond any diagnostic control.

Skin tests and other immunological tests (Table 3)

No single laboratory test can replace clinical diagnosis of food allergy by elimination and challenge. There are, however, valuable laboratory methods to prove pathological immune reactions in patients with proven intolerance to a given food (see Definition). Skin-prick testing and serum determination of specific IgE antibodies deserve special mention.

Out of different skin tests, the prick technique using defined, standardized food antigens is acceptable to minimize non-specific irritant reactions and to avoid severe systemic reactions. Skin-prick testing is reliable in immediate food allergy, in particular with wheat, milk and soy. There are, however, many false-positive skin-prick tests without any clinical significance (Sampson and Albergo, 1984; Dreborg, 1991) and skin-prick tests, in many cases, might just be useful in helping to exclude immediate-type food allergy. Skin-prick testing is not reliable in young children with delayed reactions, malabsorption and enteropathy. Over-interpretation of positive skin tests in GI food allergy is still a major source of confusion with respect to diagnosis and dietary consequences.

Another indicator of immediate immune reactions towards food is the appearance of specific IgE antibodies in serum (Dannaeus and Johansson, 1979; Björksten et al, 1983; Sampson and Albergo, 1984; Firer et al, 1987; Adler et al, 1991; Kemeny et al, 1991; Høst et al, 1992; Raesaenen et al, 1992). However, blood tests like this do not necessarily reflect changes at GI, dermatological and respiratory organ levels. Nevertheless, IgE antibodies are instrumental in producing immediate food allergic reactions (cf. Basics). Consequently, the diagnostic value of IgE antibodies towards cow's milk, egg, peanuts, soy and fish is well established, whereas other specificities are not well documented (Metcalfe et al, 1991). There is no justification of multiple food specific IgE antibody tests (Adler et al, 1991) instead of individually selected IgE antibody determinations by radio-allergosorbent test (RAST). RAST is approximately as sensitive as skin-prick testing. Again, there are many false-positives. By no means does a high RAST class exclude clinical tolerance to a given food. This is particularly true in children with no history of food allergy at all. The possibility remains that high concentration IgE food antibodies indicate sensitization, with clinical reactivity only developing after further follow-up (Hattevig et al, 1987). Comparison of immunological laboratory tests with regard to their diagnostic value did not show superiority of the skin-prick test or RAST over clinical diagnosis based on defined challenge.

Other immunological tests have been proposed and advocated by 'enthusiasts or for commercial reasons' (Metcalfe et al, 1991). For instance, serum IgG antibodies to common food antigens are a frequent finding in normal children, indicating exposure rather than sensitization. Differentiation into IgG 1 and IgG 4 shows age-dependence differences (Kemeny et al, 1991) but fails to indicate clinical sensitivity. Tests for circulating immune complexes, C_{1q} binding, for leukocyte migration inhibition, and for histamine release and metabolism have been described (Brostoff and Challacombe, 1987; Paganelli et al, 1987; Sampson et al, 1989). Most of these tests were not confirmed and should not be generally used. Many additional non-validated food allergy tests (e.g. leukocyte toxicity testing, subcutaneous and sub-lingual provocation, neutralization) have not been approved by the American Academy of Allergy and should be abandoned. The same applies to paramedical approaches trying to establish the diagnosis (Brostoff and Challacombe, 1987; Metcalfe et al, 1991).

Gastroenterological tests

The GI tract has been investigated both functionally and morphologically to establish the connection between local immune reactions and GI clinical symptoms from the diagnostic view. Gastroenterological methods appear justified in infants with chronic diarrhoea and failure to thrive and in children with chronic bloody diarrhoea and atopic family history. GI biopsies are not justified in most children with immediate food allergic reactions.

Gastric biopsy is diagnostic in eosinophilic gastroenteropathy (see above). Intra-gastric provocation under endoscopic control produced data on morphology and local mast cell degranulation consistent with clinical diagnosis. However, the method has not been used widely and appears not to be suitable in children.

Small intestinal biopsy has been widely applied to the study of children with food-induced enteropathy (Kuitunen et al, 1973; Phillips et al, 1979; Rosekrans et al, 1980; Walker-Smith, 1992). Since small intestinal mucosal lesions are widely variable, it is not possible to establish a morphology-based definition of intestinal food allergy. Morphometry and immunohistochemistry are of some help to describe more precisely local changes. In severe cases, small intestinal biopsy usually shows severe lesions. In these cases (usually small infants), small intestinal biopsy is mandatory, also for differential diagnosis (e.g. coeliac disease, lymphangiectasia, congenital microvillus atrophy).

If there is chronic bloody diarrhoea in young infants with a family history positive for atopic disease, rectosigmoidoscopy and biopsy have to be done to identify food-allergic colitis. This is also mandatory for differential diagnosis of chronic inflammatory bowel disease. Histologically, inflammatory colon changes can be distinguished (Jenkins et al, 1984).

Tests of gut function, such as sugar absorption studies and stool analysis for loss of protein (α_1-antitrypsin clearance) and blood are non-invasive GI diagnostic tools. Their diagnostic value in GI food allergy is, at most, complementary (Savilahti et al, 1992).

MANAGEMENT

Elimination diet

Once the diagnosis of GI food allergy has been established, the preferred therapy is dietary elimination of the food allergen identified (Table 4). Indiscriminate routine use of elimination diets without firm diagnosis is a widespread malpractice. Instead, co-operation between the children with food allergy and their families, dieticians and physicians is necessary to come to practical dietary solutions on a firm diagnostic basis. Dietary demands of a growing child, with potential initial deficiencies due to the severity and duration of symptoms, have to be met. Dietary manuals may be consulted to find the individualized, optimal diet (Brostoff and Challacombe, 1987; Pike et al, 1989; Metcalfe et al, 1991; David, 1992; Symposium proceedings, 1992). The setting up of an elimination diet must be accompanied by counselling of parents and by dietary follow-up (Committee report, 1991; Carroll et al, 1992). In any case, therapy must not be worse than the disease.

Breast-milk is the first choice in very young infants without lactose intolerance. Since minute amounts of food proteins can be transmitted to

Table 4. Therapy.

Elimination diet
  Infants
    Breast milk
    Hydrolysate formula
    (casein, whey, soy, collagen)
  Children
    Exclusion diet
    Oligoantigenic diet
    Elementary diet

Drugs
  In polyvalent allergy, respiratory symptoms
    Disodium cromoglycate, DSCG
    Ketotifen
    Inhalant drugs (beta-mimetics, steroids)
  In anaphylaxis
    Epinephrine kit

the infant via mother's milk, the mothers themselves should keep to an elimination diet avoiding cow's milk, hen's egg and fish. This possibility appears to apply exclusively to highly-sensitized infants. In the majority of cases, if breastfeeding is still possible, this is the optimal treatment.

If breastfeeding is not possible, and in severely ill infants with enteropathy and lactose intolerance, there are different artificial formula solutions to the problem of cow's milk allergy and other food allergies early in life. Complete milk protein hydrolysates, e.g. Pregestimil®, Nutramigen® (Mead Johnson) and Alimentum® (Ross Laboratories) from casein; and Alfaré® (Nestlé) from whey, have been used successfully (Sampson et al, 1991; Symposium proceedings, 1992). Infant formulas, however, promoted as 'hypo-allergenic' have to be clinically tested in milk allergic patients beforehand to assess their relative allergenic potential. Single cases have been reported with an intolerance towards casein hydrolysate formula (Rosenthal et al, 1991). Partially hydrolysed formulas are definitely not suitable for the treatment of cow's milk allergy. A complete hydrolysate formula prepared from soy and bovine collagen (Pregomin®, Milupa) is absolutely free of cow's milk and lactose. The same applies to elementary diets prepared from amino-acid solutions. Elementary and semi-elementary formula prepar-ations are balanced in trace elements and vitamins, and are thus suitable for exclusive infant nutrition. They should be prescribed and controlled like a medical drug.

Full soy formula is not recommended in young infants with severe enter-opathy, since secondary soy allergy has been described in as many as 30–50% of infants with severe cow's milk allergy. Soy formula (Nutrilon®, Cow and Gate; Prosobee®, Mead Johnson; Wysoy®, Wyeth; Humana SL®, Lactopriv®, Töpfer; Milupa SOM®, Multival Plus®, Abbott) is useful for cow's milk elimination in older children with food allergy without failure to thrive and without severe GI lesions.

In school children, single foods once identified to cause allergy can be avoided easily in many cases. One has to be aware of unlisted food components (e.g. milk proteins in margarine). A dietician with expertise in food allergy should be consulted to meet daily requirements (e.g. calcium in cow's milk-free diet). Cross-reactions have to be considered, for instance between celery and spices, between cinnamon and avocado, asparagus and garlic. Food declaration (e.g. plant proteins from different sources, hydro-lysed soy and wheat proteins in sweets) is an enormous help. Follow-up of nutritional status and dietary survey are necessary (Paganus et al, 1992). Deficiencies in trace elements like zinc and iron and low intake of substances like riboflavin and carnitin are not uncommon.

In difficult cases with polyvalent food allergy or non-identified food allergens, an oligoantigenic diet is used for diagnostic purposes (see above). If there is clinical improvement, single food challenge is started. If a reaction is observed, the newly-introduced food is eliminated again and a second challenge is done for confirmation. In general, however, most patients are allergic to only one or two foods, so dietary elimination does not have to be too restrictive. Use of elemental diets which are badly palatable and have a bitter taste is only rarely necessary.

Dietary counselling not only must raise awareness towards nutritional inadequacies but also to hidden ingredients in processed foods and towards the possibility of life-threatening reactions, in particular in children known to react anaphylactically, e.g. towards peanuts, since accidental ingestion with potential fatal consequences is not uncommon (Sampson et al, 1992). Patients have to be trained to self-administer emergency medication such as epinephrine. In most cases, optimal compliance can be reached by long-term surveillance.

Medical therapy

Most cases of GI food allergy can be treated by elimination diets alone. In polyvalent allergy, however, and in respiratory symptoms, medical treatment might be indicated. Disodium cromoglycate (DSCG) has been found unreliable, e.g. in atopic dermatitis, although DSCG might help to prevent respiratory symptoms and an asthmatic response to food challenge (Onorato et al, 1986). Application of DSCG should be restricted to cases in which dietary control is not achieved, in particular with respiratory symptoms. Oral ketotifen has been advocated by some but there are no well-controlled long-term studies. Steroids are certainly indicated in the rare syndrome of eosinophilic gastroenteritis.

Other forms of immune therapy such as hyposensitization (Egger et al, 1992) and immunomodulation have been reported. Some single successful reports still await confirmation. It is premature, at present, to put peanut allergic patients on 'rush immunotherapy', based on these preliminary papers.

Emergency medications include epinephrine (0.01 mg/kg, as a 1:1000 aqueous solution) preferably in the form of self-injecting devices (Epipen Junior®, Center Laboratories; Ana-Kit®, Hollister-Stier Laboratories). In addition, adrenalin can be administered by inhalation. Emergency kits should contain steroids, oral antihistamines, and volume expander solutions. Detailed medical treatment of anaphylactic shock and non-GI food allergy are well beyond the scope of this chapter.

Prevention (Table 5)

Epidemiological insight into the development of food allergy and atopical diseases has provided us with some potential of prevention, or at least postponement of symptoms. The current conflict between medical knowledge and economical interest of infant food producers has been recently summarized (Björksten and Kjellman, 1991; Symposium proceedings, 1992; Aggett et al, 1993).

First of all, identification of infants at risk to develop food allergy and/or atopy later in life is necessary. This is accomplished by family history (e.g. one parent or sibling positive for atopy). Only in high-risk infants have preventive effects of infant nutrition been shown, whereas in unselected groups there was no benefit. After several well-controlled studies (Kajosaari and Saarinen, 1983; Hattevig et al, 1989; Zeiger et al, 1989, 1992; Chandra

Table 5. Prevention.

Identification of infants at risk
  Family history of atopy
  Cord blood IgE ≥0.9 kU/litre

Dietary prevention
  Proven effect
    Exclusive breast feeding (4–6 months)
    In high risk infants (maternal diet)
    Alternative: hydrolysate formula
    Late introduction of solids (>6 months)
    Avoidance of cow's milk, egg (12–24 months)
  No effect
    Maternal diet, pregnancy

Other epidemiological factors
  Parental smoking
  Pets, molds, mites
  Respiratory infections

and Hamed, 1991; Halken et al, 1992; Sigurs et al, 1992; Vandenplas et al, 1992a) the following dietary preventive measures have been proven to be effective:

(i)   exclusive breast-feeding for 4–6 months, with mothers on a diet restrictive of cow's milk, egg and fish;

(ii) as an alternative, hydrolysate formula;

(iii) late introduction of solid foods after 6 months;

(iv) avoidance of cow's milk and egg for the first 12–24 months.

Studies show that not only complete but also partial hydrolysates are effective (e.g. Aletemil HA® and Beba HA®, Nestlé; Aptamil Hypo-antigen®, Milupa; Humana HA®, Profylac® ALK).

Contrary to these measures, maternal diet during pregnancy was not shown to have any benefit. Preventive effects were seen after an observation period of up to 48 months, in particular with respect to GI and skin symptoms, whereas respiratory symptoms and bronchial asthma were not consistently influenced. Practicability of combined prevention programmes (e.g. Zeiger et al, 1989, 1992) is restricted, compliance is not guaranteed, and socio-economic factors add to the many practical difficulties.

Other epidemiological factors for the development of atopical disease have to be considered in any preventive programme, such as discontinuation of parental smoking, elimination of pets, molds, mites, and restriction of respiratory infections (e.g. by avoidance of early day-care centres). Thus, dietary preventive measures alone are insufficient, since dietary exposure is not the sole factor for the development of atopic disease. It is conceivable that the problem of atopy, which appears to rise in significance in well-developed countries cannot be controlled by dietary measures alone (e.g. season of birth is another factor of influence). Nevertheless, it might be useful to postpone food allergic symptoms in small infants, thus preventing severe early deficiencies in growth and development.

Natural history and prognosis

GI food allergy of the paediatric age group is, most often, a temporary disease. Prospective studies on natural history of food allergy have shown that many children outgrow their clinical sensitivity (Sampson and Scanlon, 1989; Bishop et al, 1990; James and Sampson, 1992; Schrander et al, 1992; Hill et al, 1993). Thus, tolerance of the offending food antigen was achieved after 1–4 years of allergen avoidance. Initial IgE food antibody values, completeness of allergen avoidance and specificity of the food antigen appeared to influence natural history. As a consequence, re-challenge testing for food allergy should be done after 12–18 months for cow's milk, hen's egg, soy and wheat; after 2–3 years for nuts; and after 3 years for peanut and fish (Sampson and Scanlon, 1989). After 3 years, approximately 80% of confirmed food allergic symptoms disappeared (Bock, 1987). However, patients with allergies to peanut, nuts and fish rarely lose their reactivity and, as a consequence, mostly have to stick to life-long elimination diets. This group of patients is particularly threatened by severe anaphylactic reactions after inadvertent ingestion of the antigen.

GI food allergy has changed in clinical patterns over the last decades from severe to milder cases. Malnutrition due to cow's milk allergy, for instance, is rare today. Food allergy may change in symptoms from GI to respiratory levels, intra-individually, during later childhood. It might be influenced by preventive nutritional measures in the years to come. Thus, Gerrard's verdict that food allergy, at least cow's milk allergy in infants, might be a problem of our century and that it 'should in its turn become a historical curiosity' (Gerrard et al, 1973) does not appear timely. GI food allergy probably will pose questions for many more paediatric generations to come.

SUMMARY

The GI tract is not only the target of allergic reactions to food, but also serves as a vehicle for delivery of food antigens to cause reactions at distant sites such as the skin and respiratory system. Food allergy is defined as a reproducible clinical reaction towards a food component, based on a pathological immune reaction. Most important food antigens are proteins from cow's milk, soy and hen's egg. Pathogenesis involves macromolecular uptake and loss of immunological tolerance. A genetic disposition to develop atopical disease is encountered in most, but not all, forms of GI food allergy. Gastrointestinal symptoms range first (50–80%), followed by skin (20–40%) and respiratory reactions (10–25%). Systemic anaphylaxis and shock are a considerable life-threatening potential. Diagnosis of food allergy is clinical, involving elimination and challenge protocols. Immunological tests, above others skin-prick testing and detection of specific IgE food antibodies, help to establish the diagnosis. Other tests, for instance gastric, intestinal and colonic biopsies are valuable tools in differential diagnosis. Elimination of the offending food is the principle of dietary therapy. Medical therapy is restricted to respiratory symptoms and polyvalent allergy. A note of caution has to be made on the uncritical use of elimination diets without appropriate diagnosis: deficiency syndromes and malnutrition may be a consequence. Prognosis of GI food allergy, in most cases, is good, requiring re-challenge after 2–3 years. In some cases, GI clinical reactivity turns into respiratory symptoms after infancy. In infants at risk to develop atopical disorders and food allergy, preventive measures are suitable to reduce and postpone symptoms. In this respect, dietary steps are as important as other epidemiological interventions.

REFERENCES

Adler BR, Assadullahi T, Warner JA & Warner JO (1991) Evaluation of a multiple food specific IgE antibody test compared to parental perception, allergy skin tests and RAST. *Clinical and Experimental Allergy* **21:** 683–688.

Aggett PJ, Haschke F, Heine W et al (1993) Comment on antigen-reduced infant formulae. *Acta Paediatrica Scandinavica* **82:** 314–319.

Bahna SL & Heiner DC (1980) *Allergies to Milk.* New York: Grune & Stratton.

Berezin S, Schwarz SM, Glassman M et al (1989) Gastrointestinal milk intolerance of infancy. *American Journal of Diseases of Children* **143:** 361–362.

Bernhisel-Broadbent J & Sampson HA (1989) Cross-allergenicity in the legume botanical family in children with food hypersensitivity. *Journal of Allergy and Clinical Immunology* **83:** 435–440.

Bishop JM, Hill DJ & Hosking CS (1990) Natural history of cow milk allergy: Clinical outcome. *Journal of Pediatrics* **116:** 862–867.

Björksten B & Kjellman N-IM (1991) Does breast feeding prevent food allergy? *Allergy Proceedings* **12:** 233–239.

Björksten B, Ahlstedt S, Björksten F et al (1983) Immunoglobulin E and immunoglobulin G4 antibodies to cow's milk in children with cow's milk allergy. *Allergy* **38:** 119–124.

Bock SA (1987) Prospective appraisal of complaints of adverse reactions to foods in children during the first 3 years of life. *Pediatrics* **79:** 683–688.

Bock SA & Atkins FM (1990) Patterns of food hypersensitivity during sixteen years of double-blind, placebo-controlled food challenges. *Journal of Pediatrics* **117:** 561–567.

Bousquet J, Neukirch F, Noyola A & Michel F-B (1992) Prevalence of food allergy in asthma. *Pediatric Allergy and Immunology* **3/4:** 206–213.

Brandtzaeg P, Bengtsson U, Halstensen TS et al (1991) Mucosal immunology and food antigens. In Müller HR & Ockhuizen T (eds) *Food Allergy and Food Intolerance. Nutritional Aspects and Development. Biblioteca Nutritio et Dieta,* pp 30–54. Basel: Karger.

Brostoff J & Challacombe SJ (1987) *Food Allergy and Intolerance.* London: Baillière Tindall.

Carroll P, Caplinger KJ & France GL (1992) Guidelines for counseling parents of young children with food sensitivities. *Journal of the American Dietetic Association* **92:** 602–603.

Chandra RK & Hamed A (1991) Cumulative incidence of atopic disorders in high risk infants fed whey hydrolysate, soy, and conventional cow milk formulas. *Annals of Allergy* **67:** 129–132.

Committee report from the Adverse Reactions to Food Committee of the American Academy of Allergy and Immunology (1991) The treatment in school of children who have food allergies. *Journal of Allergy and Clinical Immunology* **87:** 749–751.

Croner S, Kjellmann NIM, Eriksson B & Roth A (1982) IgE screening in 1701 newborn infants and the development of atopic disease during infancy. *Archives of Disease in Childhood* **57:** 364–368.

Crowe SE & Perdue MH (1992) Gastrointestinal food hypersensitivity: Basic mechanisms of pathophysiology. *Gastroenterology* **103:** 1075–1095.

Dannaeus A & Johansson SGO (1979) A follow-up study of infants with adverse reactions to cow's milk. I. Serum IgE, skin test reactions and RAST in relation to clinical course. *Acta Paediatrica Scandinavica* **69:** 377–382.

David TJ (1992) Extreme dietary measures in the management of atopic dermatitis in childhood. *Acta Dermato-Venereologica.* **176 (supplement):** 113–116.

De Blay F, Pauli G & Bessot JC (1991) Cross-reactions between respiratory and food allergens. *Allergy Proceedings* **12:** 313–317.

Dreborg S (1991) Skin test in diagnosis of food allergy. *Allergy Proceedings* **12:** 251–254.

Egger J, Stolla A & McEwen LM (1992) Controlled trial of hyposensitisation in children with food-induced hyperkinetic syndrome. *Lancet* **339:** 1150–1153.

Egger J, Carter C, Wilson J et al (1983) Is migraine food allergy? A double-blind controlled trial of oligo-antigenic diet treatment. *Lancet* **ii:** 865–869.

Firer MA, Hosking CS & Hill DJ (1987) Humoral immune response to cow's milk in children with cow's milk allergy. Relationship to the time of clinical response to cow's milk challenge. *International Archives of Allergy and Applied Immunology* **84:** 173–177.

Forsyth BWC (1989) Colic and the effect of changing milk formulas: a double-blind, multiple crossover study. *Journal of Pediatrics* **115:** 521–526.

Gerrard JW, Mackenzie JWA, Goluboff N et al (1973) Cow's milk allergy: prevalence and manifestations in an unselected series of newborns. *Acta Paediatrica Scandinavica* **234 (supplement):** 1–21.

Giampietro PG, Ragno V, Daniele S et al (1992) Soy hypersensitivity in children with food allergy. *Annals of Allergy* **69:** 143–146.

Goldman AS, Anderson DW, Sellers WS et al (1963) Milk allergy. I. Oral challenge with milk and isolated milk proteins in allergic children. *Pediatrics* **32:** 425–443.

Goldman H & Proujansky R (1986) Allergic proctitis and gastroenteritis in children. Clinical and mucosal biopsy features in 53 cases. *American Journal of Surgical Pathology* **10:** 75–86.

Goldstein GB & Heiner DC (1970) Clinical and immunological perspectives in food allergy. *Journal of Allergy and Clinical Immunology* **46:** 270–291.

Guillet G & Guillet M-H (1992) Natural history of sensitizations in atopic dermatitis. A 3-year follow-up in 250 children: Food allergy and high risk of respiratory symptoms. *Archives of Dermatology* **128:** 187–192.

Halken S, Høst A, Hansen LG & Østerballe O (1992) Effect of an allergy prevention programme on incidence of atopic symptoms in infancy. A prospective study of 159 'high-risk' infants. *Allergy* **47:** 545–553.

Hattevig G, Kjellman B & Björksten B (1987) Clinical symptoms and IgE responses to common food proteins and inhalants in the first 7 years of life. *Clinical Allergy* **17:** 571–578.

Hattevig G, Kjellman B, Sigurs N et al (1989) Effect of maternal avoidance of eggs, cow's milk and fish during lactation upon allergic manifestations in infants. *Clinical and Experimental Allergy* **19:** 27–32.

Heyman M, Grasset E, Ducroc R & Desjeux J (1988) Antigen absorption by the jejunal epithelium of children with cow's milk allergy. *Pediatrics* **24:** 197–202.

Hill SM & Milla PJ (1990) Colitis caused by food allergy in infants. *Archives of Disease in Childhood* **65:** 132–140.

Hill DJ, Firer MA, Ball G et al (1993) Natural history of cows' milk allergy in children: immunological outcome over 2 years. *Clinical and Experimental Allergy* **23:** 124–131.

Høst A & Halken S (1990) A prospective study of cow milk allergy in Danish infants during the first 3 years of life. Clinical course in relation to clinical and immunological type of hypersensitivity reaction. *Allergy* **45:** 587–596.

Høst A, Husby S, Gjesing B et al (1992) Prospective estimation of IgG, IgG subclass and IgE antibodies to dietary proteins in infants with cow milk allergy. Levels of antibodies to whole milk protein, BLG and ovalbumin in relation to repeated milk challenge and clinical course of cow milk allergy. *Allergy* **47:** 218–229.

Husby S, Høst A, Teisner B & Svehag SE (1990) Infants and children with cow milk allergy/ intolerance. Investigation of the uptake of cow milk protein and activation of the complement system. *Allergy* **45:** 547–551.

Iacono G, Carroccio A, Montalto G et al (1991) Severe infantile colic and food intolerance: a long-term prospective study. *Journal of Pediatric Gastroenterology and Nutrition* **12:** 332–335.

Isolauri E, Suomalainen H, Kaila M et al (1992) Local immune response in patients with cow milk allergy: follow-up of patients retaining allergy or becoming tolerant. *Journal of Pediatrics* **120:** 9–15.

Jakobsson I & Lindberg T (1979) A prospective study of cow's milk protein intolerance in Swedish infants. *Acta Paediatrica Scandinavica* **68**: 853–859.

Jalonen T, Isolauri E, Heyman M et al (1991) Increased beta-lactoglobulin absorption during rotavirus enteritis in infants—relationship to sugar permeability. *Pediatric Research* **30**: 290–392.

James JM & Sampson HA (1992) Immunologic changes associated with the development of tolerance in children with cow milk allergy. *Journal of Pediatrics* **121**: 371–377.

Jenkins HR, Pincott JR, Soothill JF et al (1984) Food allergy: the major cause of infantile colitis. *Archives of Disease in Childhood* **59**: 326–329.

Jewett DL, Fein G & Greenberg MH (1990) A double-blind study of symptom provocation to determine food sensitivity. *New England Journal of Medicine* **323**: 429–478.

Jones SM, Cooke SK & Sampson HA (1993) Immunological cross-reactivity among cereal-grains and grasses in children with food hypersensitivity. *Journal of Allergy and Clinical Immunology* **91**: 343.

Juvonen P, Jakobsson I & Lindberg T (1991) Macromolecular absorption and cows' milk allergy. *Archives of Disease in Childhood* **66**: 300–303.

Kajosaari M & Saarinen UM (1983) Prophylaxis of atopic disease by six months' total solid food elimination. Evaluation of 135 exclusively breast-fed infants of atopic families. *Acta Paediatrica Scandinavica* **72**: 411–414.

Kardinaal AF (1991) Epidemiology of food allergy and food intolerance. *Bibliotheca Nutritio et Dieta* **48**: 105–115.

Katz AJ, Twarog FJ, Zeiger RS & Falchuk ZM (1984) Milk-sensitive and eosinophilic gastroenteropathy: similar clinical features with contrasting mechanisms and clinical couse. *Journal of Allergy and Clinical Immunology* **74**: 72–78.

Kemeny DM, Price JF, Richardson V et al (1991) The IgE and IgG subclass antibody response to foods in babies during the first year of life and their relationship to feeding regimen and the development of food allergy. *Journal of Allergy and Clinical Immunology* **87**: 920–929.

King WP (1992) Food hypersensitivity in otolaryngology. Manifestations, diagnosis, and treatment. *Otolaryngologic Clinics of North America* **25**: 163–179.

Kosnai I, Kuitunen P, Savilahti E et al (1980) Cell kinetics in the jejunal crypt epithelium in malabsorption syndrome with cow's milk protein intolerance and in coeliac disease. *Gut* **21**: 1041–1046.

Kuitunen P, Rapola J, Savilahti E & Visakorpi JK (1973) Response to the jejunal mucosa to cow's milk in the malabsorption syndrome with cow's milk intolerance. A light and electron-microscopic study. *Acta Paediatrica Scandinavica* **62**: 585–595.

Leinhaus JL, McCaskill CC & Sampson HA (1987) Food allergy challenges: guidelines and implications. *Journal of the American Dietetic Association* **87**: 604–608.

Lindfors ATB, Danielsson L, Enocksson E et al (1992) Allergic symptoms up to 4–6 years of age in children given cow milk neonatally. A prospective study. *Allergy* (Copenhagen) **47**: 207–211.

Lothe L, Lindberg T & Jakobsson I (1982) Cow's milk formula as a cause of infantile colic: a double-blind study. *Pediatrics* **70**: 7–10.

Lucas A, Brooke OG, Morley R et al (1990) Early diet of preterm infants and development of allergic or atopic disease: randomised prospective study. *British Medical Journal* **300**: 837–840.

Machtinger S & Moss R (1986) Cow's milk allergy in breast-fed infants: the role of allergen and maternal secretory IgA antibody. *Journal of Allergy and Clinical Immunology* **77**: 341–347.

Manuel PD, Walker-Smith JA & France NE (1979) Patchy enteropathy in childhood. *Gut* **20**: 211–215.

May C (1986) Defined versus ill-defined syndromes associated with food sensitivity. *Journal of Allergy and Clinical Immunology* **78**: 144–148.

Metcalfe DD (1992) Food challenge procedures: Standardization of oral challenge and pulmonary measurements. *Pediatric Allergy and Immunology* **3/4**: 171–175.

Metcalfe D, Sampson H & Simon RA (eds) (1991) *Food Allergy*. Boston: Blackwell Scientific Publications.

Onorato J, Merland N, Terral C et al (1986) Placebo-controlled double-blind food challenge in asthma. *Journal of Allergy and Clinical Immunology* **78**: 1139–1146.

Paganelli R, Quinti I, D'Offizi GP et al (1987) Immune complexes in food allergy: a critical reappraisal. *Annals of Allergy* **59**: 157–161.

Paganus A, Juntunen-Backman K & Savilahti E (1992) Follow-up nutritional status and dietary survey in children with cow's milk allergy. *Acta Paediatrica* **81**: 518–521.

Perkkiö M, Savilahti E & Kuitunen P (1981) Morphometric and immuno-histochemical study of jejunal biopsies from children with intestinal soy allergy. *European Journal of Pediatrics* **137**: 63–69.

Phillips AD, Rice SJ, France NE & Walker-Smith JA (1979) Small intestinal intraepithelial lymphocyte levels in cow's milk protein intolerance. *Gut* **20**: 509–512.

Pike MG, Carter CM, Boulton P et al (1989) Few food diets in the treatment of atopic eczema. *Archives of Disease in Childhood* **64**: 1691–1698.

Powell GK (1978) Milk- and soy-induced enterocolitis of infancy: clinical features and standardization of challenge. *Journal of Pediatrics* **93**: 553–560.

Price CE, Rona RJ & Chinn S (1990) Associations of excessive irritability with common illnesses and food intolerance. *Pediatric and Perinatal Epidemiology* **4**: 156–160.

Raesaenen L, Lehto M & Reunala T (1992) Diagnostic value of skin and laboratory tests in cow's milk allergy/intolerance. *Clinical and Experimental Allergy* **22**: 385–390.

Rona RJ & Chinn S (1987) Parents' perceptions of food intolerance in primary school children. *British Medical Journal* **294**: 863–866.

Rosekrans PCM, Meijer CJLM, Cornelisse CJ et al (1980) Use of morphometry and immuno-histochemistry of small intestinal biopsy specimens in the diagnosis of food allergy. *Journal of Clinical Pathology* **33**: 125–130.

Rosenthal E, Schlesinger Y, Birnbaum Y et al (1991) Intolerance to casein hydrolysate formula. Clinical aspects. *Acta Paediatrica Scandinavica* **80**: 958–960.

Sampson HA & Albergo R (1984) Comparison of results of skin tests, RAST, and double-blind, placebo-controlled food challenges in children with atopic dermatitis. *Journal of Allergy and Clinical Immunology* **74**: 26–33.

Sampson HA & Scanlon SM (1989) Natural history of food hypersensitivity in children with atopic dermatitis. *Journal of Pediatrics* **115**: 23–27.

Sampson HA & Metcalfe DD (1992) Food allergies. *Journal of the American Medical Association* **20**: 2840–2844.

Sampson HA, Broadbent KR & Bernhisel-Broadbent J (1989) Spontaneous release of histamine from basophils and histamine-releasing factor in patients with atopic dermatitis and food hypersensitivity. *New England Journal of Medicine* **321**: 228–232.

Sampson HA, Mendelson L & Rosen JP (1992) fatal and near-fatal anaphylactic reactions to food in children and adolescents. *New England Journal of Medicine* **327**: 380–384.

Sampson HA, Bernhisel-Broadbent J, Yang E & Scanlon SM (1991) Safety of casein hydroly-sate formula in children with cow's milk allergy. *Journal of Pediatrics* **118**: 520–525.

Sanderson IR & Walker WA (1993) Uptake and transport of macromolecules by the intestine: possible role in clinical disorders (an update). *Gastroenterology* **104**: 622–639.

Savilahti E (1992) Diagnostic criteria of food allergy with predominantly intestinal symptoms. *Journal of Pediatric Gastroenterology and Nutrition* **14**: 108–112.

Savilahti E, Tuomikoski-Jaakkola P, Järvenpää A-L & Virtanen M (1993) Early feeding of preterm infants and allergic symptoms during childhood. *Acta Paediatrica Scandinavica* **82**: 340–344.

Savilahti E, Tainio VM, Salmenperae L et al (1991) Low colostral IgA associated with cow's milk allergy. *Acta Paediatrica Scandinavica* **80**: 1207–1213.

Schrander JJ, Oudsen S, Forget PP & Kuijten RH (1992) Follow up study of cow's milk protein intolerant infants. *European Journal of Pediatrics* **151**: 783–785.

Shiner M (1981) Ultrastructural features of allergic manifestations in the small intestine of children. *Scandinavian Journal of Gastroenterology* **70** (**supplement**): 49–64.

Sigurs N, Hattevig G & Kjellman B (1992) Maternal avoidance of eggs, cow's milk, and fish during lactation: Effect on allergic manifestations, skin-prick tests, and specific IgE antibodies in children at age 4 years. *Pediatrics* **89**: 735–739.

Sloper KS, Wadsworth J & Brostoff J (1991) Children with atopic eczema. I: Clinical response to food elimination and subsequent double-blind food challenge. *Quarterly Journal of Medicine* **80**: 677–693.

Strobel S (1990) Immunologically mediated damage to the intestinal mucosa. *Acta Paediatrica Scandinavica* **365** (**supplement**): 46–57.

Strobel S (1993) Epidemiology of food sensitivity in childhood—with special reference to cow's milk allergy in infancy. *Monographs in Allergy* **31:** 119–130.

Sullivan PB (1993) Cows milk induced intestinal bleeding in infancy. *Archives of Disease in Childhood* **68:** 240–245.

Suomalainen H, Isolauri E, Kaila M et al (1992) Cow's milk provocation induces an immune response to unrelated dietary antigens. *Gut* **33:** 1179–1183.

Symposium proceedings. (1992) Adverse reactions to foods in infancy and childhood. *Journal of Pediatrics* **121:** 1–126.

Vandenplas Y, Hauser B, Van den Borre C et al (1992) Effect of a whey hydrolysate prophylaxis of atopic disease. *Annals of Allergy* **68:** 419–424.

Vandenplas Y, Bahna SL, Bousquet J et al (1992b) Extraintestinal manifestations of food allergy in infants and children. *Nutrition Research* **12:** 161–177.

Verkasalo M, Kuitunen P & Savilahti E (1981) Changing pattern of cow's milk intolerance. *Acta Paediatrica Scandinavica* **70:** 289–295.

Waldmann TA, Wochner RD, Laster L & Gordon RS (1967) Allergic gastroenteropathy. A cause of excessive gastrointestinal protein loss. *New England Journal of Medicine* **276:** 761–769.

Walker-Smith JA (1982) Cow's milk intolerance as a cause of postenteritis diarrhoea. *Journal of Pediatric Gastroenterology and Nutrition* **1:** 163–173.

Walker-Smith JA (1992) Gastrointestinal food allergy in childhood—current problems. *Nutrition Research* **12:** 123–135.

Webb EL, Fiedler ER, Villacis BF et al (1992) Abnormal psychological profiles in persons reporting food allergies. *Journal of Allergy and Clinical Immunology* **89:** 193.

Wilson N & Scott A (1989) A double-blind assessment of additive intolerance in children using a 12 day challenge period at home. *Clinical and Experimental Allergy* **19:** 267–272.

Zeiger RS, Heller S, Mellon MH et al (1989) Effect of combined maternal and infant food-allergen avoidance on development of atopy in early infancy: A randomized study. *Journal of Allergy and Clinical Immunology* **84:** 72–89.

Zeiger RS, Heller S, Mellon MH et al (1992) Genetic and environmental factors affecting the development of atopy through age 4 in children of atopic parents: A prospective random-ized study of food allergen avoidance. *Pediatric Allergy and Immunology* **3:** 120–127.

Ziegler EE, Fomon SJ, Nelson SE et al (1990) Cow milk feeding in infancy: Further observa-tions on blood loss from the gastrointestinal tract. *Journal of Pediatrics* **116:** 11–18.

8

Recognizing inflammatory bowel disease

BARBARA S. KIRSCHNER

The inflammatory bowel diseases (IBD), ulcerative colitis (UC) and Crohn's disease (CD) are among the most important causes of chronic gastrointestinal dysfunction during childhood and adolescence. In most cases, the two disorders can be differentiated by the clinical course, and radiological, endoscopic and microscopic features described below. Some children have an atypical form of colitis which is designated indeterminate colitis. Children with these diseases experience a wide range of gastrointestinal and extraintestinal manifestations (Kirschner, 1988a). An awareness of the multisystemic nature of IBD will enable the practitioner to recognize more readily these conditions.

DIFFERENTIATING ULCERATIVE COLITIS AND CROHN'S DISEASE

Ulcerative colitis

The rectum is inflamed in 95% of patients with UC. Depending upon the extent of disease, colitis is classified as proctitis, rectosigmoiditis, disease of the left colon, extensive colitis or pancolitis. Two-thirds of children with UC have pancolitis. The endoscopic appearance varies from erythema and mild friability (grade 1) to extensive ulcers, exudate and spontaneous bleeding (grade 3). A characteristic feature is the absence of normal mucosa between areas of disease.

Microscopically, UC is characterized by acute and chronic inflammation of colonic mucosa with goblet cell depletion, distortion of crypt architecture and crypt abscesses. Inflammatory changes rarely extend into deeper layers of the bowel wall except with toxic megacolon.

Crohn's disease

In contrast to UC, CD can involve any segment of the gastrointestinal tract, from the mouth to the anus. Aphthoid ulcers (small superficial ulcerations over Peyer's patches) are thought to be the earliest lesion. The cellular infiltrate contains predominantly chronic inflammatory cells, sometimes forming epithelioid granulomas. Focally inflamed mucosa with aphthoid or linear ulcers is often seen next to normal mucosa resulting in the term 'skip lesions'. The inflammatory process is transmural, involving all layers of bowel wall from the mucosa to the serosa. Extension through the serosa may lead to sinus tracts or fistulas between bowel and adjacent tissues such as other loops of bowel, bladder, vagina, the abdominal wall or perineal area.

The frequency of disease involvement is: diffuse small bowel (20%); terminal ileum alone (20%); ileocolonic (34–52%); isolated colitis (10–30%); and anorectal (6%). Endoscopic evaluation of paediatric patients documented that oesophageal, gastric and duodenal Crohn's disease is more common than previously appreciated (Mashako et al, 1989; Schmidt-Sommerfeld et al, 1990). Perianal skin tags, fissures, and fistulas should strongly suggest the diagnosis of CD.

EPIDEMIOLOGIC ASPECTS

In Scotland, Crohn's disease in children increased three-fold between 1968 and 1983 (Barton et al, 1989). The onset of symptoms may begin at any age with rare cases beginning in infancy (Chong et al, 1986; Gryboski, 1993). The most significant risk factor for developing IBD is a positive family history (Gilat et al, 1987). In that international study, 20% of children with IBD had an affected family member—parent (9%), grandparent (8%) or sibling (4%). Other factors including formula intolerance, tendency toward infectious gastroenteritis, breast-feeding, or stressful life events such as parental death, divorce, severe parental disease or disability did not influence the frequency of IBD. The importance of genetic factors is further supported by the strong concordance of UC or CD within families. Toyoda et al (1993) reported a positive association between UC and genes HLA DR2 and CD with HLA DR1/DQw5. Jews have a two–four-fold higher risk and Asians a lower risk than the general population (Calkins and Mendeloff, 1986). Recently, perinuclear antineutrophilic cytoplasmic antibody (p-ANCA) has been shown to have a higher association with ulcerative colitis and primary sclerosing cholangitis than with Crohn's disease, and has proved to be a useful marker for distinguishing these disorders (Yang et al, 1992).

There is no evidence that underlying personality disturbances predispose children to develop IBD. The greater prevalence of emotional disturbance in children with IBD compared with healthy children is thought to result from chronic disease (Steinhausen and Kies, 1982; Engström and Lindquist, 1991).

PATHOGENESIS OF IBD

Genetic predisposition and complex disordered regulation of the mucosal immune system are thought to contribute to the pathogenesis of IBD. Under experimental conditions, intestinal epithelial cells of IBD patients induce proliferation of lamina propria T-cells while normal epithelial cells suppress the immune response (Mayer and Eisenhardt, 1990). Mucosal immunoglobulin secretion is increased and alterations in cytokine, prostaglandin or leukotriene production may also be important.

Infectious agents may have a pivotal role in causing IBD, based on the association of pathogens with the onset (Willoughby et al, 1989; Kirschner, 1993) and relapse (Kangro et al, 1990; Gryboski, 1991) of disease. A slow-growing strain of mycobacterium (*M. linda*) has been isolated from several patients although its significance remains unclear (Chiodini et al, 1984).

The observation that elemental (Morin et al, 1980; Sanderson et al, 1987; Giaffer et al, 1991) and polymeric formulas (Rigaud et al, 1991) and food elimination diets (Alun Jones et al, 1985) decrease disease activity in CD, suggests that food antigens may play a role in this disease.

CLINICAL PRESENTATION

Intestinal signs and symptoms

Ulcerative colitis

The most characteristic features of UC are blood mixed with stool and lower abdominal cramping during defecation. Episodes may be mild, moderate, or severe depending upon stool frequency, amount of abdominal tenderness, fever, and haemoglobin and albumin concentrations (Werlin and Grand, 1977). A rare complication of UC is toxic megacolon (colon diameter > 6.0 cm). Air insufflation during barium enema or colonoscopy, anticholinergic medications, and hypokalaemia predispose children with moderate or severe disease to this potentially life-threatening situation. Perforation and sepsis may occur under these circumstances. Fortunately, toxic megacolon develops in only 2% of children with pancolitis.

Crohn's disease

The subtle nature of the intestinal signs of CD may cause the diagnosis to be delayed for months to years (Burbige et al, 1975). Complaints often correspond to the site of disease. Ileocaecal involvement is seen in the majority of children (80%) and is usually associated with obstructive symptoms occurring at mealtime. Despite complaints of pain in the periumbilical region, direct palpation often elicits fullness or tenderness in the right lower quadrant. Diffuse small bowel disease is usually accompanied by diarrhoea and anorexia. Lactose intolerance and other forms of malabsorption are most prevalent in this group (Kirschner et al, 1981b). The symptoms of Crohn's disease of the colon mirror those of UC with bloody stools and pain associated with defecation. Active perianal inflammation manifest by skin tags, deep anal fissures, and perianal fistula should alert the physician to the diagnosis of Crohn's disease.

Systemic and extra-intestinal findings

Systemic and extra-intestinal manifestations of IBD occur in both UC and CD. When these features precede or overshadow gastrointestinal symptoms, the diagnosis of IBD is often delayed.

Weight loss

Failure to gain weight at a normal rate and weight loss are among the commonest systemic signs of IBD in children. In our patient population, 87% of children with CD lost weight, averaging 5.7 kg. Weight loss is less common in ulcerative colitis (68%) and of a reduced magnitude (4.1 kg).

Arthralgias and arthritis

Arthralgias and arthritis occur commonly in children with IBD (Lindsey and Schaller, 1974; Passo et al, 1986). Arthritis is usually pauciarticular affecting large joints such as knees, ankles and hips. Attacks tend to coincide with intestinal activity and subside with treatment of the intestinal disease. Joint deformity rarely develops although granulomatous synovitis and joint destruction have been reported in adults. Refractory joint complaints may require nonsteroidal anti-inflammatory therapy. Ankylosing spondylitis develops in a minority of children with CD, especially those positive for HLA B_{27} (Passo et al, 1986). This form of arthritis is unaffected by the response of intestinal disease, and progresses despite reduction of intestinal symptoms.

Fever

Fever is noted in approximately 40% of children with IBD. Low grade fever may occur more frequently but go unrecognized.

Delayed growth and sexual maturation

Growth impairment is defined as a reduced growth velocity (cm/year) or a fall in height percentile for age. It is less common in children with newly-diagnosed UC (5–10%) than CD (30%) (Kirschner et al, 1978). Prepubertal children may be particularly affected (Kanof and Bayless, 1985; Kirschner, 1990). It is important to emphasize that active disease interferes with growth independently of corticosteroids.

Malabsorption

Malabsorption (as detected by quantitative faecal fat and d-xylose and vitamin B_{12} absorption) does not occur in most growth-impaired children in the absence of intestinal resection (Layden et al, 1976; Kelts et al, 1979; Kirschner et al, 1981a). Protein-losing enteropathy is demonstrable by measuring faecal α_1-antitrypsin (Thomas et al, 1983).

Growth-promoting peptides

Early studies suggested that growth hormone (GH) was reduced in growth-impaired children with IBD. Subsequently, normal GH levels were demonstrated following provocative stimulation tests (Tenore et al, 1977) although spontaneous nocturnal secretion is subnormal in some children (Farthing et al, 1981). Somatomedin C or insulin-like growth factor I (IGF-I) is a GH-dependent peptide modulated by nutritional status. Low levels in poorly growing children with IBD, rise during intensive medical and nutritional therapy and may modulate the changes in growth velocity (Kirschner and Sutton, 1986).

Nutritional deficiency

Chronic reduction in calorie intake is the most likely cause of the growth failure (Kirschner, 1988b). Children with active CD ingest 1764 kJ/day (420 kcal/day) less than healthy-matched controls (Thomas et al, 1993). Improved linear growth usually follows nutrition support whether supplied as oral formula supplements (Kirschner et al, 1981a), continuous or nocturnal nasogastric infusion of liquid formulas (Morin et al, 1980; Navarro et al, 1982; Aiges et al, 1989; Belli et al, 1988) or total parenteral nutrition in the hospital (Layden et al, 1976; Kelts et al, 1979) and at home (Strobel et al, 1979).

Delayed sexual maturation

Delayed or arrested sexual maturation often accompanies impaired linear growth. In postmenarchal patients, secondary amenorrhoea may follow periods of poor weight gain or weight loss. When menarche does arrive, it does not necessarily herald the cessation of linear growth. Growth potential after menarche depends on the age of menarche in children with IBD. Children whose menarche begins < 13 years of age grow an average of 10.6 cm following menarche while those with menarche after 16 years grow only 2.3 cm (Kirschner et al, 1993).

Mucocutaneous lesions

Oral aphthoid ulcers are frequently multiple and usually appear during periods of active IBD. Cutaneous lesions include erythema nodosum, pyoderma gangrenosum, and diffuse papulonecrotic eruptions. These develop when the intestinal disease is active, either at disease onset or during exacerbations. Resolution coincides with disease remission although pyoderma gangrenosum may be refractory and require intensive local care and systemic therapy.

Renal disease

The urinary tract is the site of several complications of IBD. Renal calculi develop in about 6% of patients, being composed predominantly of uric acid in UC and oxalate in CD. Renal colic may be preceded by painless microscopic haematuria. Additional potential risks in CD are hydroureter, hydronephrosis or pyelonephritis due to ureteral compression by an inflammatory mass, enteric-vesicular fistulas and rarely, renal insufficiency caused by secondary amyloidosis.

Hepatobiliary disease

The liver and biliary system are affected in 4% of children with IBD (Lloyd-Still and Cahan, 1987). Sclerosing cholangitis, the commonest hepatic complication, occurs almost exclusively in children with UC and may precede overt colonic symptoms. Most patients experience pruritus, elevated alkaline phosphatase and blood levels of perinuclear antineutrophil cytoplasmic antibody (p-ANCA). Medical therapy and colectomy do not prevent progression. Chronic active hepatitis should be excluded in children with abnormal liver tests.

Ocular complications

Ophthalmological disease develops in some children with IBD. Uveitis, iritis, and episcleritis are observed in approximately 4% of patients with UC but increase to 13% in children with Crohn's colitis. Corticosteroids enhance the risk of posterior subcapsular cataracts and raised intraocular pressure, but individual susceptibility may also affect the frequency of these complications (Tripathi et al, 1992).

DIAGNOSING ULCERATIVE COLITIS AND CROHN'S DISEASE
(See Table 1)

Ulcerative colitis

Excluding enteric infection

Enteric pathogens must be excluded before making a diagnosis of UC. Infectious agents to be ruled out by appropriate stool examination include: *Salmonella, Shigella, Campylobacter, Yersinia, Aeromonas, Clostridium difficile, Giardia lamblia*, and *Entamoeba histolytica. Escherichia coli* 0157:H7 causes haemorrhagic colitis and should be identified if facilities are available (Karmali et al, 1983; Neill et al, 1987).

Endoscopic evaluation

Colonoscopy with biopsy establishes the diagnosis, severity and extent of inflammation. Bowel preparation and endoscopic examination should be performed with extreme caution in patients with severe disease to avoid precipitating toxic megacolon. Conscious sedation with meperidine (1–2 mg/kg) and midazolam (0.1–0.3 mg/kg) is generally used to ensure comfort and diminish anxiety about future examinations (Rossi, 1988).

Table 1. Approach to the diagnosis of IBD in children.

Test	Expected result
Physical examination	Height and weight curve abdominal perianal findings
Haematologic tests	
CBC, differential	↑ WBC, ↑ Bands
Platelet count	Anaemia, microcytic indices
Acute phase reactants	
Erythrocyte sedimentation rate	Elevated
C-Reactive protein; orosomucoid	Elevated
Serum albumin	Reduced
Stool examinations	
Occult blood and leukocytes	Usually present with colitis, often negative, small bowel C.D.
Stool culture; ova and parasites	Negative
Endoscopic evaluation	Oesophagogastroduodenoscopy for upper GI symptoms Colonoscopy: rectal bleeding, abnormal stools
Radiologic studies	Upper GI/SB follow-through or enteroclysis Barium enema (double contrast)

X-ray studies

Colon X-rays are infrequently used to diagnose UC following the availability of endoscopy, since colonic mucosa may appear normal, radiologically, early in the course. When a barium enema is needed to assess the extent of disease or to exclude strictures, double contrast (air–barium) examinations are recommended because they provide greater mucosal detail. Spiculation, mucosal irregularity, and loss of haustration can be visualized (Figure 1). Small bowel studies are important in equivocal cases to exclude the possibility of CD.

Blood tests

Selected blood tests are useful in screening patients for IBD and monitoring the course of disease (Campbell et al, 1982; Kirschner, 1988a; Holmquist et al, 1989). These include: blood count with complete differential, platelet count, serum iron and iron-binding capacity, total protein, albumin, erythrocyte sedimentation rate (ESR), C-reactive protein (CRP), orosomucoid and platelet count. The percent band forms, platelet count and ESR are often elevated in active UC. Rectal bleeding with anaemia and low platelet count suggests the possibility of other disorders such as haemolytic uraemic syndrome, idiopathic thrombocytopenic purpura or leukaemia.

Crohn's disease

The sequence of diagnostic studies in CD varies depending upon the most likely site of disease. In the absence of rectal bleeding, blood tests and small

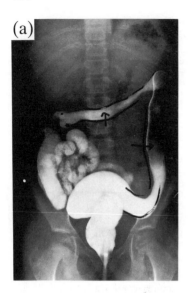 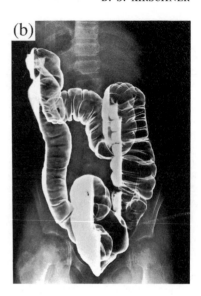

Figure 1(a). Barium enema showing continuous loss of haustrations and rigidity of the descending and transverse colon in a child with chronic nonspecific ulcerative colitis.
(b) Air contrast barium enema illustrating normal haustral pattern.

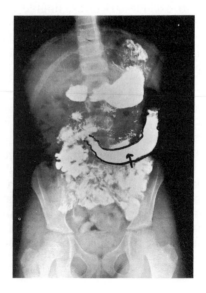

Figure 2. Small bowel X-ray showing focal narrowing and deformity of a jejunal loop in a child with growth failure and chronic anaemia secondary to Crohn's disease.

bowel X-rays often precede endoscopic evaluation. The ESR and CRP are elevated in most children (Kirschner, 1988a; Holmquist et al, 1989). Haemoglobin, serum albumin and iron concentrations are often low. Enteric infections (especially *Yersinia enterocolitica*) must be excluded. After blood and stool screening tests, radiological and endoscopic examinations are scheduled as indicated.

Endoscopic evaluation

Where possible, the diagnosis of CD should be confirmed by histology, especially if there is suspected gastroduodenal or colonic disease. Microscopic features of CD are often present in biopsies from normal-appearing mucosa. When disease cannot be reached endoscopically, the diagnosis rests on physical findings, laboratory tests, and typical X-ray changes.

Radiological assessment

Small bowel enema (enterolysis) is superior to routine follow-through examinations for diagnosing CD (Ratcliffe, 1983; McFarlane et al, 1986). The important diagnostic features are mucosal nodularity and irregularity, oedematous valvulae, ulcerations, and reverse peristalsis. Narrowed intestinal segments with proximal dilation occur with advanced disease (Figures 2–4).

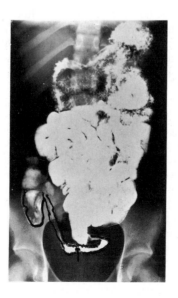

Figure 3. Small bowel series illustrating focal rigidity and mucosal irregularity suggestive of ulceration in the terminal ileum.

Table 2. Drug therapy for children with IBD.

Aminosalicylates	
Oral sulphasalazine	50–75 mg/kg/day divided p.c. 3–4 times a day
Mesalamine (5-aminosalicylate)*	30–50 mg/kg/day divided p.c. 2–3 times a day
Topical mesalazine enema	2–4 g bedtime
Mesalazine suppository	0.5 g bedtime
Corticosteroids	
Oral prednisone	1–2 mg/kg/day
	Alternate-day vs discontinuation
Intravenous methylprednisolone	1–1.5 mg/kg/day
Rectal hydrocortisone foam	100 mg bedtime
Methylprednisolone enema	20–40 mg 1–2 times a day
Metronidazole	10–15 mg/kg/day divided after meals
6-Mercaptopurine	1.0–1.5 mg/kg/day
Azathioprine	1.5–2.0 mg/kg/day
Cyclosporin A	Highly selected cases
	2.0 mg/kg i.v. b.i.d.
	4–6 mg/kg p.o. b.i.d.

* New 5-ASA preparations may be substituted as indicated in patients with sulpha sensitivity or side effects from sulphasalazine.

MEDICAL THERAPY (see Table 2)

Ulcerative colitis

The ability to predict the outcome of an individual child is hampered by the knowledge that the intensity of the initial attack does not predict the severity of future attacks (Michener et al, 1979; Mir-Madhjessi et al, 1986). Pancolitis is thought to augur a severe clinical course. However, Gryboski (1993) recently reported that although 89% of 38 children with UC developed pancolitis, only two patients required colectomy during 2–19 years of follow-up.

Mild ulcerative colitis

Children with mild UC have < five stools per day, minimal abdominal tenderness, and no significant anaemia, hypoalbuminaemia, or fever. Sulphasalazine (SASP) or mesalazine (5-aminosalicylate; 5-ASA) preparations constitute the first line of therapy (Barden et al, 1989). The active ingredient, 5-ASA, acts topically to diminish inflammation in the colon, possibly by inhibiting prostaglandin and leukotriene metabolism, inhibiting interleukin-1 and IgG production and reducing reactive oxygen molecules. Side effects due to SASP are frequent and include headache, gastrointestinal distress, haemolytic anaemia, and pruritic rash. Mesalamine, which does not contain sulpha, causes less side effects in most patients. Topical 5-ASA or corticosteroid foam or enemas administered at bedtime reduces tenesmus, bleeding or stool frequency.

Moderate activity

Children with moderately severe disease have > five stools daily, cramping with defecation, abdominal tenderness, fever, anaemia, and hypoalbuminaemia. The intensity of these symptoms justifies the use of corticosteroids. Oral prednisone dose is recommended at 1–2 mg/kg/day, in divided doses (every 8–12 h). Once clinical improvement occurs, the frequency is changed to a single morning dose. SASP or 5-ASA is added as tolerated. The addition of topical corticosteroid or 5-ASA preparations promotes healing in the left colon. Many paediatric gastroenterologists restrict roughage (raw fruits and vegetables, seeds, nuts, popcorn) and potential colonic irritants (barbecue sauce, pepper, etc.) when the disease is active. The elimination of dairy products is unnecessary except in lactose intolerant children. Acetaminophen may be prescribed but antispasmodics are avoided to prevent possible toxic megacolon.

Severe disease

Children with severe disease have systemic toxicity, marked abdominal tenderness, cramping, anaemia (Hb < 9.0 g/dl), hypoalbuminaemia, and fever. The abdomen should be palpated frequently to detect early signs of toxic megacolon or perforation (increasing distension, tenderness or hypoactive bowel sounds). An abdominal X-ray should be obtained to assess the diameter of the colon if these findings are present. The clinical course is also monitored by the following blood tests: blood count (with attention to the per-cent band forms), platelet count, serum albumin, serum electrolytes (especially potassium), magnesium, calcium and others as clinically indicated. Blood should be typed and crossed for potential transfusion.

Medical intervention for these children consists of intravenous fluids, medications, and nutritional support, and avoidance of anticholinergic drugs. Intravenous corticosteroids (either methylprednisolone 1.0–2.0 mg/kg/day or hydrocortisone 10 mg/kg/day) in divided doses are the mainstay of therapy. Although antibiotics are of unproven efficacy, coverage for *Clostridium difficile* with intravenous vancomycin or metronidazole is often administered. Albumin infusions may be required to maintain intravascular volume due to enteric protein losses. Nutrition support by peripheral or central veins is often needed to reverse ongoing weight loss and provide nutrients concurrently with drug therapy. The majority of children who respond to this regimen do so within 12 days, although some continue to improve (Seashore et al, 1982; Gold et al, 1993).

Immunosuppressive medications (azathioprine and 6-mercaptopurine) are effective in 70% of children with steroid-dependent or refractory disease although remission may not occur for several weeks (Verhave et al, 1990). Cyclosporin A (CyA) may induce rapid resolution within 1–2 weeks even after other medical therapies have failed (Kirschner et al, 1989; Lichtiger and Present, 1990). Because experience with CyA in children with severe UC is limited, its therapeutic role awaits further study.

For those patients who enter remission, maintenance therapy with SASP or 5-ASA is effective in suppressing the emergence of disease activity (Dissanayke and Truelove, 1973; Barden et al, 1989). Daily prednisone is gradually tapered and continued on an alternate-day regimen or discontinued (Sadeghi-Nejad and Senior, 1968).

Crohn's disease

Because large-scale drug treatment studies are rarely performed in children with IBD, information regarding drug efficacy is often derived from studies in adult patients. The National Cooperative Crohn's Disease Study (NCCDS) in the United States compared prednisone, sulphasalazine, azathioprine and placebo over a 17-week period (Summers et al, 1979). Prednisone induced remission more rapidly and consistently than sulphasalazine. Sulphasalazine was ineffective against small bowel disease but useful against colonic disease. Newer mesalamine preparations which are released throughout the small bowel appear to be more effective (Griffiths et al, 1993). Metronidazole is active against perianal (Bernstein et al, 1980) and colonic (Ursing et al, 1982) disease. Children must be questioned regarding signs of peripheral neuropathy (numbness and paraesthesiaes) and the dosage lowered or stopped if these symptoms develop (Duffy et al, 1985). The European Cooperative Crohn's Disease Study (ECCDS) compared sulphasalazine, prednisone, a combination of both, and placebo over a 2-year period (Malchow et al, 1984). Prednisone was most effective in small bowel and ileocolonic disease, whereas the combination of prednisone and sulphasalazine was beneficial in colon disease. Patients with recurrently

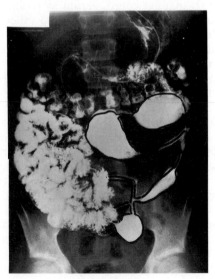

Figure 4. Radiograph of the small intestine demonstrating advanced Crohn's disease. Features include multiple stenotic segments, pseudodiverticuli (outpocketing proximal to narrowed segments), creating symptoms of partial small bowel obstruction and dilatation of the small bowel.

active disease had a lower relapse rate if given continuous low-dose methyl-prednisolone (alone or with SASP) compared with SASP alone or placebo.

Immunosuppressive therapy with azathioprine or 6-mercaptopurine (6-MP) induces remission in 67% of patients with CD compared with 8% with placebo (Present et al, 1989). Recently, the combination of predniso-lone and azathioprine was shown to induce a more rapid remission in active Crohn's disease than prednisolone alone (Ewe et al, 1993). Because of the potential risk of lymphoma, leukopenia, and pancreatitis, these medications are usually reserved for children who are steroid-dependent, have extensive non-resectable disease, or those with prior resections (Verhave et al, 1990; Markowitz et al, 1990). Side effects are minimal and most children tolerate these drugs without requiring drug withdrawal.

For mild disease, sulphasalazine or mesalamine (5-ASA) preparations may be sufficient. Controlled-release 5-ASA (Pentasa®) may be effective when disease involves the proximal small intestine while delayed-release pH-dependent preparations (Asacol®, Salofalk®, Rowasa®, Claversal®) reduce symptoms in ileocolonic disease.

Once remission has occurred, the benefits of maintenance therapy are less well documented in CD than UC. Many paediatric gastroenterologists continue maintenance levels of SASP or 5-ASA, alternate-day prednisone (Whitington et al, 1977), or azathioprine or 6-MP in an attempt to decrease the frequency of relapse.

NUTRITION SUPPORT

Ulcerative colitis

Total parenteral nutrition (TPN) is less effective in inducing remission in UC (40%) than CD (70%) (Elson et al, 1980). Jarnerot et al (1985) correlated the response to intensive therapy with the extent and severity of disease. Remission was greater in mild attacks (91%) than severe episodes (51%) and poorest in patients with pancolitis (47%). A paediatric study of adoles-cents with severe colitis (14 UC, 5 CD) showed that 32% initially improved but only 5% were still in remission at 2 years (Werlin and Grand, 1977). Seashore et al (1982) evaluated the course of 22 children on TPN, eight of whom had UC with pancolitis. Four of the eight (50%) improved within 1 week but the others required colectomy. The authors were unable to identify risk factors for predicting response to aggressive medical manage-ment. Recently, Gold et al (1993) reported a long-term beneficial response in 80% of children who received similar therapy for more than 2 weeks.

Crohn's disease

Nutrition support is clearly effective primary and adjunctive therapy for CD. Elemental and polymeric formulas whether given orally (Kirschner et al, 1981a; O'Morain et al, 1984) or by nasogastric infusion (Morin et al, 1980; Sanderson et al, 1987; Belli et al, 1988) and parenteral nutrition (Kelts et al, 1979; Strobel et al, 1979) decrease symptoms, increase weight gain and reverse growth failure. Relapse often occurs when concurrent drug therapy is not provided (Morin et al, 1980; Strobel et al, 1979; Seidman et al, 1986, 1993). The recommended intake of calories, protein, and specific nutrients varies with age, sex, degree of undernutrition, and extent of disease and enteric losses. Calorie intakes of 60–80 kcal/kg are usually necessary to meet the recommended dietary allowance for age (Kirschner, 1988b). TNP is reserved for children unresponsive to enteral therapy.

SURGERY

Ulcerative colitis

Prior to the 1970s, approximately 50% of children with UC underwent proctocolectomy within 5 years of diagnosis (Binder et al, 1973). By the 1970s, the likelihood of proctocolectomy in children with UC had decreased from 50 to 25% within 5 years of diagnosis (Michener et al, 1979). Colectomy is indicated for persistent toxicity, uncontrollable bleeding, suspected perforation or abscess, toxic megacolon, growth failure, medical intractability with dependence corticosteroids. Epithelial dysplasia and long duration of disease are associated with an increased risk of colon cancer and are additional factors for considering colectomy. Surveillance colonoscopy is used to monitor mucosal histology.

Recently described surgical procedures eliminate the need for a permanent ostomy (Telander, 1993). The Kock pouch is an intra-abdominal pouch created from 30 cm of terminal ileum which is emptied by inserting a catheter through the abdominal wall through a nipple valve. Technical difficulties make this procedure less popular than when first described. The most widely performed procedure in young patients with UC is the creation of an ileal pouch within the pelvis which is anastomosed to the anus (Martin et al, 1977; Telander et al, 1990). A temporary ileostomy is used for 8–12 weeks until healing has occurred. Postoperative problems include some degree of nocturnal faecal incontinence, frequent stools, an increased risk of small bowel obstruction (15%) and chronic or recurrent inflammation ('pouchitis') (Telander, 1993). Metronidazole or topical anti-inflammatory preparations usually control symptoms. About 10% of patients with chronic pouchitis are subsequently diagnosed with Crohn's disease.

Crohn's disease

Most children with CD eventually require surgery with 69% within the first 8 years after diagnosis (Farmer and Michener, 1979) and 87% by 15 years (Puntis et al, 1984). Indications include obstruction, fistula formation with possible perforation, refractory disease including growth failure, perianal complications and toxic megacolon. Patients with ileocolonic disease have more surgery (91%) than patients with small intestinal (65%) or coloanorectal (58%) disease. Recurrent disease after surgery is frequent, approaching

57% in one series within 6 years of follow-up (Wesson and Schandling, 1981). This may interfere with the full recovery of growth potential (Homer et al, 1977).

PROGNOSIS

Ulcerative colitis

The long-term prognosis of 336 children with UC was reported by Michener et al (1979). Children diagnosed early in the course of their disease were thought to have an improved quality of life although chronic symptoms persisted in 60–70%. Proctocolectomy was performed in 26% because of refractory disease. Colonic cancer developed in nine patients, all of whom had pancolitis. The earliest cancer was detected 11 years after the diagnosis of UC when the patient was 19 years old. The youngest patient with colonic cancer was 16 years of age. Greenstein et al (1979) emphasized that long latent periods without active disease were noted in half of their patients with UC-associated cancer.

Crohn's disease

Farmer and Michener (1979) reviewed the long-term course of 513 children diagnosed with CD before age 20. Surgery was frequent (67%) and mortality increased (12%). Most deaths occurred in the first 5 years and were caused by perforation with abscess, toxic megacolon with sepsis or malnutrition. In our experience, mortality has been considerably lower. There have been no hospital deaths in almost 300 children diagnosed with CD since 1975. Two children died at home, one from fungal sepsis from an infected TPN catheter and the second from unrecognized intestinal perforation. Early surgical intervention in children with progressive disease and the broad range of available antibiotics may have improved the outcome.

SUMMARY

Children with IBD present with a variety of gastrointestinal signs and symptoms and extraintestinal manifestations. Recognizing individual differences in the severity and extent of disease will enable the practitioner to recommend an appropriate approach to diagnosis and therapeutic intervention. In most instances, paediatricians work with gastroenterologists to provide individualized medical, nutritional, and emotional support to this challenging group of patients.

REFERENCES

Aiges H, Markowitz J, Rosa J et al (1989) Home nocturnal supplemental nasogastric feedings in growth retarded adolescents with Crohn's disease. *Gastroenterology* **97**: 905–910.

762 B. S. KIRSCHNER

Alun Jones V, Workman E, Freeman AH et al (1985) Crohn's disease: maintenance of remission by diet. *Lancet* 2: 177–180.

Barden L, Lipson A, Pert P, Walker-Smith JA (1989) Mesalazine in childhood inflammatory bowel disease. *Alimentary Pharmacological Therapy* 3: 597–603.

Barton JR, Gillon S & Ferguson A (1989) Incidence of inflammatory bowel disease in Scottish children between 1968 and 1983: marginal fall in ulcerative colitis, three-fold rise in Crohn's disease. *Gut* 30: 618–622.

Belli DC, Seidman E, Bouthillier L et al (1988) Chronic intermittent elemental diet improves growth failure in children with Crohn's disease. *Gastroenterology* 94: 603–610.

Bernstein LH, Frank MS, Brandt LJ & Boley S (1980) Healing of perineal Crohn's disease with metronidazole. *Gastroenterology* 79: 357–365.

Binder V, Bonnevie O, Gertz TCL et al (1973) Ulcerative colitis in children: Treatment, course and prognosis. *Scandinavian Journal of Gastroenterology* 8: 161–167.

Burbige EJ, Huang SS & Bayless TM (1975) Clinical manifestations of Crohn's disease in children and adolescents. *Pediatrics* 55: 866–870.

Calkins BM & Mendeloff AI (1986) Epidemiology of inflammatory bowel disease. *Epidemiological Review* 8: 60–91.

Campbell CA, Walker-Smith JA, Hindocha P & Adinolfi M (1982) Acute phase proteins in chronic inflammatory bowel disease. *Journal of Pediatric Gastroenterology and Nutrition* 1: 193–200.

Chiodini RJ, VanKruiningen HJ, Thayer WR et al (1984) Possible role of mycobacteria in inflammatory bowel disease. 1. An unclassified mycobacterium species isolated from patients with Crohn's disease. *Digestive Diseases and Sciences* 29: 1073–1079.

Chong SKF, Blackshaw AJ, Morson BC et al (1986) Prospective study of colitis in infancy and early childhood. *Journal of Pediatric Gastroenterology and Nutrition* 5: 352–358.

Dissanayake AS & Truelove SE (1973) A controlled therapeutic trial of long-term maintenance treatment of ulcerative colitis with sulfasalazine. *Gut* 14: 923–926.

Duffy LF, Daum F, Fisher SE et al (1985) Peripheral neuropathy in Crohn's disease patients treated with metronidazole. *Gastroenterology* 88: 681–684.

Elson CO, Layden TJ, Nemchausky BA et al (1980) An evaluation of total parenteral nutrition in the management of inflammatory bowel disease. *Digestive Diseases and Sciences* 25: 42–48.

Engström I & Lindquist BL (1991) Inflammatory bowel disease in children and adolescents: a somatic and psychiatric investigation. *Acta Paediatrica Scandinavica* 80: 640–647.

Ewe K, Press AG, Singe CC et al (1993) Azathioprine combined with prednisolone or monotherapy with prednisolone in active Crohn's disease. *Gastroenterology* 105: 367–372.

Farmer RG & Michener WM (1979) Prognosis of Crohn's disease with onset in childhood or adolescence. *Digestive Diseases and Sciences* 24: 752–757.

Farthing MJG, Campbell CA, Walker-Smith et al (1981) Nocturnal growth hormone and gonadotrophin secretion in growth retarded children with Crohn's disease. *Gut* 22: 933–938.

Giaffer MH, Nann P & Holdsworth CD (1991) Long-term effects of elemental and exclusion diets for Crohn's disease. *Alimentary Pharmacological Therapy* 5: 115–125.

Gilat T, Hacohen D, Lilos P & Langman MJS (1987) Childhood factors in ulcerative colitis and Crohn's disease. An international cooperative study. *Scandinavian Journal of Gastroenterology* 22: 1009–1024.

Gold DM, Levine JJ & Pettei MJ (1993) Prolonged medical therapy for severe ulcerative colitis. *Gastroenterology* 104: A708.

Greenstein AJ, Sachar DB, Pucillo A et al (1979) Cancer in universal and left-sided ulcerative colitis: Factors determining risk. *Gastroenterology* 77: 290–294.

Griffiths A, Koletzko S, Sylvester F et al (1993) Slow-release 5-aminosalicylic acid therapy in children with small intestinal Crohn's disease. *Journal of Pediatric Gastroenterology and Nutrition* 17: 186–192.

Gryboski JD (1991) Clostridium difficile in inflammatory bowel disease relapse. *Journal of Pediatric Gastroenterology and Nutrition* 13: 39–41.

Gryboski JD (1993) Ulcerative colitis in children 10 years or younger. *Journal of Pediatric Gastroenterology and Nutrition* 17: 24–31.

Holmquist L, Ahren C & Fällström SP (1989) Relationship between results of laboratory tests and inflammatory activity assessed by colonoscopy in children and adolescents with ulcerative colitis and Crohn's disease. *Journal of Pediatric Gastroenterology and Nutrition* **9**: 187–193.

Homer DR, Grand RJ & Colodny AH (1977) Growth, course, and prognosis after surgery for Crohn's disease in children and adolescents. *Pediatrics* **59**: 717–725.

Jarnerot G, Rolny P & Sandberg-Gertzen H (1985) Intensive intravenous treatment of ulcerative colitis. *Gastroenterology* **89**: 1003–1005.

Kangro HO, Chong SKF, Hardiman A et al (1990) A prospective study of viral and mycoplasma infections in chronic inflammatory bowel disease. *Gastroenterology* **98**: 549–553.

Kanof MD & Bayless TM (1985) Decreased height velocity in Crohn's disease. *Gastroenterology* **95**: 1523–1527.

Karmali MA, Petric M, Lim C et al (1983) *Escherichia coli* cytotoxin, haemolytic-uremic syndrome, and haemorrhagic colitis. *Lancet* **2**: 1299–1300.

Kelts DG, Grand RJ, Shen G et al (1979) Nutritional basis of growth failure in children and adolescents with Crohn's disease. *Gastroenterology* **76**: 720–727.

Kirschner BS, Voinchet O & Rosenberg IH (1978) Growth retardation in children with inflammatory bowel disease. *Gastroenterology* **75**: 504–511.

Kirschner BS, Klich JR, Kalman SS et al (1981a) Reversal of growth retardation in Crohn's disease with therapy emphasizing oral nutritional restitution. *Gastroenterology* **80**: 10–15.

Kirschner BS, DeFavaro MV & Jensen W (1981b) Lactose malabsorption in children and adolescents with inflammatory bowel disease. *Gastroenterology* **81**: 829–832.

Kirschner BS & Sutton MM (1986) Somatomedin-C levels in growth-impaired children and adolescents with chronic inflammatory bowel disease. *Gastroenterology* **91**: 830–836.

Kirschner BS (1988a) Inflammatory bowel disease in children. *Pediatric Clinics of North America* **35**: 189–209.

Kirschner BS (1988b) *Enteral nutrition in inflammatory bowel disease*. Report of the 94th Ross Conference on Pediatric Research, Enteral Feeding: Scientific basis and clinical applications. Columbus, OH: Ross Laboratories.

Kirschner BS, Whitington PF & Malfeo-Klein R (1989) Experience with cyclosporin A (CyA) in severe non-specific ulcerative colitis (UC). *Pediatric Research* **25**: 117A.

Kirschner BS (1990) Consequences for growth and development in chronic inflammatory bowel disease. *Acta Paediatrica Scandinavica* **366**: 98–104.

Kirschner BS, Uebler N & Sutton MM (1993) Growth after menarche in pediatric patients with chronic inflammatory bowel disease. *Gastroenterology* **104**: A629.

Kirschner BS (1993) Does acute infection trigger chronic inflammation in pediatric patients with chronic inflammatory bowel disease? *Gastroenterology* **104**: 725A.

Layden T, Rosenberg J, Nemchausky B et al (1976) Reversal of growth arrest in adolescents with Crohn's disease after parenteral alimentation. *Gastroenterology* **70**: 1017–1026.

Lichtiger S & Present DH (1990) Preliminary report: cyclosporin in treatment of severe active ulcerative colitis. *Lancet* **336**: 16–19.

Lindsey CB & Schaller JG (1974) Arthritis associated with inflammatory bowel disease in children. *Journal of Pediatrics* **84**: 16–20.

Lloyd-Still JD & Cahan J (1987) Liver disease associated with childhood inflammatory bowel disease (IBD) (abstract) *Hepatology* **7**: 1088.

McFarlane PL, Miller V & Ratcliffe JF (1986) Clinical and radiological diagnosis of Crohn's disease in children. *Journal of Pediatric Gastroenterology and Nutrition* **5**: 87–92.

Malchow H, Ewe K, Brandes JW et al (1984) European cooperative Crohn's disease study (ECCDS): Results of drug treatment. *Gastroenterology* **86**: 249–266.

Markowitz J, Rosa J, Grancher K et al (1990) Long-term 6-mercaptopurine treatment in adolescents with Crohn's disease. *Gastroenterology* **99**: 1347–1355.

Martin LW, LeCoultre C & Schubert WK (1977) Total colectomy and mucosal proctectomy with preservation of continence in ulcerative colitis. *Annals of Surgery* **186**: 477–480.

Mashako MNL, Cezard JP, Navarro J et al (1989) Crohn's disease lesions in the upper gastrointestinal tract: correlation between clinical, radiological, endoscopic, and histological features in adolescents and children. *Journal of Pediatric Gastroenterology and Nutrition* **8**: 442–446.

Mayer L & Eisenhardt D (1990) Lack of induction of suppressor T cells by intestinal epithelial cells from patients with inflammatory bowel disease. *Journal of Clinical Investigation* **86**: 1255–1260.

Michener WM, Farmer RG & Mortimer EA (1979) Long-term prognosis of ulcerative colitis with onset in childhood or adolescence. *Journal of Clinical Gastroenterology* 1: 301–305.

Mir-Madhjessi SH, Michener WM & Farmer RG (1986) Course and prognosis of idiopathic ulcerative proctosigmoiditis in young patients. *Journal of Pediatric Gastroenterology and Nutrition* 5: 570–576.

Morin CL, Roulet M, Roy CC & Weber A (1980) Continuous elemental enteral alimentation in children with Crohn's disease and growth failure. *Gastroenterology* 79: 1205–1210.

Navarro J, Vargas J, Cesard JP et al (1982) Prolonged constant rate elemental enteral nutrition in Crohn's disease. *Journal of Pediatric Gastroenterology and Nutrition* 1: 541–546.

Neill MA, Tarr PI, Clausen CR et al (1987) Escherichia coli 0157:H7 as a predominant pathogen associated with the hemolytic uremic syndrome: a prospective study in the Pacific Northwest. *Pediatrics* 80: 37–40.

O'Morain C, Segal A & Levi AJ (1984) Elemental diet as primary treatment of acute Crohn's disease: A controlled trial. *British Medical Journal* 288: 1859–1862.

Passo MH, Fitzgerald JF & Brandt KD (1986) Arthritis associated with inflammatory bowel disease in children. Relationship of joint disease to activity and severity of bowel lesion. *Digestive Diseases and Sciences* 31: 492–497.

Present DH, Meltzer SJ, Krumholz MP et al (1989) 6-Mercaptopurine in the management of inflammatory bowel disease: short and long-term toxicity. *Annals of Internal Medicine* 111: 641–649.

Puntis J, McNeish AS & Allan RN (1984) Long term prognosis of Crohn's disease with onset in childhood and adolescence. *Gut* 25: 329–336.

Ratcliffe JKF (1983) The small bowel enema in children: a description of a technique. *Clinical Radiology* 34: 287–289.

Rigaud D, Cosnes J, LeQuintrec Y et al (1991) Controlled trial comparing two types of enteral nutrition in treatment of active Crohn's disease: enteral v polymeric diet. *Gut* 32: 1492–1497.

Rossi T (1988) Endoscopic examination of the colon in infants and children. *Pediatrics Clinics of North America* 35: 331–356.

Sadeghi-Nejad A & Senior B (1968) The treatment of ulcerative colitis in children with alternate-day corticosteroids. *Pediatrics* 43: 840–845.

Sanderson IR, Udeen S, Davies PSW et al (1987) Remission induced by an elemental diet in small bowel Crohn's disease. *Archives of Disease in Childhood* 61: 123–127.

Schmidt-Sommerfeld E, Kirschner BS & Stephens JK (1990) Endoscopic and histologic findings in the upper gastrointestinal tract of children with Crohn's disease. *Journal of Pediatric Gastroenterology and Nutrition* 11: 448–454.

Seashore JH, Hillemeier AC & Gryboski JD (1982) Total parenteral nutrition in the management of inflammatory bowel disease in children: A limited role. *American Journal of Surgery* 143: 504–507.

Seidman EG, Bouthillier L, Weber AM et al (1986) Elemental diet versus prednisone as primary treatment of Crohn's disease (abstract). *Gastroenterology* 90: A1625.

Seidman E, Griffiths A, Issenman R & Canadian Collaborative Pediatric Crohn's Disease Study Group (1993) Semi-elemental (S–E) diet vs prednisone in pediatric Crohn's disease. *Gastroenterology* 104: A778.

Steinhausen H-C & Kies H (1982) Comparative studies of ulcerative colitis and Crohn's disease in children and adolescents. *Journal of Child Psychiatrics* 23: 33–42.

Strobel CT, Byrne WJ & Ament ME (1979) Home parenteral nutrition in children with Crohn's disease: An effective management alternative. *Gastroenterology* 77: 272–279.

Summers RW, Switz DM, Sessions JT Jr et al (1979) National cooperative Crohn's disease study: Results of drug treatment. *Gastroenterology* 77: 847–869.

Telander RL, Spencer M, Perrault J et al (1990) Long-term follow-up of the ileoanal anastomosis in children and young adults. *Surgery* 108: 717–723.

Telander RL (1993) Surgical management of inflammatory bowel disease in children. *Problems in General Surgery* 10: 136–146.

Tenore A, Berman WF, Parks JS et al (1977) Basal and stimulated growth hormone concentrations in inflammatory bowel disease. *Journal of Clinical Endocrinology and Metabolism* 44: 622–628.

Thomas DW, Sinatra FR & Merritt RJ (1983) Fecal a-1-antitrypsin excretion in young people with Crohn's disease. *Journal of Pediatric Gastroenterology and Nutrition* 2: 491–496.

Thomas AG, Taylor F & Miller V (1993) Dietary intake and nutritional treatment in childhood Crohn's disease. *Journal of Pediatric Gastroenterology and Nutrition* **17**: 75–81.

Toyoda H, Wang S-J, Yang H-Y et al (1993) Distinct associations of the HLA class II genes with inflammatory bowel disease. *Gastroenterology* **104**: 741–748.

Tripathi RC, Kipp MA, Tripathi BJ et al (1992) Ocular toxicity of prednisone in pediatric patients with inflammatory bowel disease. *Lens and Eye Toxicity Research* **9**: 469–482.

Ursing B, Alm T, Barany F et al (1982) A comparative study of metronidazole and sulfasalazine for active Crohn's disease: The cooperative Crohn's disease study in Sweden. II Result. *Gastroenterology* **83**: 550–562.

Verhave M, Winter HS & Grand RJ (1990) Azathioprine in the treatment of children with inflammatory bowel disease. *Journal of Pediatrics* **117**: 809–814.

Werlin SL & Grand RJ (1977) Severe colitis in children and adolescents: diagnosis, course, and treatment. *Gastroenterology* **73**: 828–832.

Wesson DE & Shandling B (1981) Results of bowel resection for Crohn's disease in the young. *Journal of Pediatric Surgery* **16**: 449–452.

Whitington PF, Barns HV & Bayless TM (1977) Medical management of Crohn's disease in adolescence. *Gastroenterlogy* **72**: 1338–1344.

Willoughby JMT, Rahman AFM & Gregory MM (1989) Chronic colitis after Aeromonas infection. *Gut* **30**: 686–690.

Yang H, Rotter JI, Toyoda H et al (1992): Ulcerative colitis: a genetic heterogeneous group defined with genetic (DR2) and subclinical markers (antineutrophilic cytoplasmic antibodies). *Gastroenterology* **102**: A716.

9

Gastro-oesophageal reflux: presentation, evaluation and management

EBERHARD SCHMIDT-SOMMERFELD

Gastro-oesophageal reflux (GOR) is the retrograde flow of gastric contents into the oesophagus due to relaxation of the lower oesophageal sphincter (LOS). It is a physiological phenomenon and occurs in normal individuals several times during the day particularly postprandially (Jolley et al, 1981;

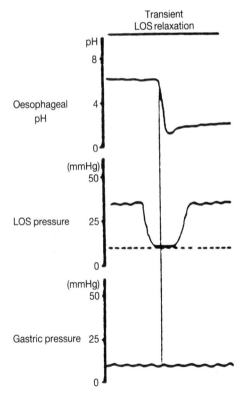

Figure 1. Gastro-oesophageal reflux (GOR) due to transient relaxation of the lower oesophageal sphincter (LOS; from Dodds et al, 1982). Reproduced with permission of *The New England Journal of Medicine* **307**: 1547, 1982).

Baillière's Clinical Paediatrics—
Vol. 2, No. 4, November 1994
ISBN 0–7020–1866–X

Kaye, 1977), but rarely at night during sleep. It is caused by spontaneous, transient relaxations of the LOS which occur without swallowing, without oesophageal body peristalsis and without increase in abdominal pressure (Figure 1). An excessively frequent rate of spontaneous LOS-relaxations is currently believed to be the most important abnormality underlying pathological reflux (Cucchiara et al, 1993). Following a reflux episode, a normal oesophagus rapidly clears more than 90% of the refluxate through peristalsis. The remaining acid on the oesophageal walls is neutralized by swallowed saliva (Figure 2). Both intact motility and flow of saliva prevent damage to the oesophageal mucosa from reflux.

Studies of large numbers of healthy infants by pH-monitoring suggest that normal infants may reflux more frequently and have longer acid-clearing time than normal older children or adults (Vandenplas et al, 1991b). Especially during the postprandial period, the reflux frequency may be higher in infancy compared with later in life. This is difficult to prove by pH-metry due to the buffering capacity of infant formulas (Vandenplas and Sacre, 1987).

Regurgitant reflux is much more common in healthy infants than in healthy older children or adults (Gryboski et al, 1963). This may be due to

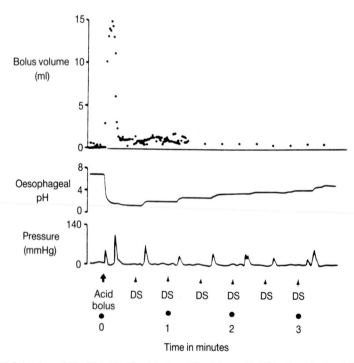

Figure 2. Injection of 15 ml labelled (technetium-99 sulphur colloid) hydrochloric acid into the oesophagus. All but about 1 ml of acid is cleared from the oesophagus (upper panel) by the first peristaltic contraction (lower panel) while the distal oesophageal pH (middle panel) remains unchanged. Then, the pH normalizes stepwise with subsequent dry swallows (DS, saliva; from Helm et al, 1984). Reproduced with permission of *The New England Journal of Medicine* **310:** 285, 1994.

the relatively smaller oesophageal capacity (1.2 versus 2.6 ml/kg body wt) and the larger volume of intake (150 versus 50 ml/kg body wt/day) of infants compared with adults. Infants have been shown to develop a circadian variation of GOR by about 6 weeks of age with less time spent below pH 4 during the nocturnal sleep period (Dreizzen et al, 1990), particularly during deep sleep (Jeffery and Heacock, 1991). The type of feeding may also influence physiological reflux. For example, healthy breast-fed neonates were found to have shorter reflux episodes than formula-fed infants (Heacock et al, 1992). This may be related to faster gastric emptying of breast milk.

CLINICAL MANIFESTATIONS OF GASTRO-OESOPHAGEAL REFLUX DISEASE (GORD)

Since GOR is physiological, pathological GOR or GORD needs to be defined clinically by history and/or investigation. Table 1 summarizes the clinical presentation of GORD.

Regurgitation

Regurgitation can be regarded as a symptom of GORD. However, its very common occurrence in otherwise healthy infants makes it a symptom of questionable pathologic significance and abnormal regurgitation in infancy has not been clearly defined clinically. For this reason, infants symptomatic with regurgitation but otherwise normal have been included in the description of pH-probe data from a large normal population of infants (Vandenplas et al, 1991b). On the other hand, although less frequent, excessive regurgitation may cause failure to thrive. If this occurs, the diagnosis of GORD should only be made after careful consideration of the differential

Table 1. Clinical presentation of GORD.

Excessive regurgitation
  Failure to thrive

Oesophagitis
  Infants
    Irritability with feedings
    Arching, 'colic'
    Haematemesis, anaemia
  Children
    Heartburn
    Chest or abdominal pain
    Dysphagia, odynophagia
    Haematemesis, anaemia
    Sandifer's syndrome

Respiratory disorders
  Aspiration pneumonia
  Bronchospasm (asthma)
  Laryngospasm (apnoea, stridor)
  Hoarseness

diagnosis which includes central nervous system disturbances, metabolic diseases, intestinal obstruction, allergy and malabsorption/maldigestion syndromes.

Oesophagitis

Oesophagitis is the central pathologic anatomic substrate of GORD. The degree of damage of the lower oesophagus is a function of the nature of the refluxate (acid, bile, pepsin, trypsin), the duration of exposure of the oesophageal mucosa to the refluxate, and the susceptibility of the mucosa to damage.

Histology

Reflux oesophagitis is defined by histological criteria (Figure 3). While polymorphonuclear and eosinophilic infiltration of the lamina propria and epithelium, and erosions and ulcerations are unequivocal morphological findings in oesophagitis, the pathological significance of the more subtle changes of increased basal cell layer thickness and elongation of vascular papillae (Ismail-Beigi et al, 1970) is controversial. Such changes have been found in the distal oesophagus of a large percentage of asymptomatic adult volunteers (Weinstein et al, 1975). It is unknown whether such mild changes are also found in asymptomatic children. It has been suggested that an increased papillary diameter, ingrowth of capillaries into the epithelium and extravasation of red cells into the epithelium may be more reliable histological signs of early reflux oesophagitis than basal cell layer thickness (Geboes et al, 1980). Thus, histological signs of oesophagitis should be evaluated critically to avoid overdiagnosis particularly in infants with non-specific symptoms.

Barrett's oesophagus

Columnar-lined epithelium in the oesophagus is of special clinical importance because of its malignant potential. Three types of metaplastic oesophageal mucosa have been described: fundic, cardiac (transitional) and specialized (villous; Speckler and Goyal, 1986). It has recently been suggested (Hassall, 1993) that the diagnosis of Barrett's oesophagus should only be made if goblet cell containing specialized epithelium is present. This is the only epithelium known to have malignant potential. Cardiac mucosa which is normally present in the distal 3 cm of the oesophagus may be a precursor of Barrett's oesophagus if it is found more proximally. Fundic mucosa found above the diaphragm is thought to originate in a hiatus hernia in most instances. Since most patients with Barrett's oesophagus also have a hiatus hernia, multiple biopsies at different levels of the oesophagus with careful documentation of the histological map are essential for the correct diagnosis. The youngest patient with unequivocal Barrett's oesophagus (goblet cell metaplasia) was 5 years old (Qualman et al, 1990). Ten paediatric patients (age 11–25 years) were reported to have developed adenocarcinoma of the oesophagus (Hassall et al, 1993). Complete regression of

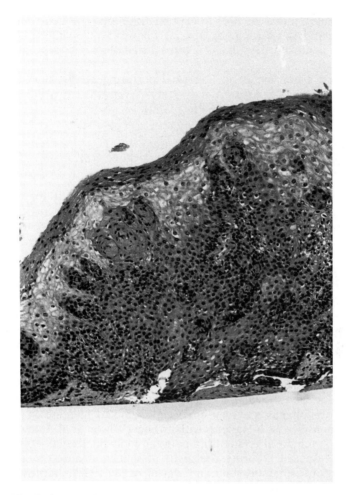

Figure 3. Histological oesophagitis: increased basal cell layer thickness, elongation of vascular papillae with increased diameter and dilated capillaries (courtesy of Dr Barbara Kirschner).

Barrett's oesophagus has never been convincingly documented, but partial regression following anti-reflux surgery has been described (Hassall and Weinstein, 1992).

Symptoms

Haematemesis and anaemia are symptoms of severe oesophagitis and occur in all age groups. Other symptoms in infants are less specific and difficult to differentiate from such common problems as 'colic', sleeplessness, irritability, and severe parental anxiety. However, an infant that becomes irritable soon after the initiation of feeding is more likely to have oesophagitis.

Older children may be able to express symptoms like heart burn, chest pain, difficulty swallowing (dysphagia) or pain with swallowing (odynophagia) as adults do. Dysphagia is often a sign of an oesophageal stricture due to GORD.

Sandifer's syndrome is an abnormal posturing of the head and neck following a period of paroxysmal dystonic movements (torticollis, opisthotonus) due to oesophagitis (Sutcliffe, 1969).

Respiratory disorders

Aspiration

Aspiration of gastric content during GOR may cause respiratory disease if protecting mechanisms like swallow reflex, cord closure or arytenoid–epiglottic approximation fail. This is particularly common in neurologically impaired and severely retarded patients (Sondheimer and Morris, 1979) and in those with depressed consciousness (Huxley et al, 1978). Patients with repaired oesophageal atresia (Parker et al, 1979), bronchopulmonary dysplasia (BPD; Hrabovsky and Mullet, 1986) and asthma have also been considered high risk for recurrent aspiration pneumonia. However, inhalation of gastric contents during GOR is difficult to distinguish from neural-mediated reflex bronchospasm. Studies of patients with reflux-related respiratory symptoms may have overestimated aspiration as the only cause.

Asthma

There is now good evidence that reflux of acidic gastric content into an inflamed oesophagus may cause a vagal-mediated increase in bronchial hyper-responsiveness in patients with asthma (Wilson et al, 1985; Herve et al, 1986). A temporal relationship between individual reflux episodes and wheezing, especially during the night, has been demonstrated by pH-monitoring in asthmatic children (Martin et al, 1982). Improvement of bronchospastic symptoms following anti-reflux therapy has been documented (Berquist et al, 1981). This improvement was most pronounced when GORD was most severe (Gustafsson et al, 1992). Moreover, acid but not saline infusion into the oesophagus (modified Bernstein test) may cause bronchoconstriction in asthmatic patients, particularly if oesophagitis is present.

Chest pain in children with asthma has also been related to GORD with oesophagitis.

Apnoea

The relationship between GOR and life-threatening events, such as obstructive or central apnoea, is a much debated issue (Byrne, 1989). Herbst et al (1979) have demonstrated a temporal relationship between reflux and obstructive apnoea in former premature infants with BPD using pH-monitoring, a nasal thermistor and thoracic impedance (Figure 4). An

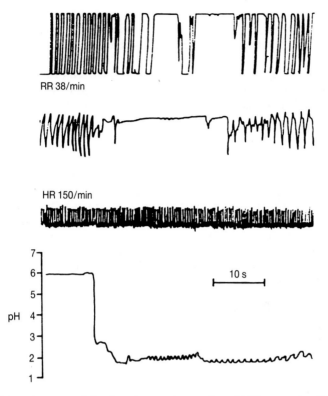

RR 38/min

HR 150/min

Figure 4. Obstructive apnoea following a decrease in oesophageal pH in premature infants with bronchopulmonary dysplasia. From top to bottom: impedance pneumotachogram, nasal thermistor measuring airflow, electrocardiogram, oesophageal pH. Reproduced with permission from Herbst et al (1979).

apnoea episode could be elicited by acid infusion into the oesophagus. Spitzer et al (1984) described a specific syndrome of postprandial, obstructive apnoea with staring or startled expression, rigid posturing followed by hypotonia, plethora, cyanosis or pallor, absence of tonic–clonic movements and absence of coughing, gagging or choking in 15 full-term infants. In most of these infants, a temporal relationship between obstructive apnoea and GOR could be demonstrated. Central apnoea was not found. Regurgitation of stomach contents, which has also been associated with obstructive apnoea, was only seen in a minority of cases.

A systematic study of a large number of infants evaluated for apnoea did not reveal a higher incidence of central or obstructive apnoeic episodes during GOR periods compared with periods without GOR (Walsh et al, 1981). However, brief episodes of obstructive apnoea occurred frequently at the onset of GOR suggesting that GOR may trigger obstructive apnoea. A recent study of former premature infants could not demonstrate a temporal relationship between acid reflux and obstructive or mixed apnoeas during wakefulness or sleep (Ajuriaguerra et al, 1991).

In conclusion, a relationship between GOR and obstructive apnoea has clearly been demonstrated in a number of infants. However, such phenomenon may be difficult to prove and its incidence is unknown. In contrast to obstructive apnoea, central apnoea is generally not related to GOR (Ariango et al, 1982; Kahn et al, 1992) although 'respiratory dysfunction' with repeated irregular short apnoeic episodes (less than 15 s) has been observed with GOR in term as well as preterm infants (Vandenplas et al, 1989b).

Hoarseness

Hoarseness, a well-described symptom of GOR in adults, has recently been described in an 8-year-old girl with reflux oesophagitis (Putnam and Orenstein, 1992). The symptom resolved with anti-reflux therapy. Fibreoptic examination of the upper airway may demonstrate erythema and/or oedema of the posterior larynx (reflux laryngitis).

EVALUATION OF GORD

There is no uniform test to diagnose GORD. The type of evaluation depends entirely on the question being asked by the clinician (Table 2). The diagnosis of reflux with regurgitation as the leading symptom is made clinically and does not require specialized evaluation. However, if regurgitation is associated with other symptoms, such as bilious vomiting (duodenal stenosis, malrotation) electrolyte imbalance (pyloric stenosis), acidosis (metabolic disease), lack of weight gain (gastric outlet obstruction, cystic fibrosis), signs of oesophagitis (Table 1), or respiratory symptoms (Table 1), then further investigation is needed.

Barium study

A barium examination of the upper gastrointestinal tract is not helpful in the diagnosis of GORD except in the case of an extremely decreased LOS

Table 2. Evaluation for GORD.

Question to ask	Test performed
Are there structural abnormalities in the upper GI-tract?	Upper GI barium study, ultrasound
Is there a delay in gastric emptying?	Scintigram, ultrasound
Does aspiration occur?	Chest X-ray, scintigram, barium swallow, bronchoscopy
Is oesophagitis (Barrett's oesophagus) present?	Endoscopy and biopsy
Are specific symptoms causally related to GOR?	pH-monitoring, Bernstein test
Is a hiatus hernia present?	Barium swallow, endoscopy
Is the quantity of acid GOR abnormal?	pH-monitoring
Is there a motility disorder?	Barium swallow, manometry

pressure. This is because (a) postprandial reflux is physiological; (b) barium is an unphysiological substance, and (c) the time of observation is limited. However, barium studies are indispensable in detecting structural abnormalities of the upper gastrointestinal tract or motility disorders of the oesophagus, e.g. achalasia.

Manometry

Oesophageal motility disorders are best diagnosed by manometry. Manometry has also been used for studying the mechanisms of GORD, but is not useful clinically unless LOS pressures are permanently very low (below 5 mm/Hg) as may be the case in severe oesophagitis or in neurologically impaired children.

Ultrasound

Ultrasound techniques have been used for the detection of GOR. As the barium study, ultrasound examination is limited to a short period of time after feeding, but it will detect postprandial reflux under more physiological conditions. Recently, ultrasound has also been used to measure gastric emptying time (Carroccio et al, 1992).

Scintigraphy

Scintigraphy using meals labelled with technetium-99 sulphur colloid can monitor GOR over a period of 1 h following ingestion. It has the advantage that the rate of gastric emptying can be measured at the same time and aspiration of labelled material can be detected in delayed images of the lungs. However, scintigraphy is rather insensitive in detecting aspiration.

Biopsy

The diagnosis of oesophagitis can only be made by oesophageal biopsy with or without endoscopy. Blind oesophageal suction biopsy may provide a larger specimen for more reliable histological evaluation than endoscopic grasp biopsy (Whitington and Orenstein, 1984). However, combined endoscopy and biopsy is the preferable approach because inspection of the oesophageal, gastric, and duodenal mucosa provides important additional information. The extent and severity (erythema, friability, erosions, ulcerations, stricture) of oesophagitis can be evaluated. This is particularly helpful if histological findings are equivocal (see above under Oesophagitis). In addition, infectious oesophagitis, gastritis or peptic ulcers can be differentiated from reflux oesophagitis. As mentioned earlier, the diagnosis of oesophageal metaplasia requires careful histological mapping and avoidance of taking biopsies from a hiatus hernia. This is only possible if biopsies are taken under direct vision.

Acid perfusion

Oesophageal acid perfusion (Bernstein test) is a well-established method used in adults to investigate whether oesophagitis is the cause of chest pain. It may also be used in children to investigate whether reflux is related to other symptoms such as stridor, bronchospasm or laryngospasm. Despite its potential, this test has not been widely publicized for clinical use in paediatrics.

Twenty-four hour pH-monitoring

Twenty-four hour pH-monitoring enables quantitative measurement of exposure of the distal oesophageal mucosa to acid over a 24 h period. It is only an indirect measure of GOR. It does not register non-acid reflux and does not yield information about the volume of the refluxate. Comparison of reflux tests, such as barium swallow, scintigraphy or ultrasound, with pH-monitoring are not meaningful since these tests evaluate different components of reflux (postprandial versus inbetween meals; Shay et al, 1991; Vandenplas et al, 1992). Moreover, correlation of 24 h pH-monitoring with histological oesophagitis is relatively poor (Black et al, 1990). This is not surprising since (a) components of the refluxate other than acid (e.g. bile, pepsin, trypsin) cause damage of the oesophagus; and (b) individual patients may have a different mucosal resistance to acid exposure. It follows that pH-monitoring cannot be regarded as the 'gold standard' of GORD evaluation in paediatrics as has often been suggested. However, pH-monitoring has produced a wealth of physiological and clinical information. Its main advantages are that it yields information over an extended period of time and that symptoms of oesophagitis or respiratory events can be linked

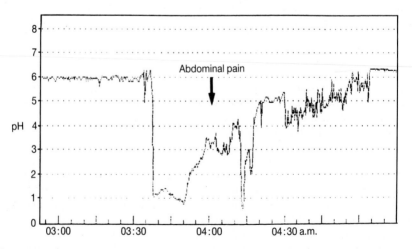

Figure 5. Oesophageal pH-tracing of a 9 year old white male with reflux oesophagitis: The patient wakes up at 4 a.m. following a prolonged reflux episode and complains of abdominal pain.

temporally to reflux episodes. Monitoring over a 24 h period makes it possible to differentiate acid reflux occurring during the day (while awake) from that occurring during the night (while asleep). GOR during sleep may be of greater clinical significance since it is associated with a longer acid-clearance time (Figure 5; Sondheimer, 1989). In addition, positional therapy and the effect of medications on GORD can be evaluated using pH-monitoring.

Quantification

For the quantification of acid reflux by pH-monitoring, the availability of normal data is crucial (Table 3). Traditionally, the following parameters are

Table 3. Normal values for 24 h pH-monitoring.

	Infants < 1 year old* ($n = 509$)	Adults† ($n = 42$)
Time pH < 4 (%)	< 10 (4)	< 7 (2.6)
Episodes/24 h	< 72 (27)	—
Episodes > 5 min/24 h	< 9 (3)	< 2 (0)
Longest episode (min)	< 41 (12)	< 12 (4.5)

* From Vandenplas et al (1991b): numbers represent the 95th and (50th) percentiles.
† From Schindlbeck et al (1987): numbers represent the 'optimal threshold' (value that yields optimal sensitivity and specificity) and (median) values.

used to quantify acid reflux: number of episodes per 24 h; percent time with pH below 4; number of episodes longer than 5 min; and time of longest episode. The latter two parameters are a reflection of the ability of the oesophagus to clear acid. The percent time spent with pH below 4 is a function of both number of episodes and acid clearance. The area under the pH 4 curve is used less but also takes into account the degree of acidity and may predict oesophagitis more accurately (Vandenplas et al, 1989a).

If pH-monitoring is used to quantify acid GOR, the following confounding factors, unique in the paediatric age group, must be considered: age, type and frequency of feeding, and sleep/awake proportion.

Age-related normal data

Meaningful interpretation of pH-monitoring requires the availability of normal age-related data. Ideally, every pH-monitoring laboratory should establish its own age-related normal values in order to correct for technical differences of the procedure. (One of the most important technical details is the site of the probe in the oesophagus; Sondheimer and Haase, 1988.) However, unlike in adulthood where volunteers can be studied, ethical considerations prohibit invasive tests in healthy children. Therefore, in many studies involving children, control groups are either small or infants and older children are not separated (Euler and Byrne, 1981), or differentiation between abnormal and normal is made retrospectively on the basis of pH-monitoring results. The latter approach is unlikely to produce normal data representative of a general population of children. Fortunately, a large number of healthy thriving infants has been studied in Belgium as part of a screening programme for sudden infant death syndrome (Vandenplas et al, 1991b). Regurgitation was considered normal, but treatment for GOR was a criteria for exclusion from the study. It was found that pH-data were not normally distributed and therefore, percentiles for the reflux parameters (instead of mean and sd) were established (Table 3). The 95th percentile of the percent time spent below pH 4 fluctuated between 13, at 1 month old, and 8 at the end of the first year of life. It is believed that beyond the first year of life through childhood, reflux parameters shift toward adult values (Table 3). However, further true normal data are needed for age groups older than 1 year.

Feedings

The type and frequency of feedings influences pH-probe results. It has been shown that gastric acid is partially neutralized by infant formula for up to 2 h after feeding (Vandenplas and Sacre, 1987). This makes the detection of postprandial acid reflux difficult in this age group. Therefore, apple juice, clear liquids or acidified formulas have been used to demonstrate postprandial reflux. However, such feeding regimens are unphysiological for the infant and may be emptied differently from the stomach than regular formulas. In addition, postprandial reflux can be regarded as a physiological phenomenon in most infants and its evaluation may be of limited clinical significance. The pH-monitoring results may be obscured if children are continuously fed a formula during the study which neutralizes gastric acid. Therefore, it is advisable in this situation to switch to bolus feeding for the purpose of the study. Intervals between feedings should be at least 3 h in order to be able to detect acid reflux between feedings.

Sleep–awake rhythm

An additional variable to be considered in interpreting pH-data is the sleep–awake rhythm. In healthy newborn infants, the number of reflux episodes is highest in wakefulness, lower in active sleep and rare in quiet sleep. On the other hand, reflux episodes are longest during active sleep (Jeffery and Heacock, 1991). In addition, 'drift onset' reflux episodes with a gradual decrease in pH have been observed during sleep (Sondheimer and Hoddes, 1992). The clinical significance of this reflux phenomenon is unknown. More research is needed to establish the importance of different reflux patterns during wakefulness and sleep in the evaluation of pathological reflux in children.

Symptoms related to GOR

Although quantification of GOR by pH-monitoring may be useful, simply defining a patient as having pathological reflux does not mean that such reflux is causative of the symptoms that led to the evaluation. Therefore, the most important indication for pH-monitoring is the association of reflux episodes with symptoms like coughing, sneezing, wheezing, apnoea, irritability, chest or abdominal pain (Figure 5), heartburn and vomiting. Careful recording of these symptoms, preferably by a parent, is essential. A device built into the system that can be pressed to mark an event is helpful. Exact recording of the time of the event and of the termination of the study is crucial in evaluating temporal relationships between GOR and symptoms. For documentation of obstructive apnoea related to GOR, pneumocardiographic data including those from a nasal thermistor must be temporally linked to pH-monitoring (Figure 4).

Alkaline reflux

Reflux of alkaline gastroduodenal material may cause damage to the oesophagus due to the presence of bile acids and pancreatic enzymes (Lillemoe et al, 1983). Little information on alkaline reflux in children is available. Alkaline reflux may be responsible for oesophagitis found in a subgroup of patients exhibiting a 'normal' pH-study (Malthaner et al, 1991). The diagnosis of alkaline reflux has been made through evaluation of episodes of pH above 7 in the oesophagus (Vandenplas and Loeb, 1991). The diagnosis may be more reliable if oesophageal and gastric pH are monitored at the same time (Angulo et al, 1992). However, the clinical usefulness of this approach has not been established.

MANAGEMENT

In the majority of infants who regurgitate excessively without other associated symptoms, abnormal GOR can be diagnosed on the basis of the history and a therapeutic trial of conservative management, with or without a prokinetic drug (Table 4). In the postprandial period, infants should be either held upright or placed prone. The sitting position should be avoided. Elevation of the head of the bed for infants in the prone position, which requires a harness, has not been proven to be effective (Orenstein, 1990). Therefore, such restriction does not appear to be justified. If oesophagitis is suspected, specific evaluation (Table 2) which can help to determine the indication for acid-reducing therapy is desirable. Most infants with abnormal reflux will out-grow their problems by 1–2 years of age. Surgical intervention is rarely needed before age 2 except in severely neurologically-impaired patients.

Prokinetic drugs

Prokinetic agents generally raise basal LOS-pressure, improve oesophageal clearance and speed gastric emptying. Metoclopramide, a dopamine antagonist, is used by many paediatric gastroenterologists as the initial

Table 4. Management of GORD.

Conservative
Infants
Postprandial position: prone, upright
Thickening of formula (1 tbsp dry rice cereal per 1–2 oz)
Older children
Fasting before bedtime
Head of bed elevated
Weight loss (if obese)
Avoid carbonated drinks, caffeine, alcohol, smoking, tomato
products, chocolate
Pharmacologic
Prokinetic
Metoclopramide (0.1–0.15 mg/kg/dose q.i.d. 30 min before
meals and at bedtime)
Bethanechol (0.1–0.3 mg/kg/dose t.i.d.)
Cisapride (0.3 mg/kg/dose t.i.d.)
Acid-reducing
Cimetidine (5–10 mg/kg/dose q.i.d.)*
Ranitidine (1–2 mg/kg/dose t.i.d.)
Omeprazole†
Antacids (0.5–1.0 ml/kg/dose—maximum 30 ml—after meals
and at bedtime)
Sucralfate slurry (infants: 0.1–0.2 g; children: 0.5–1 g q.i.d. after
meals and at bedtime)
Surgical
Nissen fundoplication

* Inhibits hepatic metabolism of diphenylhydantoin and theophylline
(blood levels must be monitored).
† Dosage not established in children.

agent. However, the margin between effective dose and undesirable side effects is narrow. Parents should be informed about the possible occurrence of extrapyramidal symptoms in which case the drug should be discontinued.

Bethanechol, a cholinergic drug, was the first prokinetic agent used in children (Moroz et al, 1976). However, it may exacerbate bronchospasm and therefore should not be used in children who have respiratory disease.

Cisapride, a new agent which releases acetylcholine from postganglionic nerve endings of the myenteric plexus, has been shown to be effective in children. It improves clinical symptoms of GOR, histological oesophagitis, gastric emptying and all pH-parameters except the number of reflux episodes (Cucchiara et al, 1990; Vandenplas et al, 1991a; Iacono et al, 1992). Due to its reported minimal side effects, it holds promise to become the drug of choice for the treatment of GORD in children.

Acid reduction

Therapy of oesophagitis with H2-blockers is well established (e.g. cimetidine and ranitidine). Antacid preparations in small frequent doses provide short-term relief. Sucralfate, a synthetic carbohydrate is absorbed to inflamed tissue thus decreasing mucosal contact with gastric acid and promoting healing of oesophagitis. Omeprazole, a new agent that blocks the proton pump of the parietal cell, has been recently administered to 15 children with refractory severe oesophagitis (Gunasekaran and Hassall, 1993). All patients had hiatus hernia or repaired oesophageal atresia. Most of them were neurologically handicapped and two had metaplasia. The dosage ranged from 0.7 to 3.3 mg/kg/day and was titrated upward according to pH-monitoring results. All patients showed improvement of symptoms and oesophagitis diminished in most cases. Mildly elevated serum transaminases and elevated fasting gastrin levels were common. The observed hypergastrinaemia is of concern in long-term treatment with omeprazole because of the potential formation of carcinoid in the stomach.

Surgery

The most commonly used surgical approach to GORD is the Nissen fundoplication. It is required if medical therapy fails. Since infants will usually outgrow their reflux problem, surgery is rarely necessary in this age group. It is limited to those with severe neurological impairment (Byrne et al, 1982), peptic stricture, and repaired oesophageal atresia (Ashcraft et al, 1977). Some infants with BPD may also benefit from anti-reflux surgery (Giuffre et al, 1987). In older children without neurological or oesophageal anatomic abnormalities, GORD with oesophagitis tends to relapse after discontinuation of medical therapy (Treem et al, 1991). In these cases, risks and benefits of surgery need to be weighed against those of long-term medical treatment. Surgery should be considered particularly in cases of unequivocal Barrett's oesophagus (see under Oesophagitis).

Gastrostomy and fundoplication

Neurologically handicapped children frequently require anti-reflux surgery. They also frequently require a gastrostomy tube for feeding purposes. Whether gastrostomy placement should always be combined with an anti-reflux procedure in this patient population has been debated. Proponents of such an approach have argued that the incidence of GORD is high and may even increase following gastrostomy placement (Berezin et al, 1986). On the other hand, the complication rate of anti-reflux surgery is considerably increased in neurologically impaired children (Byrne et al, 1982). Therefore, it was proposed that placement of a percutaneous endoscopic gastrostomy (PEG) for feeding purposes, with subsequent addition of an anti-reflux procedure if necessary, is a reasonable approach (Byrne, 1990). We currently evaluate all candidates for a PEG for GORD using 24 h pH-monitoring. If reflux is excessive or if respiratory symptoms are obviously related to GOR, we prefer a combined anti-reflux procedure and gastrostomy placement. Laparoscopic Nissen fundoplication has recently been performed in children (Lobe et al, 1993). It remains to be seen whether this approach will have an impact on the indications for anti-reflux procedures in neurologically handicapped children.

Complications

Although surgical success rates are remarkable, both short- and long-term complications following anti-reflux surgery are common. Long-term problems include gas bloating, inability to burp or vomit, delayed gastric emptying, and dysphagia (Harnsberger et al, 1983). Dumping syndrome after anti-reflux surgery is probably underdiagnosed (Caulfield et al, 1987). It should be suspected in children with postprandial irritability and diarrhoea. The diagnosis is made by scintigraphic demonstration of rapid initial gastric emptying and an abnormal oral glucose tolerance test. Dietary manipulation with reduction of disaccharides and addition of uncooked corn starch and long chain triglycerides to the formula is rewarding (Khoshoo et al, 1991).

SUMMARY

Gastro-oesophageal reflux (GOR) is a physiological phenomenon. Normal infants reflux more frequently and have a longer acid-clearing time than normal older children or adults.

GOR disease (GORD) presents as excess regurgitation, oesophagitis or respiratory disease. In infants with regurgitant reflux and failure to thrive, the diagnosis of GORD should only be made after careful consideration of the differential diagnosis which includes central nervous system disturbances, metabolic diseases, intestinal obstruction, allergy and malabsorption/maldigestion syndromes. Oesophagitis is defined histologically, but the pathological significance of the subtle changes of increased basal cell layer thickness and elongation of vascular papillae is controversial. Columnar lined epithelium in the oesophagus is of special clinical importance because of its malignant potential. The diagnosis of Barrett's oesophagus should only be made if goblet cell containing specialized epithelium is present. Acid reflux into an inflamed oesophagus may cause a vagal-mediated increase in bronchial hyperresponsiveness in patients with asthma. A relationship between GOR and obstructive apnoea has clearly been demonstrated. However, such phenomenon may be difficult to prove and its incidence is unknown. Central apnoea is generally not related to GOR.

There is no uniform test to diagnose GORD and the type of evaluation depends entirely on the question being asked by the clinician. Barium studies are indispensable in detecting structural abnormalities of the upper gastrointestinal tract. Combined endoscopy and biopsy is the preferable approach to diagnose oesophagitis. Twenty-four hour pH-monitoring enables quantitative measurement of exposure of the distal oesophagus to acid. The availability of normal data is crucial for interpretation. Confounding factors like age and type and frequency of feeding must be considered. Establishing temporal relationships between GOR and symptoms is the main indication for pH-monitoring.

Management of GORD consists of conservative measures, prokinetic and acid-reducing drugs and surgery. Cisapride may become the prokinetic drug of choice for the treatment of GORD. Omeprazole has been used successfully as an acid-reducing drug in children. Nissen fundoplication is required if medical therapy fails but is rarely necessary in children less than 2 years of age. Neurologically handicapped children requiring a feeding gastrostomy should be evaluated for GORD to assess whether a simultaneous anti-reflux procedure is indicated.

REFERENCES

Ajuriaguerra M, Radvanyi-Bouvet M, Muon C & Moriette G (1991) Gastroesophageal reflux and apnea in prematurely born infantas during wakefulness and sleep. *American Journal of Diseases of Children* **145:** 1132–1136.

Angulo JM, Gorostiaga L & Tovar JA (1992) 24-hour simultaneous esophagogastric pH-metry in children. *Cir Pediatrics* **5:** 160–165.

Ariango RL, Guilleminault C, Baldwin R et al (1982) Movement and gastroesophageal reflux in awake term infants with 'near miss' SIDS, unrelated to apnea. *Journal of Pediatrics* **100:** 894–897.

Ashcraft KW, Goodwin C, Amoury RA et al (1977) Early recognition and aggressive treatment of gastroesophageal reflux following repair of esophageal atresia. *Journal of Pediatric Surgery* **12:** 317–321.

Berezin S, Schwarz SM & Newman LJ (1986) Gastroesophageal reflux secondary to gastrostomy tube placement. *American Journal of Diseases of Children* **140:** 699–701.

Berquist WE, Rachelefsky GS, Kadden M et al (1981) Gastroesophageal reflux-associated recurrent pneumonia and chronic asthma in children. *Pediatrics* **68:** 29–35.

Black DD, Haggitt RC, Orenstein SR et al (1990) Esophagitis in infants: morphometric histologic diagnosis and correlation with measures of gastroesophageal reflux. *Gastroenterology* **98:** 1408–1414.

Byrne WJ (1989) Reflux and related phenomena. *Journal of Pediatric Gastroenterology and Nutrition* **8:** 283–285.

Byrne WJ (1990) A reevaluation of the role of anti-reflux procedures in severely neurologically handicapped children requiring a gastrostomy for feeding (letter). *Journal of Pediatric Gastroenterology and Nutrition* **11:** 141–144.

Byrne WJ, Euler AR, Ashcraft E et al (1982) Gastroesophageal reflux in the severely retarded who vomit: Criteria for and results of surgical intervention in twenty-two patients. *Surgery* **81:** 95–98.

Carroccio A, Jacono G, Li Voti G et al (1992) Gastric emptying in infants with gastroesophageal reflux. *Scandinavian Journal of Gastroenterology* **27:** 799–804.

Caulfield, ME, Wyllie R, Firor MV & Michener W (1987) Dumping syndrome in children. *Journal of Pediatrics* **110:** 212–215.

Cucchiara S, Staiaho A, Boccieri A et al (1990) Effects of cisapride on parameters of oesophageal motility and on the prolonged intraesophageal pH test in infants with gastroesophageal reflux disease *Gut* **31:** 21–25.

Cucchiara S, Bortolotti M, Minella R & Auricchio S (1993) Fasting and postprandial mechanism of gastroesophageal reflux in children with gastroesophageal reflux disease. *Digestive Disease and Science* **38:** 86–92.

Dodds WJ, Dent J, Hogan WJ et al (1982) Mechanisms of gastroesophageal reflux in patients with reflux esophagitis. *New England Journal of Medicine* **307:** 1547–1552.

Dreizzen E, Escourrou P, Odievre M et al (1990) Esophageal reflux in symptomatic and asymptomatic infants; Postprandial and circadian variations. *Journal of Pediatric Gastroenterology and Nutrition* **10:** 316–321.

Euler AR & Byren WY (1981) Twenty-four hours esophageal intraluminal pH probe testing. A comparative analysis. *Gastroenterology* **80:** 959–963.

Geboes K, Desmet V, Vantrappen G et al (1980) Vascular changes in the esophageal mucosa—an early histologic sign of esophagitis. *Gastrointestinal Endocopy* **26:** 29–32.

Giuffre RM, Rubin S & Mitchell I (1987) Anti-reflux surgery in infants with bronchopulmonary dysplasia. *American Journal of Diseases of Children* **141:** 648–651.

Gryboski JD, Thayer WR & Spiro HM (1963) Esophageal motility in infants and children. *Pediatrics* **31:** 382–395.

Gunasekaran TS & Hassall EG (1993) Efficacy and safety of omeprazole for severe gastroesophageal reflux in children. *Journal of Pediatrics* **123:** 148–154.

Gustafsson PM, Kjellman NI & Tibbling L (1992) A trial of ranitidine in asthmatic children and adolescents with or without pathological gastro-oesophageal reflux. *European Respiratory Journal* **5:** 201–206.

Harnsberger JK, Corey JJ, Johnson DJ et al (1983) Long-term follow-up of surgery for gastroesophageal reflux in infants and children. *Journal of Pediatrics* **102:** 505–508.

Hassall E (1993) Barrett's esophagus: new definitions and approaches in children. *Journal of Pediatric Gastroenterology and Nutrition* **16:** 345–364.

Hassall E & Weinstein WM (1992) Partial regression of childhood Barrett's esophagus after fundoplication. *American Journal of Gastroenterology* **87:** 1506–1512.

Hassall E, Dimmick JE & Magee JF (1993) Adenocarcinoma in childhood Barrett's esophagus. Case documentation and the need of surveillance in children. *American Journal of Gastroenterology* **88:** 282–288.

Heacock HJ, Jeffery HE, Baker JL & Page M (1992) Influence of breast versus formula milk on physiological gastroesophageal reflux in healthy, newborn infants. *Journal of Pediatric Gastroenterology and Nutrition* **14:** 41–46.

Helm JF, Dodds WJ, Pelc LR et al (1984) Effect of esophageal emptying and saliva on clearance of acid from the esophagus. *New England Journal of Medicine* **310:** 284–288.

Herbst JJ, Minton SD & Book LS (1979) Gastroesophageal reflux causing respiratory distress and apnea in newborn infants. *Journal of Pediatrics* **95:** 763–768.

Herve O, Denjean A, Juan R et al (1986) Intraesophageal perfusion of acid increases the bronchomotor response to methacholine and to isocapnic hyperventilation in asthmatic subjects. *American Review of Respiratory Disease* **134:** 986–989.

Hrabovsky EE & Mullett MD (1986) Gastroesophageal reflux and the premature infant. *Journal of Pediatric Surgery* **21:** 583–587.

Huxley EJ, Viroslav J, Gray WR et al (1978) Pharyngeal aspiration in normal adults and patients with depressed consciousness. *American Journal of Medicine* **64:** 564–568.

Iacono G, Carroccio A, Montalto G et al (1992) Evaluation of the effectiveness of cisapride in the treatment of gastroesophageal reflux. *Minerva Pediatrics* **44:** 613–616.

Ismail-Beigi F, Morton PF & Pope CE (1970) Histologic consequences of gastroesophageal reflux in man. *Gastroenterology* **58:** 163–174.

Jeffery HE & Heacock HJ (1991) Impact of sleep and movement on gastroesophageal reflux in healthy, newborn infants *Archives of Disease in Childhood* **66:** 1136–1139.

Jolley SG, Herbst JJ, Johnson DJ et al (1981) Postcibal gastroesophageal reflux in children. *Journal of Pediatric Surgery* **16:** 487–490.

Kahn A, Rebuffat E, Sottiaux M et al (1992) Lack of temporal relation between acid reflux in the proximal esophagus and cardiorespiratory events in sleeping infants. *European Journal of Pediatrics* **151:** 208–212.

Kaye MD (1977) Postprandial gastroesophageal reflux in healthy people. *Gut* 18: 709–712.

Khoshoo V, Reifen RM, Gold BD et al (1991) Nutrional manipulation in the management of dumping syndrome. *Archives of Disease in Childhood* **66:** 1447–1448.

Lillemoe KD, Johnson LF & Harmon JW (1983) Alkaline esophagitis: A comparison of the ability of components of gastroduodenal contents to injure the rabbit esophagus. *Gastroenterology* **85:** 621–628.

Lobe, TE, Schropp KP & Lunsford K (1993) Laparoscopic Nissen fundoplication in childhood. *Journal of Pediatric Surgery* **28:** 358–360.

Malthaner RA, Newman KD, Parry R et al (1991) Alkaline gastroesophageal reflux in infants and children. *Journal of Pediatric Surgery* **26:** 986–990.

Martin ME, Grunstein MM & Larsen GL (1982) The relationship of gastroesophageal reflux to nocturnal wheezing in children with asthma. *Annals of Allergy* **49:** 318–322.

Moroz SP, Espinoza J, Cumming WA et al (1976) Lower esophageal sphincter function in children with and without gastroesophageal reflux. *Gastroenterology* **71:** 236–241.

Orenstein SR (1990) Prone positioning in infant gastroesophageal reflux: Is elevation of the head worth the trouble? *Journal of Pediatrics* **117:** 184–187.

Parker AF, Christie DL & Cahill JL (1979) Incidence and significance of gastroesophageal reflux following repair of esophageal atresia and tracheoesophageal fistula and the need for anti-reflux procedures. *Journal of Pediatric Surgery* **14:** 5–8.

Putnam PE & Orenstein SR (1992) Hoarseness in a child with gastroesophageal reflux. *Acta Pediatrica* **81:** 635–636.

Qualman SJ, Murray RD, McClung J & Lucas J (1990) Intestinal metaplasia is age related in Barrett's esophagus. *Archives of Pathological and Laboratory Medicine* **114:** 1236–1240.

Schindlbeck NE, Heinrich C, König A et al (1987) Optimal thresholds, sensitivity, and specificity of long-term PH-metry for the detection of gastro-oesophageal reflux disease. *Gastroenterology* **93:** 85–90.

Shay SS, Eggli D & Johnson LF (1991) Simultaneous esophageal pH monitoring and scintigraphy during the postprandial period in patients with severe reflux esophagitis. *Digestive Disease and Science* **36:** 558–564.

Sondheimer JM (1989) Clearance of spontaneous gastroesophageal reflux in awake and sleeping infants. *Gastroenterology* **97:** 821–826.

Sondheimer JM & Morris BA (1979) Gastroesophageal reflux among severely retarded children. *Journal of Pediatrics* **94:** 710–714.

Sondheimer JM & Haase GM (1988) Simultaneous pH recordings from multiple esophageal sites in children with and without distal gastroesophageal reflux. *Journal of Pediatric Gastroenterology and Nutrition* **7:** 46–51.

Sondheimer JM & Hoddes E (1992) Gastroesophageal reflux with drifting onset in infants: a phenomenon unique to sleep. *Journal of Pediatric Gastroenterology and Nutrition* **15:** 418–425.

Speckler SJ & Goyal RK (1986) Barrett's esophagus. *New England Journal of Medicine* **315:** 361–371.

Spitzer AR, Boyle JT, Tuchman DN et al (1984) Awake apnea associated with gastro-esophageal reflux: a specific clinical syndrome. *Journal of Pediatrics* **104:** 200–205.

Sutcliffe J (1969) Torsion spasms and abnormal posture in children with hiatus hernia. Sandifer's syndrome. *Progressive Pediatric Radiology* **2:** 190–197.

Treem WR, Davis PM & Hyamas JS (1991) Gastroesophageal reflux in the older child: Presentation, response to treatment and long-term follow-up. *Clinica Pediatrics (Phila)* **30:** 435–440.

Vandenplas Y & Sacre L (1987) Continuous 24-hour esophageal pH monitoring in 285 asymptomatic infants 0–15 months old. *Journal of Pediatric Gastroenterology and Nutrition* **6:** 220–224.

Vandenplas Y & Loeb H (1991) Alkaline gastroesophageal reflux in infancy. *Journal of Pediatric Gastroenterology and Nutrition* **12:** 448–452.

Vandenplas Y, Franckx-Goossens A, Pipeleers-Marichal M et al (1989a) Area under pH4: Advantages of a new parameter in the interpretation of esophageal pH monitoring data in infants. *Journal of Pediatric Gastroenterology and Nutrition* **9:** 34–39.

Vandenplas Y, Deneyer M, Verlinden M et al (1989b) Gastroesophageal reflux incidence and respiratory dysfunction during sleep in infants: Treatment with Cisapride. *Journal of Pediatric Gastroenterology and Nutrition* **8:** 31–36.

Vandenplas Y, de Roy C & Sacre L (1991a) Cisapride decreases prolonged episodes of reflux in infants. *Journal of Pediatric Gastroenterology and Nutrition* **12:** 44–47.

Vandenplas Y, Goyvaerts M, Melven R & Sacre L (1991b) Gastroesophageal reflux, as measured by 24-hour pH-monitoring, in 509 healthy infants screened for risk of sudden infant death syndrome. *Pediatrics* **88:** 834–840.

Vandenplas Y, Derde MP & Piepsz A (1992) Evaluation of reflux episodes during simultaneous esophageal pH monitoring and gastroesophageal reflux scintigraphy in children. *Journal of Pediatric Gastroenterology and Nutrition* **14:** 256–260.

Walsh JK, Farrell MK, Keenen WJ et al (1981) Gastroesophageal reflux in infants; Relation to apnea. *Journal of Pediatrics* **99:** 197–201.

Weinstein WM, Bogoch ER & Bowes KL (1975) The normal esophageal mucosa: A histologic reappraisal. *Gastroenterology* **68:** 40–44.

Whitington PF & Orenstein SR (1984) Manometric guidance in suction biopsy of the esophagus in children. *Journal of Pediatric Gastroenterology and Nutrition* **3:** 535–538.

Wilson NM, Charrette L, Thomson AH & Silverman M (1985) Gastroesophageal reflux and childhood asthma. *Thorax* **40:** 592–597.

10

A new look at recurrent abdominal pain in children by subdivision of patients into symptomatic subgroups: simplifying the role of endoscopy in the diagnostic evaluation

J. TIMOTHY BOYLE

In the hands of a trained specialist, fibreoptic endoscopy is generally a safe and effective diagnostic procedure for the evaluation of a wide variety of gastro-intestinal problems. The technique permits examination of the oesophagus, the stomach, the first and second portions of the duodenum, and the entire colon. The indications for endoscopy are broad, and the diagnostic accuracy and therapeutic potential are high (Caulfield et al, 1989; Steffen et al, 1989; Bines and Winter, 1990; Moyer and Gryboski, 1990; Morrisey and Reichel-derfer, 1991a,b). The value of diagnostic accuracy, however, is only relevant if it is consistently associated with improvement in patient outcome. At present, not enough controlled prospective data are available on the indications for endoscopy in the evaluation of recurrent abdominal pain in children to justify a consensus with which most experts could subscribe.

'Recurrent abdominal pain' (RAP) is a common description which has evolved from the seminal definition by Apley of intermittent abdominal pain in children between the ages of 4 and 16 years which persists for greater than 3 months duration, and affects normal activity (Apley, 1975). RAP has been reported to occur in 10–15% of children between the ages of 4 and 14 years (Pringle et al, 1966; Oster, 1972; Apley, 1975; Faull and Nicol, 1986). Although exact prevalence figures are unknown, functional abdominal pain is by far the most common aetiology of RAP in children. The modifier 'functional' is used if no specific structural, infectious, inflammatory, or biochemical cause for the abdominal pain can be determined. Current speculation is that functional abdominal pain represents a disturbance of gastrointestinal (GI) motility provoked by physical and/or psychological stress (Zighelboim and Talley, 1993).

Since the majority of patients will have functional pain, the optimal management of the patient who presents with recurrent abdominal pain remains controversial. Basically the physician is presented with two options: (1) empirical therapy after a minimum of screening tests; or (2) immediate comprehensive investigation (including endoscopy) to reassure both the patient and physician and treat specific disease. In the absence of outcome

Baillière's Clinical Paediatrics—
Vol. 2, No. 4, November 1994
ISBN 0–7020–1866–X

data, such as patient function, cost of visits, and cost of medications, a pattern has evolved in practice in which the paediatrician or family physician employs empirical therapy for the patient with an initial episode of RAP. More comprehensive investigation ensues when a family with a child with an initial or recurrent episode of RAP directly consults or is referred to a gastroenterologist.

An alternative approach is to choose therapy or investigation based on the clinical presentation. Children with recurrent abdominal pain tend to exhibit one of three clinical presentations: (1) isolated paroxysmal abdominal pain; (2) abdominal pain associated with symptoms of dyspepsia; and (3) abdominal pain associated with altered bowel pattern. Since the exact aetiology and pathogenesis of the pain are unknown, and no specific diagnostic markers exist for any group, functional abdominal pain in general is too often perceived as a diagnosis of exclusion. It is the clinical presentation together with a well-structured medical history and physical examination which usually indicates that functional abdominal pain is the likely diagnosis in an individual child presenting with recurrent abdominal pain. Rather than a shotgun approach to rule out all potential infectious, inflammatory, structural, and biochemical causes of a particular pain presentation, diagnostic evaluation should be driven by pertinent signals in the history and physical examination.

The purpose of this chapter is to focus on the diagnostic evaluation and management of functional abdominal pain by subdividing patients into symptomatic subgroups. The format will be to describe the clinical presentation of each subgroup and to discuss the differential diagnosis of each clinical presentation. The criteria for a positive diagnosis of functional pain will be presented with special emphasis on the role of endoscopy in the diagnostic evaluation. Finally, the management of functional pain in each subgroup will be discussed.

RECURRENT ISOLATED PAROXYSMAL ABDOMINAL PAIN

Clinical presentation of isolated functional abdominal pain

Isolated paroxysmal abdominal pain tends to occur in children younger than 10 years of age. By definition, the pain varies in severity. Onset is usually gradual. Pain episodes last less than 1 h in 50% of patients, and less than 3 h in the vast majority. Continuous pain has been described in less than 10% of patients. The patient may look well while vocalizing the presence of pain. During severe attacks, the child may exhibit a variety of motor behaviours including doubling over, grimacing, crying, and clenching or pushing on the abdomen. Parents describe the child as miserable and appearing pale or listless during episodes of pain.

The child is often unable to describe the nature of the pain (stabbing, burning, dull). Even when asked to locate the point of maximal pain with one finger, the child will usually use his or her whole hand and radiate around the periumbilical area. Radiation to the back, chest, or legs is rare.

The parent or young child is usually unable to describe a temporal relationship to meals, activity, stress, or bowel movements. The pain rarely awakens the child from sleep, but it is not uncommon for pain to occur in the evening and affect the ability of the child to fall asleep.

Extraintestinal symptoms are common including headache, pallor, dizziness, and fatigability. Parents may report 'fever' between 99 and 100°F (Apley, 1975).

In addition to the clinical features of the pain and associated symptoms, functional paroxysmal pain is characterized by a constellation of historical features that facilitate recognition of the syndrome.

1. Concurrent physical or psychosocial stress factors. Examples of physical stress include viral infection, lactose intolerance, or menses. Examples of psychosocial stressful life events include death or separation of a family member, physical illness or chronic handicap in parents or siblings, school problems, poverty or financial problems, or a recent geographical move.
2. A positive family history for irritable bowel syndrome, peptic ulcer, previous appendectomy, or migraine headaches (Apley, 1975).
3. A characteristic reinforcement response to the pain behaviour by parents, school, and primary physician (Miller and Kratochwill, 1979). Reinforcement responses include social attention, rest periods during pain episodes, missed school, medication, escalating diagnostic tests, and hospitalization. The characteristic parental response following a report of pain includes requesting the child to lie down on a couch or bed, providing TV, toys, books, drinks, or food to distract the child: and administering some type of symptomatic therapy, either tactile, such as massaging the abdomen or using a heating pad, or medication, such as acetaminophen, ibuprofen, or anticholinergic agent.

Differential diagnosis of recurrent abdominal pain presenting as isolated paroxysmal abdominal pain

Table 1 lists the major differential conditions of chronic paroxysmal abdominal pain in children.

Obstructive symptoms include recurrent episodes of acute crampy, paroxysmal periumbilical pain, particularly after meals, episodic vomiting, abdominal distension, and altered bowel pattern. Weight loss, chronic occult blood loss, and iron deficiency anaemia are common. Potential aetiologies of recurrent small bowel obstruction that can present with progressive abdominal pain over a period of weeks include Crohn's disease, malrotation with volvulus, intussusception caused by a specific lead point (i.e. Meckel's diverticulum, polyp, duplication, lymphoid hyperplasia), adhesions following previous abdominal surgery, small bowel lymphoma, endometriosis, tuberculosis, vascular disorders such as polyarteritis nodosa and mesenteric-vein thrombosis with ischaemia, eosinophilic gastroenteritis, and angioneurotic oedema. Crohn's disease should be suspected when pressure tenderness is localized to the right lower quadrant, a fullness or

Table 1. Differential conditions of recurrent abdominal pain presenting as isolated paroxysmal abdominal pain.

I.	Obstructive disorders
	1. Crohn's disease
	2. Malrotation w/wo volvulus
	3. Intussusception with lead point
	4. Postsurgical adhesions
	5. Small bowel lymphoma
	6. Endometriosis
	7. Infection (tuberculosis, *Yersinia*)
	8. Vascular disorders
	9. Eosinophilic gastroenteritis
	10. Angioneurotic oedema
II.	Appendiceal colic
III.	Dysmenorrhoea
IV.	Musculoskeletal disorders
V.	Ureteropelvic junction obstruction
VI.	Abdominal migraine, epilepsy
VII.	Acute intermittent porphyria
VIII.	Psychiatric disorders
IX.	Functional abdominal pain

mass effect is appreciated on abdominal examination, and extraintestinal symptoms such as fever, rash, or joint pains are present. Ninety percent of patient's with Crohn's disease will have an elevated sedimentation rate (Gryboski and Spiro, 1978). Rare disorders such as polyarteritis nodosa, intestinal ischaemia, eosinophilic gastroenteritis, and angioneurotic oedema can be indistinguishable from Crohn's disease on clinical grounds. Suspicion of polyarteritis nodosa rests on evidence of extraintestinal disease, particularly renal involvement (Camilleri et al, 1983). Mesenteric-vein obstruction should be considered in adolescents using oral contraceptives. Clinically, it can present gradually with progressive abdominal pain over a period of weeks (Grendell and Ocknea, 1982). Pneumatosis is usually a late finding. The clinical presentation of eosinophilic gastroenteritis depends on the depth of the infiltration by the eosinophilic process. Submucosal disease can become manifest with abdominal pain and signs of obstruction (Whitington and Whitington, 1988; Wershil and Walker, 1992). Any region of the GI tract can be involved. Angioneurotic oedema can be heralded by recurrent episodes of pain in the absence of cutaneous or oropharyngeal oedema (Weinstock et al, 1987). Family history is usually positive for allergy. Abdominal pain associated with pseudo-obstruction is rarely colicky in nature. The most characteristic physical finding in pseudo-obstruction is abdominal distention (Faulk et al, 1978).

Appendiceal colic, caused by inspissated casts of faecal material within the appendix, should be suspected in patient's recurrent acute episodes of crampy right lower quadrant or periumbilical pain, and right lower quadrant pressure tenderness demonstrated on several examinations (Schisgall, 1980).

Ureteropelvic junction (UPJ) obstruction is well known to present with recurrent episodes of periumbilical, crampy pain, but in all cases reported in the literature to date, the pain has been associated with vomiting (Byrne et al, 1985).

Typical dysmenorrhoea consists of cramping, dull, midline, or generalized lower abdominal pain at the onset of a menstrual period. The pain may coincide with the start of bleeding, or precede the bleeding by several hours. Gynaecological disorders associated with secondary dysmenorrhoea include endometriosis, partially obstructed genital duplications, ectopic pregnancy, and adhesions following pelvic inflammatory disease. Cystic teratoma has been described in prepubertal patients presenting with right or left lower quadrant pain. The vast majority of such patients have a palpable abdominal mass (Ahmed, 1975). Benign ovarian cysts in adolescent females do not cause recurrent abdominal pain.

Muscle pain is usually well-localized and sharp, and may be triggered by exercise or change in body position. It is usually located near the insertion of the rectus muscle or oblique muscles into the costal margins or iliac crest. Slipping-rib syndrome is a sprain disorder which may be confused with intra-abdominal conditions (Porter, 1985). The symptoms are sharp or dull pain in one of the upper abdominal quadrants 'under the ribs, frequently accompanied by a sensation of something rubbing in the anterior costal area. Another localized musculofascial problem, exacerbated by exercise, is a linea alba hernia, which is midline, and may be either infra- or supra-umbilical (Bugensten and Phibbs, 1975). The anatomic defect is detected in the midline while the child performs sit-up exercises. Discitis, which is really an osteomyelitis of the vertebral end plate, may present as a combination of back and abdominal pain. The condition is usually associated with intermittent fever, elevated white count, and elevated sedimentation rate (Leahy et al, 1984).

Abdominal migraine (Prensky, 1976), epilepsy (Zarline, 1984), and acute intermittent porphyria (AIP) (Stein and Tschudy, 1970) are disorders characterized by the temporal association of paroxysmal abdominal pain and a wide variety of central nervous system symptoms including headache, dizziness, weakness, syncope, confusion, memory loss, confusion, hallucinations, seizures, and transient blindness. Both disorders are classically associated with nausea and vomiting. AIP is often precipitated by low intake of carbohydrate, or by specific drugs such as barbiturates or sulphonamides.

Psychic abdominal pain, triggered by environmental stress or critical life setbacks, is by definition a conversion reaction. Several factors suggest a conversion reaction including patient's age at onset greater than 12 years, an hysterical personality (dramatic, exhibitionist, labile, excitable, egocentric, seductive), and a parent who is clinically depressed (Maloney, 1980).

The inclusion of a number of disorders in the differential of RAP has been confusing because of the tendency in the literature to describe pain in isolation from associated symptoms. Thus, parasitic infections and carbohydrate intolerance are probably not primary causes of paroxysmal abdominal pain in the absence of associated symptoms such as diarrhoea, nausea, bloating, and increased flatulence. Also, while one retrospective report has described abdominal pain as the sole presenting symptom of peptic ulcer in children (Drumm et al, 1988), the authors described only presenting symptoms, and did not even address pain location, associated symptoms, or relationship of the pain to eating. The majority of reviews of peptic ulcer and gastritis describe a clinical presentation in which abdominal pain is located in the epigastric area, and associated with meals, vomiting, evidence of GI blood loss, or a positive family history within a second-degree relative (Silverman and Roy, 1983; Tomomasa et al, 1986). Until further evidence is described, peptic ulcer should not be included routinely in the differential of isolated paroxysmal abdominal pain.

Criteria for a positive diagnosis of functional abdominal pain in a patient with chronic isolated paroxysmal abdominal pain

Criteria for a positive diagnosis of functional abdominal pain in patients who present with recurrent paroxysmal abdominal pain include a characteristic history, negative physical examination (except for abdominal pressure tenderness), and negative results of a few routine laboratory studies including a complete blood count, an erythrocyte sedimentation rate, and urinalysis to screen for inflammatory bowel disease and urinary tract infection.

The most valuable diagnostic test in a patient with symptoms suggesting obstruction is an upper GI series and small bowel follow through. The X-ray request should specifically ask the radiologist to rule out peptic ulcer, malrotation, thickening of intestinal folds, and terminal ileitis. Rare conditions such as lymphoma, angioneurotic oedema, mesenteric vein thrombosis with ischaemia, eosinophilic gastroenteritis, and pseudo-obstruction will also be picked up by an upper GI series. Barium enema should be considered in patients with chronic right lower quadrant pain to evaluate the appendix. Filling defects, focal globular or diffuse distention of the appendix, or retained barium in the appendix 72 h after contrast study should raise the question of appendiceal colic (Schisgall, 1980). Meckel's diverticulum should not be included in the differential diagnosis of chronic abdominal pain unless there are signs of obstruction, or GI bleeding. Abdominal ultrasound has a low diagnostic yield, but may pick up rare cases of ureteropelvic obstruction, or cystic teratoma of the ovary.

When the patient's medical evaluation indicates probable functional pain, the clinician must be particularly careful to ensure that the extent of the work-up is based on clinical judgment arising from the history, physical examination, and screening test results, not on the parents insistence or urgent request for diagnostic studies. Acting against medical judgment can lead to a cycle of increasingly invasive and expensive tests. Such testing usually only reinforces the patient's sick role and pain behaviour.

Role of endoscopy in the evaluation of chronic isolated paroxysmal abdominal pain

Endoscopy has no role in the diagnostic evaluation of the paediatric patient with isolated paroxysmal abdominal pain who fulfills diagnostic criteria for functional abdominal pain.

Treatment of functional paroxysmal abdominal pain

Management begins with a positive diagnosis, education, and establishment of realistic expectations of treatment. It is important to emphasize that the pain is real, and is caused most likely by an increased intensity of intestinal motor activity in response to a wide variety of psychophysiological stressful stimuli. The concept of visceral hypersensitivity can be used to explain why some children may experience pain even with normal amounts of stress (Zighelboim and Talley, 1993). The potential genetic vulnerability in those families with a strong history of pain should be stated (Apley, 1975). The objective of management of isolated paroxysmal abdominal pain is to prevent the pain from becoming a state of social dysfunction. The goal of management cannot be total freedom from pain and associated symptoms, but maintaining good physical health and normal activity for the patient's age. Consultants may be needed in selected cases to confirm the diagnosis, to recommend or reinforce treatment strategies, or to address suspected significant psychosocial disturbances.

The therapy of isolated paroxysmal functional pain is directed toward environmental and dietary modification. The first goal is to identify, clarify, and reverse stresses that may trigger pain. Equally important is to reverse environmental reinforcement of the pain behaviour. Parents and school must be engaged to support the child rather than the pain. Life style must be normalized regardless of the presence of pain. Regular school attendance is essential. School officials must be encouraged to be responsive to the pain behaviour, but not to let it disrupt attendance, class activity, or performance expectations. At home, parents need to foster more independent dealing with the pain on the part of the child. Dietary modifications that may lessen pain symptoms include restriction of dairy products or lactase supplementation therapy in children with documented lactose intolerance (Barr et al, 1979; Lebenthal et al, 1981; Wald et al, 1982), or restriction of gas-forming foods like legumes. Because of its safety, a trial of fibre is reasonable in all patients with functional abdominal pain although the efficacy of this treatment has not been proved (Feldman et al, 1985; Klein, 1988). Synthetic fibre supplements such as methylcellulose, psyllium, and polycarbophil may cause less bloating than natural fibre supplements because of improved solubility. Long-term compliance is always a problem. Because other dietary carbohydrates may be malabsorbed and act as provocative stimuli of pain, restriction of excessive intakes of carbonated beverages (fructose), dietary starches (corn, potato, wheat, oats), or sorbitol-containing products (sorbitol is used as a vehicle for oral medication, a sugar substitute in sweets, an ingredient in toothpaste, and a plasticizer in gelatin capsules) is reasonable.

Drug therapy of functional abdominal pain is controversial since there is no convincing evidence that any specific therapy is effective in treating any one of the three symptom complexes. However, an individual patient may benefit from treatment directed at alleviating the predominant symptom. Oral anticholinergic agents (e.g. dicyclomine (Bentyl®) or hyoscyamine (Levsin®)) are often effective in providing pain relief, particularly if used on a p.r.n. basis in conjunction with dietary fibre. Since many patients are hypersensitive to anticholinergics, it is very important to start out with a small dose, and titrate up to ensure an adequate anticholinergic dose. As a basic guideline, if the patient does not experience dryness of the mouth, then it isn't a therapeutic dose of the drug. If anticholinergic medication is used for treatment of severe exacerbations of pain, a sublingual dose form should be considered to provide more rapid relief. Patients with predictable postprandial abdominal pain may be helped by anticholinergic agents taken 30 min before meals so that the maximum effect occurs when the symptoms are expected.

Alternative therapies that may benefit selected patients include psycho-therapy, hypnotherapy, and biofeedback. Consultation with a child psychiatrist or psychologist is indicated if there is concern regarding extreme internalizing behaviour (anxiety, depression, low self-esteem), modelling or imitation of family pain behaviour, maladaptive family coping mechanisms, or failure of initial attempts at environmental modification to result in return to a normal life-style.

RECURRENT ABDOMINAL PAIN ASSOCIATED WITH DYSPEPSIA

Clinical presentation of functional dyspepsia

The symptoms of dyspepsia in association with chronic abdominal pain suggest upper gastrointestinal tract dysfunction (Talley and Phillips, 1988). Abdominal pain is often localized to the epigastrium, right or left upper quadrants. In younger children, however, pain is more likely to be peri-umbilical. There is often a temporal relationship between meal ingestion and symptoms. In some cases the rhythmicity between food ingestion and symptoms may be delayed, resembling that of classical ulcer disease. In others, the pain develops immediately or shortly after eating, and persists for 3–4 h simulating gallbladder or pancreatic dysfunction. Nausea, heartburn, oral regurgitation, early satiety, postprandial abdominal bloating and/or distention, and excess gas with or without increased belching or flatulence, are common associated problems. A history of occasional vomiting is not uncommon, but vomiting as a rule is not an important component of the clinical presentation.

Functional dyspepsia is usually associated with the same signs of environ-mental reinforcement of pain behaviour described above for isolated paroxysmal pain.

Differential diagnosis of recurrent abdominal pain associated with dyspepsia

Table 2 lists the diagnoses that need to be considered in patients with chronic abdominal pain and dyspepsia. The differential conditions are divided into those associated with upper GI inflammation, motility disorders, and other candidate disorders.

Table 2. Differential conditions of recurrent abdominal pain associated with symptoms of dyspepsia.

I.   Associated with upper GI inflammation
    1. Gastro-oesophageal reflux disease (GORD)
    2. Peptic ulcer
    3. *Helicobacter pylori* gastritis
    4. NSAID (nonsteroidal anti-inflammatory drug) ulcer
    5. Crohn's disease
    6. Eosinophilic gastroenteritis
    7. Menetrier's disease
    8. Cytomegalovirus (CMV) gastritis
    9. Parasitic infection (*Giardia, Blastocystis hominis*)
    10. Varioliform gastritis
    11. Lymphocytic gastritis/coeliac disease
    12. Henoch–Schonlein purpura
II. Motility disorders
    1. Idiopathic gastroparesis
    2. Biliary dyskinesia
    3. Intestinal pseudo-obstruction
III. Other disorders
    1. Obstructive disorders from Table 1
    2. Chronic pancreatitis
    3. Chronic hepatitis
    4. Chronic cholecystitis
    5. Ureteropelvic junction obstruction
    6. Abdominal migraine
    7. Psychiatric disorders

Gastro-oesophageal reflux disease (GORD) may result from a primary disorder of lower oesophageal sphincter dysfunction, or develop secondary to anatomical, inflammatory, or motility disorders which affect gastric emptying (McCallum, 1990; Traube, 1990). The most common pain symptom produced by GORD is heartburn, defined as a retrosternal burning discomfort which radiates toward the head. The pain can vary widely in quality such that the patient will often use such descriptive terms as 'gas pains', 'indigestion', 'burpiness', 'pressure'. Typically, heartburn is aggravated by lying in the recumbent position, and ingesting large fatty meals, tomato products, chocolate, or citrus drinks with high acid content. Regurgitation of sour or bitter gastric contents is a common complaint of patients with GORD. However, regurgitation alone must not be confused with oesophagitis. Nausea or vomiting are uncommon symptoms of GORD unless there are associated abnormalities of gastric emptying. Dysphagia or odynophagia, together with heartburn should definitely point towards a diagnosis of GORD. Extra-oesophageal symptoms of GORD in older children may include chronic sore throat, otalgia, paroxysms of coughing or wheezing, and laryngitis (Boyle, 1989).

Abdominal pain is by far the most frequent presenting symptom of chronic peptic ulcer disease in children (Silverman and Roy, 1983; Tomomasa et al, 1986; Drumm et al, 1988). Pain from the stomach and duodenum is visceral and referred to the epigastrium although a number of reviews have stressed the point that children younger than 10 years of age generally describe the pain as periumbilical. As with oesophagitis, the pain can vary widely in quality, so that the patient may describe the pain as 'burning', or 'pressure'. Only about 50% of patients will associate the pain with eating, either relieved or aggravated by meals. It is not uncommon for ulcer pain to awaken a patient at night. The most common associated symptoms are nausea and vomiting. Vomiting usually follows meals and relieves the pain in the majority of patients. Evidence of GI blood loss is not uncommon, manifested by positive stool guaiac. About 25% of patients will have a first-degree relative with peptic ulcer. An identifiable stress factor may also be identified in 40% of patients.

It is now recognized that *Helicobacter pylori*, a ubiquitous spiral bacterium, is present in almost all adults with duodenal ulcer, most with gastric ulcer, and virtually all patients with histological evidence of gastritis (Peterson, 1991). Subsequent studies have shown that incidence of infection in children increases with age, is inversely related to socio-economic class, and increases in families where an adult either has had an ulcer or documented *H. pylori* infection (Farrell, 1993). *Helicobacter pylori* is most likely transmitted from person to person, although infection from a common exogenous source has not been completely ruled out (Peterson, 1991). It is well established that *H. pylori* is associated with peptic ulcer disease in children. However, only one-third of paediatric patients with endoscopically proven peptic ulcer have been reported to have infection with *H. pylori*. Obviously, other factors are involved in the pathogenesis of peptic ulcer disease in children (Farrell, 1993; Michell et al, 1993). Whether *H. pylori* gastritis is a disease in children remains controversial. A recent NIH-sponsored consensus conference (1994) concluded that there was insufficient evidence in adults to treat isolated *H. pylori* gastritis in the absence of gross ulcer. Caution must be exercised in extending this conclusion to paediatric patients in whom the inflammatory lesion tends to show chronic rather than acute cellular elements (Michell et al, 1993).

Together with *H. pylori*, nonsteroidal anti-inflammatory drugs (NSAID) are the most important exogenous factors associated with peptic ulcer. Clinically significant ulceration occurs infrequently with NSAID use. The pathogenic mechanisms distinguishing those individuals at risk have not been identified. A careful history is required to assure that NSAID consumption is detected in any patient being evaluated for recurrent abdominal pain with dyspepsia.

Gastroduodenal Crohn's disease, eosinophilic gastroenteritis (EG) (Whitington and Whitington, 1988; Wershil and Walker, 1992), Menetrier's disease (Chouraqui et al, 1981), cytomegalovirus (CMV) gastritis (Occena et al, 1993), varioliform gastritis (VG) (Couper et al, 1989), lymphocytic gastritis (DeGiacomo et al, 1994), and Henoch–Schonlein purpura (Feldt and Stickler, 1962) may all present with abdominal pain associated with dyspepsia. Menetrier's disease, CMV gastritis, and varioliform gastritis are associated with hypertrophy of rugae in the fundus and body of the stomach. Eosinophilic gastroenteritis is more likely to result in a narrowed antrum associated with thickening of the folds in the duodenum and antrum. The aetiology of EG, VG, and LG are unknown. The importance of distinguishing between the entities is based on reports of associated conditions (coeliac disease in LG (DeGiacomo et al, 1994), food hypersensitivity in EG and VG (Couper et al, 1989; Wershil and Walker, 1992), CMV in Menetrier's disease; Occena et al, 1993) which may impact on patient management. Although intervals as long as 150 days between GI symptoms and skin findings of HSP have been reported, the majority of patients exhibit classical skin lesions within 2 weeks of onset of GI symptoms (Feldt and Stickler, 1962).

Nausea, vomiting, and early satiety are classically the predominant symptoms of gastroparesis defined as altered gastric motility resulting in delayed gastric emptying. Yet, patients often complain of epigastric abdominal pain. Gastroparesis after a presumed viral illness may persist for months (Oh and Kim, 1990). Recent evidence suggests that such prolonged symptoms are associated with evidence of systemic autonomic dysfunction. Symptoms of gastroparesis are often associated with scleroderma, uraemia, reflux oesophagitis, and following elective abdominal surgery. Diabetic gastroparesis is rarely seen in the paediatric age range.

The pain of biliary colic is usually acute in onset, frequently following a meal, and usually localized to the epigastrium or right upper quadrant. In small children, however, pain may be periumbilical. Characteristically the pain rises to a plateau of intensity in 5–20 min, and resolves over 1–4 h. Referred pain is common, particularly to the back. Nausea and/or vomiting are very common associated symptoms. Chronic acalculous cholecystitis (Williamson, 1988) and biliary dyskinesia (Steinberg, 1988) are rare causes of biliary-type pain in the absence of cholelithiasis.

Chronic fibrosing pancreatitis, hereditary pancreatitis, and relapsing pancreatitis from abnormalities of pancreatic ductal anatomy are also rare causes of recurrent episodes of sharp epigastric or periumbilical pain (Brown et al, 1993). Relapsing pancreatitis should only be considered in patients with episodic pain associated with vomiting in whom biochemical or X-ray evidence of pancreatic inflammation can be documented (Brown et al, 1993).

Criteria for a diagnosis of functional dyspepsia in a patient with recurrent abdominal pain associated with dyspepsia

In terms of both sensitivity and specificity, there are no symptoms or signs which reliably distinguish functional dyspepsia from upper GI inflammatory, structural, or motility disorders (Tally et al, 1993). Thus, symptoms of dyspepsia generate a more extensive evaluation.

Criteria for a positive diagnosis of functional dyspepsia in patients with recurrent abdominal pain and dyspepsia include a characteristic history, negative physical examination (except for abdominal pressure tenderness), a laboratory evaluation which includes a normal complete blood count, erythrocyte sedimentation rate, chemistry profile, urinalysis, stool O&P, and serology for *Helicobacter pylori* (Peterson, 1991) (if available), a normal upper GI and small bowel series if vomiting is a significant part of the history, and an upper endoscopy which reveals no specific gross or histo-logical evidence of an upper GI inflammatory process. The laboratory evaluation will screen for eosinophilic gastroenteritis, inflammatory bowel disease, chronic hepatitis, chronic renal disease, parasitic disease, and *H. pylori* gastritis. An upper GI series with small bowel follow through will help to rule out gastric outlet disorder, malrotation, and inflammatory bowel disease. Serum amylase, lipase, and ultrasonography are indicated where history reveals discrete acute episodes of pain, triggered by a meal, or localized to the right or left upper quadrants. Ultrasonography will screen for gallstones, pancreatic oedema/pseudocyst, hydronephrosis secondary to UPJ obstruction, and retroperitoneal mass. Further evaluation of motility disorders such as idiopathic gastroparesis, biliary dyskinesia, enterogastric reflux, and pseudo-obstruction is only indicated in patients with atypical symptoms who do not respond to management strategies of functional dyspepsia.

The consistent presence of central nervous system symptoms associated with recurrent abdominal pain justifies neurological consultation for the evaluation of migraine, and urine porphyrin determination. The yield of such evaluation is low, however, in the absence of vomiting.

Role of endoscopy in the evaluation of recurrent abdominal pain associated with dyspepsia

Endoscopy gives the best and most specific means, not only to discover the presence of inflammation in the upper GI tract, but also to assess for severity and complication. Recognizable objective findings by gross examination include superficial erosions, ulcer, stricture, antral nodularity associated with *H. pylori* gastritis (Bunjanover et al, 1991), gastric rugal hypertrophy associated with Menetrier's disease and CMV gastritis (Chouraqui et al, 1981; Occena et al, 1993), and the small heaped-up, volcanic-like mounds with a central crater, associated with chronic varioliform gastritis (Couper et al, 1989). Subjective gross endoscopic findings including erythema, oedema, increased vascularity, and friability become meaningful only in the context of histology.

Recognizable objective histological findings include: (1) intraepithelial eosinophils or polymorphonuclear cells, based cell hyperplasia, or papillary elongation on oesophageal biopsy to indicate reflux oesophagitis (Boyle, 1989); (2) intraepithelial eosinophils in antral or duodenal biopsies indicat-ing possible eosinophilic gastroenteritis (Whitington and Whitington, 1988); (3) intraepithelial plasma cells, polymorphonuclear leukocytes, micro-erosions, crypt abscesses, and pyloric gland metaplasia with or without non-caseating granuloma suggest Crohn's disease (Schuffler and Chaffec, 1979); (4) characteristic CMV intranuclear inclusions; (5) lymphocytic infiltrate within surface and pit gastric epithelium associated with spiral bacterium on the antral epithelium indicative of *H. pylori* gastritis (Peter-son, 1991); and (6) dense lymphocytic infiltrate within surface and pit gastric epithelium associated with a uniformly flat duodenal mucosa indicative of coeliac disease (DeGiacomo et al, 1994). In the absence of ulcer, *H. pylori*, or coeliac disease, the diagnostic value of identifying superficial gastritis characterized by inflammatory infiltration of the upper lamina propria, especially in the context of grossly normal-appearing upper GI mucosa is less clear. Chronic superficial antral gastritis is extremely common in asymptomatic adults, especially with increasing age, or associated with irritable bowel syndrome (Talley and Phillips, 1988). Likewise, it is controversial whether chronic epithelial or interstitial inflammation of the duodenum ('duodenitis'), without discrete ulceration or evidence of *H. pylori*, causes symptoms of dyspepsia. There is no evidence in adult or paediatric patients that nonspecific antral gastritis or duodenitis progresses to duodenal ulcer. Until more data are available my own viewpoint is that, given a visually normal upper endoscopy, a positive diagnosis of functional dyspepsia can be made if the only histological finding is mild, nonspecific superficial antral or duodenal inflammation.

In adults, chronic abdominal pain associated with dyspepsia is often treated medically with antacids or anti-secretory drugs, with anticipation that a favourable clinical response will reflect healing of upper GI inflammation (Talley and Phillips, 1988). Endoscopy is performed only if response to treatment is poor or if symptoms recur. In children, however, I feel that the diagnostic information gained from endoscopy improves the specificity and compliance of treatment. Endoscopy should be considered as a diagnostic and management tool that can confirm diagnosis when screening studies have not suggested the patient's problem, and can alter management based on the information obtained. Although more costly at the outset, a positive diagnosis backed by endoscopy allows the primary physician to resume management of the patient, reduces medication costs, and reduces repetition of, or escalation of, testing. Future efforts should be concentrated to decrease the cost of endoscopy rather than exclude endoscopy in the initial evaluation of children with recurrent abdominal pain and dyspepsia.

Most physicians no longer perform conventional or air contrast radiological evaluation as a complementary test to upper GI endoscopic evaluation. Barium upper GI radiography should be reserved for those patients in whom vomiting is an important part of the clinical presentation, to rule out obstructive lesions.

Endoscopic retrograde cholangiopancreatography is only indicated in the evaluation of RAP with dyspepsia if there is biochemical or radiological evidence of recurrent pancreatitis, or biliary-type abdominal pain following cholecystectomy (Brown et al, 1993).

Treatment of functional dyspepsia

As with isolated paroxysmal pain, the management of functional dyspepsia begins with a positive diagnosis, education, and establishment of realistic expectations of treatment. Therapy is also based on environmental and dietary modification, and selected drug therapy. Environmental modification is the same as described for isolated abdominal pain. Psychotherapy, hypnotherapy, and biofeedback have the same supportive roles, also. Although objective data is lacking to implicate smoking with dyspepsia, parents are strongly advised to maintain a smoke-free house. Patients are also advised to avoid caffeinated beverages and nonsteroidal analgesics. A low-fat diet may help some patients, particularly those with significant nausea and upper abdominal bloating.

Uncertainty still exists regarding the role of drug therapy in patients with functional dyspepsia. Therapy is often based on classification of patients into symptomatic subgroups (Talley et al, 1993). Patients with ulcer-like dyspepsia (predominant symptoms of localized epigastric abdominal pain, occurring before meals, relieved by food, or waking at night) are treated for 4–6 weeks with H_2-receptor antagonists. Patients with dysmotility-like dyspepsia (predominant symptoms of nausea, vomiting, early satiety, and upper abdominal bloating) are treated for 4–6 weeks with prokinetic agents (i.e. metaclopromide or cisapride). In fact, there is no objective data to support such a treatment approach. Use of H_2-receptor antagonists or prokinetic agents as part of the primary therapy of functional dyspepsia will often send mixed messages about the functional nature of the problem. I choose to use short-term therapy with anticholinergic agents, similar to that described for isolated paroxysmal pain, in conjunction with environmental and dietary modification. H_2-receptor antagonists and prokinetic agents are reserved for selected patients who with follow-up continue to exhibit symptoms which affect normal activity.

RECURRENT ABDOMINAL PAIN ASSOCIATED WITH ALTERED BOWEL PATTERN

Clinical presentation of functional abdominal pain associated with altered bowel pattern

This presentation of recurrent abdominal pain mimics irritable bowel syndrome in adults (Lynn and Friedman, 1993). This presentation is more common in adolescents. The character of the abdominal pain is similar to that described for isolated paroxysmal abdominal pain. A fair percentage of patients will also have symptoms of dyspepsia. The association of the pain with altered bowel pattern, however, suggests colonic dysfunction. Abdominal pain is relieved by defecation, or associated with an irregular pattern of defecation including change in frequency or consistency of stool, straining or urgency, feeling of incomplete evacuation, passage of mucus, or a feeling of bloating or abdominal distention. Abdominal distention is a common associated symptom. Irritable bowel syndrome is usually associated with the same autonomic-type symptoms and signs of environmental stress and reinforcement of pain behaviour described above for isolated paroxysmal pain.

Differential diagnosis of recurrent abdominal pain associated with altered bowel pattern

Table 3 lists the major differential conditions of chronic abdominal pain associated with altered bowel pattern. The major symptoms in the history of patients with this presentation include pain localized away from the umbilicus, pain that interferes with normal sleep patterns, diarrhoea that awakens the patient from sleep, visible or occult blood in the stool, weight loss, and extraintestinal symptoms such as fever, rash, and joint pains. Pertinent physical findings suggesting an organic process would include abdominal mass, joint swelling, perianal fistula, fissure, or ulceration, or positive faecal occult-blood test.

Table 3. Differential conditions of recurrent abdominal pain associated with altered bowel pattern.

I.   Idiopathic inflammatory bowel disorders
1. Ulcerative colitis
2. Crohn's disease
3. Microscopic colitis with crypt distortion
4. Lymphocytic colitis
5. Collagenous colitis
II. Infectious disorders
1. Parasitic (*Giardia, Blastocystis hominis, Dientamoeba fragilis*)
2. Bacterial (*Clostridium difficile, Yersinia, Campylobacter*, TB)
III. Lactose intolerance
IV. Complication of constipation (megacolon, encopresis, intermittent sigmoid volvulus)
V. Drug induced diarrhoea, constipation
VI. Gynaecological disorders
VII. Neoplasia (lymphoma, carcinoma)
VIII. Psychiatric disorders

Abdominal pain, diarrhoea, and rectal bleeding are always listed as the most frequent presenting symptoms of inflammatory bowel disease. Tables in review articles and original reports usually list the symptoms separately making it difficult for the physician to appreciate the association between symptoms. In fact, while abdominal pain may be the presenting symptom in patients with ulcerative colitis, complete history and physical examination always reveals signs of GI bleeding. In contrast, signs of GI bleeding may only occur in 40–50% of patients with Crohn's disease (Gryboski and Spiro, 1978). Abdominal pain associated with diarrhoea is by far the most common presentation of Crohn's disease. Crohn's disease should always be suspected in patients with associated perianal skin tags, fistula, or abscess. Ninety percent of patients with Crohn's disease will have elevated sedimentation rate (Gryboski and Spiro, 1978).

Parasitic infections, particularly *Giardia lamblia, Blastocystis hominis*, and *Dientamoeba fragilis*, are the most common infections associated with chronic pain and altered bowel pattern. Chronic *Clostridium difficile* diarrhoea may be seen in children associated with crampy abdominal pain (Sutphen et al, 1983). Fever and rectal bleeding are rare. As with irritable bowel, the diarrhoea usually contains mucus. *Clostridium difficile* cytotoxin determination in the stool is diagnostic. Recurrent or chronic episodes of bacterial enterocolitis are rare. *Yersinia* enterocolitis can mimic Crohn's disease, including nodularity, mucosal thickening of the terminal ileum and colon, and the presence of aphthous ulcers (Marks et al, 1980).

'Microscopic colitis' is an umbrella term covering any case of colitis in which there is histological, but no colonoscopic or barium abnormality. Three specific subclassifications should be considered: (1) a forme fruste of chronic idiopathic inflammatory bowel disease in which intraepithelial lymphocytes and chronic inflammation of the lamina propria is associated with gland distortion (Riddel, 1988); (2) lymphocytic colitis in which the lamina propria contains an inflammatory infiltrate of plasma cells and neutrophils, and the epithelium is invaded by lymphocytes and occasional neutrophils (Lazenby et al, 1989); and (3) collagenous colitis which is histologically similar to lymphocytic colitis with the addition of subepithelial collagen table thickening (Lee et al, 1992; Gremse et al, 1993). Microscopic colitis presents with chronic watery diarrhoea, commonly associated with crampy abdominal pain. The large volume of diarrhoea (400–1200 g/day) distinguishes patients with lymphocytic or collagenous colitis from those with irritable bowel where stool weight in excess of 300 g/day is rare (Lynn and Friedman, 1993). The significance of microscopic colitis in the paediatric population remains unknown (Mashako et al, 1990).

Lactose intolerance and irritable bowel are common and may coexist (Barr et al, 1979; Lebenthal et al, 1981; Wald et al, 1982; Lynn and Friedman, 1993). Lactose intolerance should be considered as a potential primary aetiology of chronic abdominal pain in the presence of diarrhoea, bloating, and increased flatulence. More commonly, intolerance of dietary lactose, fructose, starches, or sorbitol acts as one of several physical stimuli to provoke altered intestinal function in patients with functional pain.

Criteria for a positive diagnosis of irritable bowel syndrome (IBS) in a patient with recurrent abdominal pain associated with altered bowel pattern

Bowel irregularity is essential for a diagnosis of IBS. Criteria for a positive diagnosis of functional irritable bowel in patients with recurrent abdominal pain and altered bowel function include a characteristic history, negative physical examination including rectal examination (except for abdominal pressure tenderness), and negative routine diagnostic studies including complete blood count, erythrocyte sedimentation rate, stool O&P × 3, and C. difficile toxin (if chronic diarrhoea and history of chronic antibiotic ingestion). Empiric dietary lactose restriction or lactose breath hydrogen test should be employed to rule out lactose intolerance as a primary cause of symptoms.

Role of endoscopy in the evaluation of recurrent abdominal pain associated with altered bowel pattern

Colonoscopy is indicated for patients in whom historical or physical signals suggest the possibility of an inflammatory bowel disease (Table 4). The accuracy of colonoscopy in diagnosing inflammatory conditions of the colon is superior to barium enema because of the direct visualization of the mucosal surface and the ability to obtain biopsy and culture specimens. Intubation of the terminal ileum can also aid in the diagnosis of Crohn's disease. Recognizable objective findings by gross examination with a flexible endoscope include oedema, erosions, ulceration, pseudomembranes (discrete yellow plaques on the colonic mucosa), polyps, and induced friability appreciated during withdrawal of the instrument. Oedema can be evaluated more objectively during lower endoscopy because of loss of the normal well-demarcated vascular pattern particularly in the left colon. Subjective gross endoscopic findings including erythema, increased vascularity, and spontaneous friability become meaningful only in the context of histology since they are subject to more interobserver variation in interpretation.

Table 4. Indications for colonoscopy in patients with recurrent abdominal pain and altered bowel pattern.

1. Evidence of GI bleeding
2. Profuse diarrhoea
3. Involuntary weight loss or growth deceleration
4. Iron deficiency anaemia
5. Elevated acute phase reactants (sedimentation rate, C-reactive protein, orosomucoid)
6. Extraintestinal symptoms suggestive of inflammatory bowel disease (fever, rash, joint pains, recurrent aphthous ulceration)

Recognizable objective histological findings include: (1) cryptitis, crypt abscesses, and crypt distortion with branching and drop out, suggesting ulcerative colitis or Crohn's disease; (2) noncaseating granuloma specific for Crohn's disease; (3) fibrosis and histiocyte proliferation in the submucosa suggesting Crohn's disease; and (4) epithelial and intraepithelial lymphocytes with or without subepithelial collagen thickening in lymphocytic colitis and collagenous colitis respectively. The latter should only be considered specific findings in patients with profuse diarrhoea. Mild superficial increases in interstitial lymphocytes in the absence of crypt distortion or significant diarrhoea are nonspecific, and should not dissuade the physician from making a positive diagnosis of irritable bowel syndrome.

Most physicians no longer perform conventional or air contrast radiological evaluation as a complementary test to colonoscopic evaluation, unless they are unable to examine the entire colon, and there is a strong suspicion of inflammatory bowel disease. Upper GI series with small bowel follow through is indicated in any patient undergoing evaluation of possible Crohn's disease.

Treatment of irritable bowel syndrome

The condition of most patients with irritable bowel syndrome will improve with a management approach outlined for isolated paroxysmal abdominal pain. For patients with IBS whose predominant symptom is diarrhoea, an antidiarrhoeal agent (e.g. loperamide), or the bile salt binding agent, cholestyramine, may be helpful. Treatment with the prokinetic agent, cisapride, may decrease the severity of constipation and abdominal pain in patients whose predominant symptom is constipation (Van Outryve et al, 1991). Excessive gas can be managed by advising the patient to eat slowly, to avoid chewing gum, and to avoid excessive intake of carbonated beverages, legumes, foods of the cabbage family, and foods or beverages sweetened with fructose or sorbitol (Rumessen, 1982). Simethicone or activated charcoal may help individual patients.

SUMMARY

Recurrent abdominal pain is a broad descriptive term commonly used in paediatrics to define a heterogeneous group of patients who experience episodic attacks of abdominal pain over a period of at least 3 months. The great majority of patients who seek medical attention for recurrent abdominal pain have a functional disorder thought to be triggered by a motility or sensory disturbance of the gastrointestinal tract, provoked by a variety of physical and psychological stimuli. When evaluated critically, there are three distinct clinical presentations of functional abdominal pain in children and adolescents: primary periumbilical paroxysmal abdominal pain, functional dyspepsia, and irritable bowel syndrome. There are adequate data to support the view that medical history, physical examination, and selected laboratory or endoscopic evaluation allows a positive diagnosis of each type of functional disorder.

REFERENCES

Ahmed S (1975) Ovarian cysts in childhood. *Australian and New Zealand Journal of Surgery* **45:** 398–404.

Apley J (1975) *The Child with Abdominal Pains.* London: Blackwell Scientific Publications.

Barr RG, Levine MD & Watkins J (1979) Recurrent abdominal pain in children due to lactose intolerance. A prospective study. *New England Journal of Medicine* **300:** 1449–1452.

Bines JW & Winter HS (1990) Pediatric endoscopy: colonoscopy. In Barkin J & O'Phelan CA (eds) *Advanced Therapeutic Endoscopy*, pp 309–319. New York: Raven Press Ltd.

Boyle JT (1989) Gastroesophageal reflux in the pediatric patient. *Gastroenterology Clinics of North America* **18:** 315–337.

Brown CW, Werlin SL, Geenen JE & Schmalz M (1993) The diagnostic and therapeutic role of endoscopic retrograde cholangiopancreatography in children. *Journal of Pediatric Gastroenterology and Nutrition* **17:** 19–23.

Bugensten RH & Phibbs CM (1975) Abdominal pain in children caused by linea alba hernias. *Pediatrics* **56:** 1073–1074.

Bunjanover Y, Konikoff F & Baratz M (1991) Nodular gastritis and *Helicobacter pylori*. *Journal of Pediatric Gastroenterology and Nutrition* **11:** 41–44.

Byrne WJ, Arnold WC, Stannard MW & Redman JF (1985) Ureteropelvic junction obstruction presenting with recurrent abdominal pain: diagnosis by ultrasound. *Pediatrics* **76:** 934–937.

Camilleri M, Pusey CD, Chadwick JS & Rees AJ (1983) Gastrointestinal manifestations of systemic vasculitis. *Quarterly Journal of Medicine* **52:** 141–149.

Caulfield ME, Wyllie R, Sivak Jr. MV et al (1989) Upper gastrointestinal tract endoscopy in the pediatric patient. *Journal of Pediatrics* **115:** 339–345.

Chouraqui JP, Roy CC, Brochu P et al (1981) Menetrier's disease in children: A report of a patient and review of sixteen other cases. *Gastroenterology* **80:** 1042–1047.

Couper R, Laski B, Drumm B et al (1989) Chronic varioliform gastritis in childhood. *Journal of Pediatrics* **115:** 441–444.

DeGiacomo C, Gianetti A, Negrini R et al (1994) Lymphocytic gastritis: a positive relationship with celiac disease. *Journal of Pediatrics* **124:** 57–62.

Drumm B, Rhoads JM, Stringer DA et al (1988) Peptic ulcer disease in children: etiology, clinical findings, and clinical course. *Pediatrics* **82:** 410–414.

Farrell MK (1993) Dr. Apley meets *Helicobacter pylori. Journal of Pediatric Gastroenterology and Nutrition* **16:** 118–119.

Faulk DL, Anuras S & Christensen J (1978) Chronic intestinal pseudoobstruction. *Gastroenterology* **74:** 922–931.

Faull C & Nicol AR (1986) Abdominal pain in six-year olds: an epidemiological study in a new town. *Journal of Child Psychology and Psychiatry* **27:** 251–260.

Feldman W, McGrath P, Hodgson C et al (1985) The use of dietary fiber in the management of simple, childhood, idiopathic, recurrent abdominal pain. *American Journal of Diseases of Children* **130:** 1216–1218.

Feldt RH & Stickler GB (1962) The gastrointestinal manifestations of anaphylactoid purpura in children. *Proceedings of Staff Meetings of the Mayo Clinic* **37:** 465–473.

Gremse DA, Boudreaux CW & Manci EA (1993) Collagenous colitis in children. *Gastroenterology* **104:** 906–909.

Grendell JH & Ocknea FK (1982) Mesenteric venous thrombosis. *Gastroenterology* **82:** 358–372.

Gryboski JO & Spiro HM (1978) Prognosis in children with Crohn's disease. *Gastroenterology* **74:** 807–817.

Klein KB (1988) Controlled treatment trials in the irritable bowel syndrome: a critique. *Gastroenterology* **95:** 232–241.

Lazenby AJ, Yardley JH, Giardiello FM et al (1989) Lymphocytic (microscopic) colitis: a comparative histopathologic study with particular reference to collagenous colitis. *Human Pathology* **20:** 18–28.

Leahy AL, Fogarty EE, Fitzgerald RJ & Regan BF (1984) Discitis as a cause of abdominal pain in children. *Surgery* **95:** 412–414.

Lebenthal E, Rossi TM, Nord KS & Branski D (1981) Recurrent abdominal pain and lactose absorption in children. *Pediatrics* **67:** 828–832.

Lee E, Schiller LR, Vendrell D et al (1992) Subepithelial collagen table thickness in colon specimens from patients with microscopic colitis and collagenous colitis. *Gastroenterology* **103:** 1790–1796.

Lynn RB & Friedman LS (1993) Irritable bowel syndrome. *New England Journal of Medicine* **329:** 1940–1945.

McCallum RW (1990) Gastric emptying in gastroesophageal reflux and the therapeutic role of prokinetic agents. *Gastroenterology Clinics of North America* **19:** 551–564.

Maloney MJ (1980) Diagnosing hysterical conversion reactions in children. *Journal of Pediatrics* **97:** 1016–1020.

Marks MI, Pai CH, Lafleur L et al (1980) *Yersinia enterocolitica* gastroenteritis: a prospective study of clinical, bacteriologic, and epidemiologic features. *Journal of Pediatrics* **96:** 26–31.

Mashako MNL, Sonsino E, Navarro J et al (1990) Microscopic colitis: A new cause of chronic diarrhea in children? *Journal of Pediatric Gastroenterology and Nutrition* **10:** 21–26.

Michell HM, Bohane TD, Tobias V et al (1993) *Helicobacter pylori* infection in children: Potential clues to pathogenesis. *Journal of Pediatric Gastroenterology and Nutrition* **16:** 120–125.

Miller AJ & Kratochwill TR (1979) Reduction of frequent stomach ache complaints by time out. *Behavioural Therapy* **10:** 211–218.

Morrissey JF & Reichelderfer M (1991a) Gastrointestinal endoscopy. (First of two parts). *New England Journal of Medicine* **325:** 1142–1149.

Morrissey JF & Reichelderfer M (1991b) Gastrointestinal endoscopy. (Second of two parts). *New England Journal of Medicine* **325:** 1214–1222.

Moyer MS & Gryboski JD (1990) Pediatric endoscopy: Gastroscopy. In Barkin J & O'Phelan CA (eds) *Advanced Therapeutic Endoscopy*, pp 321–333. New York: Raven Press Ltd.

NIH Consensus Conference (1994) *Helicobacter pylori* in peptic ulcer disease. *Journal of the American Medical Association* **272:** 65–69.

Occena RO, Taylor SF, Robinson CC & Sokol RJ (1993) Association of cytomegalovirus with Menetrier's disease in childhood: Report of two new cases with a review of literature. *Journal of Pediatric Gastroenterology and Nutrition* **17**: 217–224.

Oh JJ & Kim CH (1990) Gastroparesis after a presumed viral illness: clinical and laboratory features and natural history. *Mayo Clinic Proceedings* **65**: 636–642.

Oster J (1972) Recurrent abdominal pain, headache, and limb pains in children and adolescents. *Pediatrics* **50**: 429–436.

Peterson WL (1991) *Helicobacter pylori* and peptic ulcer disease. *New England Journal of Medicine* **324**: 1043–1048.

Porter GE (1985) Slipping rib syndrome: an infrequently recognized entity in children: a report of three cases and review of the literature. *Pediatrics* **76**: 810–813.

Prensky AL (1976) Migraine and migrainous variants in pediatric patients. *Pediatric Clinics of North America* **23**: 461–471.

Pringle MLK, Butler NR & Davie R (1966) *11,000 Seven Year Olds*. London: Longmans.

Riddel RH (1988) Pathology of idiopathic inflammatory bowel disease. In Kirschner JB & Shorter RG (eds) *Inflammatory Bowel Disease*, 3rd edn. Philadelphia: Lea and Febiger.

Rumessen JJ (1982) Fructose and related food carbohydrates: source intake, absorption, and clinical implications. *Scandinavian Journal of Gastroenterology* **27**: 819–828.

Schisgall RM (1980) Appendiceal colic in childhood. The role of inspissated casts of stool within the appendix. *Annals of Surgery* **192**: 687–693.

Schuffler MD & Chaffec RG (1979) Small intestinal biopsy in a patient with Crohn's disease of the duodenum. *Gastroenterology* **76**: 1009–1014.

Silverman A & Roy CC (1983) Peptic disease. In *Pediatric Clinical Gastroenterology*, 3rd edn. St. Louis: CV Mosby.

Steffen R, Wyllie R, Sivak Jr. M et al (1989) Colonoscopy in the pediatric patient. *Journal of Pediatrics* **115**: 507–514.

Stein JA & Tschudy DP (1970) Acute intermittent porphyria: a clinical and biochemical study of 46 patients. *Medicine* **49**: 1–16.

Steinberg WM (1988) Sphincter of Oddi dysfunction: a clinical controversy. *Gastroenterology* **95**: 1409–1415.

Sutphen JL, Grand RJ, Flores A et al (1983) Chronic diarrhea associated with *Clostridium difficile* in children. *American Journal of Diseases of Children* **137**: 275–278.

Talley NJ & Phillips SF (1981) Non-ulcer dyspepsia: potential causes and pathophysiology. *Annals of Intern Medicine* **108**: 865–879.

Tally NJ, Weaver AL, Tesmer DL & Zinsmeister AR (1993) Lack of discriment value of dyspepsia subgroups in patients referred for upper endoscopy. *Gastroenterology* **105**: 1378–1386.

Tomomasa T, Hsu JY, Shigeta M et al (1986) Statistical analyses of symptoms and signs in pediatric patients with peptic ulcer. *Journal of Pediatric Gastroenterology and Nutrition* **5**: 711–715.

Traube M (1990) The spectrum of the symptoms and presentations of gastroesophageal reflux disease. *Gastroenterology Clinics of North America* **19**: 607–616.

Van Outryve M, Milo R, Toussaaint J & Van Eoghan P (1991) 'Prokinetic' treatment of constipation predominant irritable bowel syndrome: a placebo-controlled study of Cisapride. *Journal of Clinical Gastroenterology* **13**: 49–57.

Wald A, Chandra R, Fisher SE et al (1982) Lactose malabsorption in recurrent abdominal pain in childhood. *Journal of Pediatrics* **100**: 65–68.

Weinstock LB, Kothari T, Sharma RN & Rosenfeld SI (1987) Recurrent abdominal pain as the sole manifestation of hereditary angioedema in multiple family members. *Gastroenterology* **93**: 1116–1118.

Wershil BK & Walker WA (1992) The mucosal barrier, IgE mediated gastrointestinal events, and eosinophilic gastroenteritis. *Gastroenterology Clinics of North America* **21**: 387–404.

Whitington PF & Whitington GL (1988) Eosinophilic gastroenteropathy in childhood. *Journal of Pediatric Gastroenterology and Nutrition* **7**: 379–385.

Williamson RCN (1988) Acalculous disease of the gallbladder. *Gut* **29**: 860–872.

Zarline EJ (1984) Abdominal epilepsy: an unusual cause of recurrent abdominal pain. *American Journal of Gastroenterology* **79**: 687–688.

Zighelboim J & Talley NJ (1993) What are functional disorders? *Gastroenterology* **104**: 1196–1201.

11

Gastrointestinal bleeding

NIZAR N. ZEIN
JEAN PERRAULT

Gastrointestinal (GI) bleeding at any age is alarming, at times frightening, and more so at a young age. Fortunately, advances in endoscopy and radiology, as well as new therapeutic modalities, permit us to pinpoint the cause of bleeding more easily and to treat it more effectively.

The majority of bleeding episodes from both upper GI (UGI) and lower GI (LGI) sources may resolve spontaneously. Nevertheless, some patients require invasive interventional techniques. The rate of hospitalization for UGI bleeding has been estimated at 150 patients per 100 000 population per year (all ages) (Gilbert, 1990). Lower GI bleeding is much less common. It is important to remember that the cornerstone of management for GI bleeding is to haemodynamically stabilize the patient before proceeding to diagnostic and therapeutic procedures.

CLINICAL PRESENTATION

Before discussing the pathophysiology of bleeding, we will define different types of GI bleeding.

Haematemesis is the vomiting of blood. The blood may be either bright red or 'coffee ground' in appearance when denatured by gastric acid. Haematemesis represents a bleeding source proximal to the ligament of Treitz. **Haematochezia** is the passage of bright red or maroon blood from the rectum. This may be pure blood, bloody diarrhoea, or blood mixed with the stool. The site of bleeding is almost always in the LGI tract, mainly in the left colon and the anorectal region. The cathartic action of blood can cause an UGI bleeding source to produce bright red blood from the rectum; in this instance, the bleeding is massive, not simply streaks. Blood from the UGI tract may appear as black or tarry, sticky, and malodorous stools called melaena. **Melaena** represents denatured blood, and suggests UGI tract bleeding, although the bleeding site may be as distal as the right colon.

Once it has been established that a child has experienced GI bleeding, localization of the bleeding site in the upper or lower GI tract is important. The vomiting of bright red blood, denatured blood, or a combination of both, strongly suggest that the site of bleeding is proximal to the ligament of

Treitz. Bright red blood that coats, but is not mixed with, the stool is most likely indicative of bleeding from the anorectal area. Blood that is darker in colour or more intimately mixed with the faeces, indicates a bleeding site higher in the intestinal tract, whereas blood alone following a bowel movement points to the perianal area or the rectum, i.e. haemorrhoids or polyp. Blood with mucus in the stool suggests an inflammatory or infectious condition. Currant jelly-like material indicates vascular congestion and hyperaemia as seen with intussusception. Black tarry stools are generally indicative of bleeding sites proximal to the ileum, or slow bleeding from the distal small bowel or right colon.

Another important distinction is the spurious bleeding due to various ingested substances, which often provokes unnecessary panic. Red food colouring as in Jell-O®, Kool-Aid®, antibiotics and other medications, and certain fruits and fruit juices like tomato, cranberry, and beets, may look like blood when vomited or passed from the rectum by a child. Bismuth, iron supplements, spinach, and dark chocolate may impart a dark coloration to the stool, often mistaken for melaena. Serratia marcescens causes a pink discoloration in nappies if some time elapses prior to their disposal (Green, 1980).

In other instances, true blood is recovered, but it does not necessarily originate from the GI tract. Blood can be swallowed during vigorous or nocturnal epistaxis, with resultant haematemesis or melaena. In the pubertal female patient with apparent haematochezia, consider the onset of menarche.

PATHOPHYSIOLOGY

Once GI bleeding occurs, a number of compensatory mechanisms are activated. These mechanisms include the increase in sympathetic activity, the release of catecholamines, adrenocorticotropic and antidiuretic hormones, aldosterone, glucocorticoids, and prostaglandins. This in turn helps to maintain haemodynamic stability and blood flow to vital organs such as the brain, in spite of the volume loss caused by the bleeding. Initially, the rapidity of blood loss may be a more important factor than the volume that is lost. An otherwise healthy patient can lose up to 30% of blood volume slowly and still survive; a rapid loss of over 30% of blood volume results in shock and, without therapy, may lead to death.

In addition to the volume of blood lost, and the rapidity of bleeding, a number of factors could also play an important role in the patient's outcome, and the effectiveness of the compensatory mechanisms mentioned above. The presence of associated medical conditions places the patient at a significantly higher risk. In one study, mortality in adult patients with no accompanying medical conditions was 1.2%, but rose to 71% when four or more associated illnesses were identified (Pimpl et al, 1987). Also, the recent ingestion of aspirin in a patient with a GI bleed may aggravate the haemorrhage since aspirin interferes with platelet adhesion in addition to causing direct mucosal injury. In a recent study of critically ill children, six factors were found to portend an important UGI haemorrhage: sepsis, renal failure, liver alterations, heart failure, glucocorticosteroids and metabolic acidosis (Lopez-Herce et al, 1992a).

In general, clinical indicators of a large initial bleed increase the morbidity and mortality (Peterson, 1990). These indicators include: haematemesis plus melaena at presentation (Wara and StØdkilde, 1985); delay or failure to clear nasogastric aspirate with lavage (McLaughlin et al, 1987); elevation of the BUN above 6.5 nmol/l (20 mg/dl); a haemoglobin drop of more than 0.45 mmol/l (3 g/dl) below normal; and tachycardia. Clinical shock carries the worst prognosis (Bornman et al, 1985) (Table 1).

Table 1. Risk factors potentially associated with increased morbidity and mortality in patients with gastrointestinal bleeding. Adapted from Pimpl et al (1987); Peterson (1990); Wara and StØdkilde (1985); McLaughlin et al (1987).

1. The presence of haematemesis plus melaena
2. Tachycardia
3. Delayed or failure to clear NG aspirate with lavage
4. BUN > 6.5 mmol/l (20 mg/dl)
5. Haemoglobin drop greater than 0.45 mmol/l (3 g/dl)
6. Associated medical conditions
7. Recent ingestion of aspirin, other nonsteroidal anti-inflammatory drugs, or anticoagulants

When more than 30% of the circulating blood volume is lost (severe blood loss), hypotension is invariably present. This in turn causes a decrease in cardiac output resulting in tissue damage. Acute renal failure may develop. The most important determining factor in the development of renal failure is the degree of vasoconstriction. Ischaemic liver injury can be reflected by tremendous elevations in transaminases, as well as an elevation of bilirubin and a marked fall in the synthetic rate of clotting factors. Decreased cardiac perfusion, aggravated by acidosis, can result in infarction at any age.

PATHOLOGY OF THE BLEEDING LESIONS

Close observation of the pathology of GI bleeding can offer an insight into the cause of the bleeding and its recurrent nature, not to mention the potential and limitation of various therapies for this common medical emergency.

Mucosal lesions

Ulcers and erosions

In the UGI tract, peptic ulcer disease is a frequent offender (Nord et al, 1981; Swain, 1990), from severe erosions and ulcerations of the oesophagus secondary to gastro-oesophageal reflux to ulceration of the antrum and/or duodenum from *Helicobacter pylori* infection. Acetylsalicylic acid is certainly the most frequently implicated medication in cases of GI tract bleeding. In this case, bleeding may arise from local erosions or diffuse gastritis, often enhanced by decreased platelet adhesiveness (Fromm, 1978; Domschke and Domschke, 1984; Levy et al, 1988). It is presumed that salicylates increase the incidence of ulcers by interruption of the gastric mucosal barrier, allowing back diffusion of hydrogen ions and erosive gastritis. The ability of salicylates to inhibit prostaglandin synthesis may also decrease the cytoprotective properties of the gastric mucosa. Nonsteroidal anti-inflammatory drugs (NSAIDs) such as indomethacin, ibuprofen, and naproxen are also known to cause mucosal injury of the UGI tract (Domschke and Domschke, 1984; Holvoet et al, 1991). These agents inhibit local production of prostaglandin in the UGI tract and have been associated with gastritis, gastric ulcers, and duodenal ulcers. More recently, an association between NSAIDs and ulcerations in the small intestine was reported (Allison et al, 1992). Whether corticosteroids have the same propensity remains debatable (Conn and Blitzer, 1976; Domschke and Domschke, 1984). A meta-analysis suggested an association between corticosteroids and peptic ulcer (Messer et al, 1983), but clinically this seems to be a rare occurrence at best. Chronic renal failure may be accompanied by bleeding from ulcerations or erosions of the GI tract (Dewayne Andrews and Papper, 1985; Zuckerman et al, 1985); these lesions seem to improve with the correction of uraemia.

As already demonstrated in adults (Schuster et al, 1984), children admitted to an intensive care unit have a propensity for UGI tract bleeding (Lacroix et al, 1986), especially with central nervous system lesions (Ross et al, 1987), or with burns (Abramson, 1964). The lesions are either ulcers (so-called stress ulcers) or erosions.

Inflammation

Inflammatory bowel disease is another important and frequent cause of bleeding, whether idiopathic (Crohn's disease, ulcerative colitis), or infectious. The bleeding is rarely massive but is often continuous from large surface areas, causing a gradual fall in the haemoglobin.

Polyps

Juvenile polyps are the most common cause of painless passage of bright red blood in and on the stool. Physical examination may demonstrate the polyp during digital examination of the rectum. Laboratory screening usually confirms occult blood positivity and occasionally, mild anaemia. A positive family history for multiple adenomatous colonic polyps may indicate familial polyposis, an autosomal-dominant condition with mild rectal bleeding in children but frequent carcinomatous changes in young adults (Silverman and Roy, 1983). The identification of mucosal pigmentation in a young patient with intestinal polyps suggests the diagnosis of Peutz–Jeghers syndrome; these hamartomatous polyps seldom progress to carcinoma.

Others

Trauma or external signs of physical abuse in a child with GI tract bleeding raise the possibility of an intramural haematoma of the intestine (Kleinman et al, 1986).

Vascular lesions

Telangiectasias

A family history of chronic occult GI bleeding, repeated blood transfusions, and/or evidence of GI haemorrhage should alert the physician to the possibility of hereditary haemorrhagic telangiectasia (Osler–Weber–Rendu disease) (Vase and Grove, 1986), an autosomal-dominant condition. In the younger child, the typical skin lesions are notoriously absent (Mestre and Andres, 1982). Epistaxis usually precedes, by a few years, the onset of GI bleeding. The incidence of GI bleeding in patients with hereditary haemorrhagic telangiectasia ranges between 13 and 30% (Smith et al, 1963), and the bleeding may be quite severe. The stomach is a common site for telangiectasia (90% of patients) (Vase and Grove, 1986).

Haemangiomas

The Klippel–Trenaunay syndrome with characteristic limb deformities is also associated with cutaneous vascular malformations of the skin and GI tract (Servelle et al, 1976; Schmitt et al, 1986). Turner syndrome can be complicated by telangiectasias or haemangiomas of the GI tract (Grumbach and Conte, 1985); moreover, these patients have an increased risk of inflammatory bowel disease (Price, 1979). The identification or past history of haemangiomata (Abrahamson and Shandling, 1973; Boley et al, 1984), or blue rubber bleb nevi (Fretzin and Potter, 1965; Wong and Lau, 1982) on the skin suggest similar lesions of the GI tract.

Vascular anomalies

The association of hypermobile joints, hyperextensible skin, and GI bleeding, favour the diagnosis of a group of inherited disorders of connective tissue, the Ehlers–Danlos syndrome, type IV in particular (Beighton et al, 1969; Pinnell and Murad, 1983). Endoscopy, and more specifically therapeutic endoscopy, has to be attempted with caution because of poor healing and the possibility of perforation (Sykes, 1984). *Pseudoxanthoma elasticum* is another inherited disorder of elastic tissue; vascular lesions with GI bleeding occur in 10% of patients, although the exact location of the haemorrhage might remain unidentified (Morgan, 1982).

Portal hypertension

Portal vein hypertension, whether caused by pre-, intra-, or suprahepatic venous obstruction is often complicated by oesophageal or gastric varices, with splenomegaly and hypersplenism. Extrahepatic portal venous obstruction (prehepatic obstruction) most commonly follows omphalitis in the neonatal period, either secondary to catheterization of the umbilical vein (Alvarez et al, 1983), or secondary to a spontaneous inflammatory process.

Intrahepatic portal venous obstruction is usually caused by liver cirrhosis; common causes include infantile cholangiopathy, hepatitis, and cystic fibrosis. Obstruction of the hepatic veins (suprahepatic venous obstruction) also causes portal hypertension. This could be a secondary phenomenon (e.g. congestive heart failure or pericarditis), or it may represent a true obstruction (Budd–Chiari syndrome). A hypercoagulable state associated with the use of birth control pills is often implicated in the latter condition (Maddrey, 1987).

Although uncommon in the first year of life, two-thirds of infants with portal hypertension experience bleeding varices before 5 years of age, and 85% do so by 10 years of age (Ament, 1990).

Coagulopathies

Historically, peptic ulcer disease and its complications accounted for one-third of deaths from haemophilia. Modern replacement therapy, and the advent of H_2 blocker agents have changed the natural history to the point where only 10–25% of patients with haemophilia now demonstrate evidence of GI bleeding at any time. Patients on anticoagulants can be at increased risk for bleeding, especially if the coagulation time is out of therapeutic range. The long list of medications that can affect coagulation factors or potentiate the effect of coumarin derivatives includes antibiotics (chloramphenicol, metronidazole, trimethroprim, and sulphamethoxazole), phenytoin, barbiturates, and salicylates (O'Reilly, 1985).

Patients with chronic liver disease not only can develop portal hypertension with oesophageal, gastric, and duodenal varices, but also may have a deficiency of many coagulation factors because of poor synthetic function; moreover, because of bile acid deficiency, these patients can malabsorb vitamin K.

Similarly, any malabsorption syndrome can be complicated by vitamin K deficiency with the potential for bleeding (Berezin et al, 1986); spontaneous bleeding from the GI tract would be unusual, but a potential bleeding site would bleed more briskly if such conditions existed.

CAUSES OF GI BLEEDING IN INFANTS AND CHILDREN ACCORDING TO AGE

Newborns (the first month of life)

Gastrointestinal bleeding in the newborn period differs from that in the older child (Tables 2 and 3). The neonates have a small circulating blood volume and an impaired ability to compensate for the bleeding (Horton and

Table 2. Differential diagnosis of upper gastrointestinal bleeding.

Newborn (birth to 1 month)	Infant (1 month to 2 years)	Child (older than 2 years)
(a) Common		
Swallowed maternal blood	Peptic ulcer	Peptic ulcer
Gastritis	Gastritis	Oesophagitis
Peptic ulcer	Oesophagitis	Mallory–Weiss tear
Nasopharyngeal bleeding	Duodenitis	Oesophageal or gastric varices
(b) Less common		
Haemorrhagic disease of infancy	Swallowed blood (e.g. epistaxis)	Swallowed blood
		Dieulafoy's lesion
Traumatic injury to oesophagus or stomach	Oesophageal or gastric varices	Foreign body erosion
	Mallory–Weiss tear	Haematobilia or haematochylia
	Vascular malformations	
	Duplication cyst	
	Foreign body erosion	

Table 3. Differential diagnosis of lower gastrointestinal bleeding.

Newborn (birth to 1 month)	Infant (1 month to 2 years)	Child (older than 2 years)
(a) Common		
Swallowed maternal blood	Anal fissure	Anal fissure
Necrotizing enterocolitis	Intussusception	Juvenile polyp
Milk-protein intolerance	Meckel's diverticulum	Meckel's diverticulum
Infectious colitis	Milk-protein intolerance	Inflammatory bowel disease
	Infectious colitis	Infectious colitis
(b) Less common		
Hirschsprung's disease	Intestinal duplications	Henoch–Schönlein purpura
Coagulopathy	Lymphonodular hyperplasia	Haemolytic–uraemic syndrome
Anal fissure		
Vascular malformations	Vascular malformations	Vascular malformations
Malrotations with volvulus	Inflammatory bowel disease	Vasculitis (SLE)*
	Juvenile polyp	Leiomyoma
		Hereditary–haemorrhagic telangiectasia

* SLE—systemic lupus erythematosus.

Coln, 1985). However, most episodes of bleeding in this age group are self-limited, allowing non-emergent evaluation and management.

Swallowed maternal blood explains 30% of the cases of GI bleeding and should be ruled out by the Apt–Downey test (Apt and Downey, 1955). A bleeding site on the nipple of a nursing mother may lead to traces of haem in the stool of a breast-fed infant.

Haemorrhagic disease of infancy is very uncommon since the prophylactic administration of vitamin K. However, a similar syndrome may be seen when the mother has received certain medications such as warfarin sodium, phenytoin, or promethazine during pregnancy.

Peptic ulcers or haemorrhagic gastritis may occur in the newborn, particularly after a stormy delivery or birth asphyxia. Even more unusual is the instance of an ulcer induced by the tip of a catheter. These ulcers are more common in the oesophagus complicating a lengthy nasogastric intubation.

Rectal bleeding in the newborn period is not a common finding. Here, as in UGI bleeding, it must be confirmed that the blood is foetal in origin and not swallowed maternal blood (melaena neonatorum). Haematochezia in the neonatal period is most commonly associated with a colitis secondary to an intolerance to milk protein. It may be a direct intolerance to cow or soy milk protein (Powell, 1978; Coello-Ramirez and Larrosa-Haro, 1984), or can be induced indirectly through breast milk in mothers drinking cow's milk (Lake et al, 1982), or possibly through transplacental sensitization (Sherman and Cox, 1982). Sigmoidoscopy may show erythema and friability of the mucosa, which return to normal within 72 h after withdrawal of the offending antigen. The patient with intolerance to cow's milk formula often is intolerant to soy protein as well (Halpin et al, 1977).

Other serious conditions presenting with blood in the stool during the newborn period include necrotizing enterocolitis, Hirschsprung's disease with enterocolitis, and malrotation with an associated volvulus (Table 3). Although necrotizing enterocolitis is generally associated with prematurity, 10% of all cases do occur in full-term infants. The first symptoms are usually seen between the third and tenth day of life, including temperature instability, apnoea, and bradycardia—all nonspecific signs of sepsis. With time, abdominal distention, increased gastric residuals, and GI bleeding in the form of guaiac positive or grossly bloody stools may then arise. The diagnosis is supported by the detection of pneumatosis intestinalis on abdominal radiographs. Malrotation with midgut volvulus is most commonly seen during this period, and constitutes a surgical emergency. If melaena is present, it signifies vascular compromise. Hirschsprung's disease may present with enterocolitis in 24% of infants and children (Teitelbaum et al, 1988).

Infectious colitis also needs to be considered in the newborn with LGI bleeding. The infectious agent is usually bacterial (e.g. *Salmonella, Shigella, Yersinia enterolitica, Campylobacter jejuni*, or *E. coli*) or parasitic (*Entamoeba histolytica, Dientamoeba fragilis*). The small amount of blood is mixed with mucus or stool. Microscopic examination of the stool reveals abundant leukocytes, and stool cultures may confirm the diagnosis.

Finally, vascular malformations of the GI tract are rare causes of GI bleeding in newborns. These are suggested when similar lesions are observed on the skin and when a thrill or bruit is either palpated or auscultated over the abdomen.

Infants and children less than 2 years

In this age group, both very benign and very serious lesions may be associated with GI bleeding. These include Mallory–Weiss tear, oesophagitis, intussusception, Meckel's diverticulum, duplication cyst, inflammatory bowel disease, and lymphonodular hyperplasia of the colon, in addition to the causes seen in neonates (see Tables 2 and 3). Mallory–Weiss tear is a laceration at the gastro-oesophageal junction resulting from forceful or prolonged vomiting (Powell et al, 1984). The diagnosis is confirmed only by endoscopy (Michel et al, 1980). Oesophagitis secondary to gastro-oesophageal reflux usually presents as occult blood in the stool. Since scintigraphy or pH-monitoring studies can only confirm the presence or absence of reflux, oesophagoscopy is the diagnostic tool of choice.

Idiopathic intussusception involves mostly the ileocaecal valve region, without a lead point identified. Sixty-five percent of cases occur before 1 year of age, and 80% by 2 years of age. The diagnosis is suggested by the sudden onset of abdominal pain, and the passage of stools mixed with blood and mucus (currant-jelly stool). A mass in the right lower quadrant may be palpated. This diagnosis is confirmed by a gentle barium enema, which may also be therapeutic.

Meckel's diverticulum is the result of incomplete obliteration of the omphalomesenteric duct, and it is usually located within 100 cm of the ileocaecal valve. It presents with either intermittent or massive painless GI bleeding. In most cases, the cause of bleeding is ectopic gastric mucosa within the diverticulum. Diagnosis is usually confirmed by performing a technetium-99 (^{99m}Tc) scan (Meckel's scan), to demonstrate the ectopic gastric mucosa. Duplications of the small intestine are uncommon. They are usually found in the ileum, and are connected with the bowel at their distal end. They may contain gastric mucosae, causing peptic ulceration of the intestine and subsequent bleeding. A Meckel's scan is often positive when ectopic mucosa is present.

Both ulcerative colitis and Crohn's disease have been reported in infants and young children. Benign nodular lymphoid hyperplasia ranks behind anal fissure and allergic colitis as a cause of bright red LGI tract bleeding in infants less than 1 year of age (Kaplan et al, 1984). The diagnosis is made by sigmoidoscopy or by air contrast radiography. Finally, anal fissures are the most common cause of LGI bleeding in this age group. In most cases, fissures are secondary to constipation. However, the paediatrician should always keep in mind that anal fissures, regardless of the age group, may be the result of sexual abuse.

Children over 2 years

Upper GI bleeding in this age group is most likely related to peptic ulcer disease, gastritis, or oesophagitis (Table 2). Less common causes include variceal bleeding in patients with portal hypertension, and Dieulafoy's lesion, a ruptured thick-walled arterial vessel with no associated ulceration (Hoffman et al, 1984).

The two conditions most likely to cause LGI bleeding in children are juvenile polyps and infectious enterocolitis; other causes are given in Table 3.

Juvenile polyps usually present as painless rectal bleeding in an otherwise healthy preschool child. They rarely occur before 1 year of age or during adolescence. Juvenile polyps account for 90% of all polyps found in children and associated malignancy (adenocarcinoma) has been reported in isolated rare instances. An air contrast barium enema is adequate for diagnosis, but colonoscopy is preferred because it allows polypectomy to be performed at the same time.

Haematochezia may be the presenting manifestation of several multisystemic diseases. These include haemolytic–uraemic syndrome which initially resembles ulcerative colitis (Craner and Burdick, 1976), and Henoch–Schönlein purpura (Byrn et al, 1976). Less common causes of LGI bleeding include leiomyoma (Nader and Margolin, 1966), arteriovenous malformations (Myer et al, 1981), and intestinal ulcers (Sunaryo et al, 1981; Testart et al, 1988).

The incidence of inflammatory bowel disease increases sharply during adolescence to become a very common cause of LGI bleeding in this age group. Finally, GI bleeding in the immune-compromised host can present a diagnostic dilemma (Berry and Perrault, 1991); opportunistic infections and neutropenic colitis need to be ruled out.

ASSESSMENT

General principles

Determining the urgency of the situation has to take priority while evaluating a patient with GI bleeding. A team approach, including a special-care nurse, paediatrician, paediatric gastroenterologist, paediatric surgeon, and intensivist, can most effectively deliver such care by integrating early stabilization and therapeutic efforts with ongoing information gathering. A brief history should be obtained immediately, and a more detailed history to follow if the clinical situation allows it. Questions regarding the patient's medical history, bleeding tendencies, and the use of any medications are important early on. A description of the bleeding episode (e.g. haematemesis, melaena, and haematochezia) will direct the diagnostic and therapeutic approach.

The initial physical examination assesses the stability of the patient; the finding of tachycardia associated with orthostatic hypotension suggests a large volume deficit (10–20% of total blood volume) and dictates a quick replacement of the lost blood, and the use of plasma expanders (e.g. lactated-ringer, plasmanate). Once the patient has been stabilized or deemed stable, a more complete examination will follow.

Confirmation of gastrointestinal bleeding

In the newborn, it is important first to determine whether red blood cells are foetal (GI bleeding) or maternal (swallowed blood). A simple bedside test was described by Apt and Downey (Apt and Downey, 1955) to differentiate foetal from maternal blood by the addition of sodium hydroxide to the blood. Foetal blood remains pink, owing to the alkaline resistance of foetal haemoglobin, whereas adult haemoglobin gives a brown colour. The test should not be performed with melaena or coffee-ground gastric contents, since the blood is already denatured. A biochemical analysis of gastric contents or the stool can provide a rapid answer to confirming the presence of blood. In gastric fluids, Gastroccult® provides the most reliable confirmation of blood, mainly because of its stability in acidic environment (Rosenthal et al, 1984). The stool analysis can be performed on a specimen retrieved by rectal examination, using orthotoluidine or guaiac; the peroxidase contained in haemoglobin leads to oxidation of the reagent, resulting in a blue discoloration. However, it is worth noting that peroxidases are present not only in human haemoglobin, but also in animal blood and in myoglobin, so that a false-positive reaction can be obtained in a patient who recently ate red meat. Also, iron preparations (Lifton and Kreiser, 1982) and certain plant peroxidases give a false-positive test, whereas large doses of ascorbic acid inhibit the reaction (Ahlquist and Beart, 1985).

More recently, we have been using a new assay, HemoQuant®. It measures quantitatively the amount of haemoglobin present per unit of stool volume. The upper limit of normal is defined as less than 2 mg of faecal haemoglobin per gram of stool. HemoQuant® is unaffected by many of the factors that interfere with guaiac testing (Ahlquist et al, 1984).

Localizing the site of bleeding

Nasogastric tubes

As soon as the presence of GI bleeding has been established, it is critical to determine the site of bleeding. Insertion of a nasogastric tube, and aspiration of the gastric contents rapidly differentiate upper from lower GI bleeding. If the aspirate is positive for blood, the site of bleeding is almost always proximal to the ligament of Treitz. However, the physician needs to remember that a negative aspirate does not exclude a bleeding site beyond the pylorus. A Sengstaken–Blakemore tube, or one of its modifications (Teres et al, 1978), can be used diagnostically in a patient bleeding acutely and profusely, especially a patient known to harbour varices. The tube is available in a paediatric size or can be adapted for a young child (Kline, 1986).

Upper GI endoscopy

It is indicated for the evaluation of haematemesis or a nasogastric tube aspirate of fresh or old blood. It is also indicated in cases of melaena, or the passage of large amounts of blood from the rectum. The introduction of fibreoptic endoscopes in the 1960s has radically changed our approach to diagnosis and management of GI bleeding. State-of-the-art, ultrathin instruments now transmit endoscopic images to TV monitors. These endoscopes permit easy oral passage with minimal patient discomfort, and maximal safety. Moreover, these instruments have the capacity for certain therapeutic interventions such as sclerotherapy of bleeding varices, cauterization of bleeding vessels, and removal of polyps. There is a clear advantage of fibreoptic endoscopy over contrast radiography in the evaluation of the patient with GI bleeding. These advantages include: the ability to visualize directly the bleeding lesion not detected by radiography (Tedesco et al, 1976; Gryboski, 1981); the determination of the bleeding lesion when more than one lesion is identified (Ament et al, 1988); and the immediate use of other diagnostic modalities if no lesion is found. When contrast radiography is used, 2 or 3 days may be required to clear the intestinal tract.

In the pre-endoscopic era, 20–50% of bleeding sites remained unidentified (Sherman and Clatworthy, 1967; Cadranel et al, 1977), compared to less than 20% at the present time (Cox and Ament, 1979; Hyams et al, 1985; Ament et al, 1988). Upper endoscopy in children is safe in expert hands (Tedesco et al, 1976; Prolla et al, 1983; Ament et al, 1988). Complications should remain below 1%, whether routine or emergency UGI endoscopy is performed. These complications could be related to sedation (thrombophlebitis or respiratory arrest), to general anaesthesia, or to the procedure itself (sore throat, aspiration pneumonia, or rare perforation) (Gryboski, 1981; Katron, 1981; Ament et al, 1988).

Lower GI endoscopy

This includes anoscopy, sigmoidoscopy, and total colonoscopy. The choice of procedure depends on the clinical situation.

(a) Anoscopy. This procedure permits a good visualization of the anal canal. It is indicated in the evaluation of bright red blood from the rectum, especially in patients with local symptoms such as painful defecation (anal fissure). It is a simple procedure and is frequently underutilized (Cucchiara et al, 1983).

(b) Flexible proctosigmoidoscopy. It is indicated in almost all cases of haematochezia where physical examination did not identify a perianal source of bleeding. The instrument ranges between 30 and 65 cm in length (Haubrich, 1985). Mild sedation for younger patients at the time of procedure and a rectal enema half an hour prior to it will allow a more comfortable and accurate examination. This procedure will permit visualization of the mucosa, and biopsies may be obtained whenever indicated. Perforation, particularly in the sigmoid colon, is a rare but well described complication.

(c) Colonoscopy. Colonoscopy is the procedure of choice in patients with LGI bleeding, unless anoscopy or sigmoidoscopy have disclosed an actively bleeding lesion. Examination of the terminal ileum if Crohn's disease is suspected, polypectomy, electrocautery, or laser treatment of a bleeding lesion are distinct advantages over barium enema (Cadranel et al, 1977; Tedesco et al, 1978; Maxfield and Maxfield, 1986). Unless there is a suspicion of intestinal obstruction or toxic megacolon, an oral lavage solution such as GoLYTELY® (Braintree Laboratories Inc.) or Colyte® (Edlaw Preparations Inc.) in a dose of 20 ml/kg/h for 4 h is used to prepare the colon. Sedation is preferable to general anaesthesia to limit the risk of perforation by allowing the patient to respond to increased pressure. A combination of meperidine (Demerol®) and midazolam (Versed®) is frequently used.

Scintigraphic studies

When applied selectively, nuclear medicine imaging offers the capability of prolonged monitoring, particularly useful in patients with intermittent bleeding. In addition, these radiopharmaceuticals help in the detection of abnormally located gastric mucosa (e.g. Meckel's diverticulum).

(a) ^{99m}Tc-pertechnetate scan (Meckel's scan). It identifies functional gastric mucosa in an ectopic location such as Meckel's diverticulum and duplications of the small intestine.

^{99m}Tc pertechnetate is injected intravenously. Images are then obtained every 5 min for 1 h. A Meckel's diverticulum is often seen as an abnormal focal collection of radioactive substances, usually in the right lower quadrant of the abdomen (Sfakianakis and Conway, 1981). It is noticed on the images taken 30–60 min after the injection of the radioactive material. On the other hand, duplications of the small intestine can be spotted anywhere in the abdominal field.

A number of reasons may give rise to a false-positive Meckel's scan (Table 4). These include any highly vascularized lesions such as arteriovenous malformations (Wesselhoeft et al, 1986), haemangioma, and

Table 4. False results with Meckel's scan.

False-positive	False-negative
1. Focal collection of radioactive material: —ureteral obstruction —sacral meningomyelocele	1. Overlap by adjacent organs: —bladder overdistention —stomach overlap
2. Vascular lesions: —haemangioma —arteriovenous malformations	2. The presence of barium in the GI tract
3. Inflammatory lesions: —Crohn's disease —intussusception	3. Lack of sufficient gastric mucosa in the diverticulum

inflammatory bowel disease. Also, false-positive results have been reported with ureteral obstruction, and meningomyelocele due to local accumulation of the radioactive substance. False-negative results do occur in cases of Meckel's diverticulum devoid of gastric mucosa, or containing less than 1 cm^2 of gastric mucosa [10% of Meckel's diverticula do not contain gastric mucosa (Majd, 1985)] and in cases of unusual location of the diverticulum behind the stomach, or bladder where the local activity of these organs will mask the activity from the diverticulum. Overall, sensitivity and specificity of Meckel's scan in detecting Meckel's diverticulum have been estimated at 85 and 95%, respectively (Cooney et al, 1982). The sensitivity can probably be enhanced with the addition of histamine H_2 receptor antagonist or pentagastrin to stimulate the technetium uptake (Treves et al, 1978; Baum, 1981).

(b) ^{99m}Tc-labelled red blood cells (bleeding scan). Patients with suspected mild or moderate LGI bleeding benefit most from this scintigraphic technique. It gives the ability to image the intermittently bleeding patient over a prolonged period of time. Although gastric and proximal small bowel bleeding lesions may be demonstrated, the high liver/spleen activity tends to obscure the upper abdomen and limits the sensitivity of the test in this region. The technique involves labelling the patient's own red blood cells with ^{99m}Tc pertechnetate. Maximal labelling is achieved in vitro (Callahan et al, 1982). Over 95% of technetium is bound to red cells, and in dog studies, it detects a bleeding rate of less than 0.1 ml/min (Datz et al, 1986). In humans, a bleeding rate greater than 0.1 ml/min is thought to give a positive scan (Smith et al, 1987). These figures compare very favourably with a minimum bleeding rate of 0.5 ml/min for positive angiography.

A positive bleeding scan may allow more selective angiographic studies, thereby decreasing the dye load. However, if the bleeding scan is negative, angiography should be delayed (Maeda and Yamashiro, 1986).

Angiography

Its main indication is to localize the bleeding site in an actively bleeding patient where endoscopy has failed. It has been estimated that a bleeding rate of 0.5 ml/min is required to have a positive test (Afshani and Berger, 1986). In chronic or intermittent GI bleeding, angiography has identified a potential bleeding site in approximately 50% of adults (Sheedy et al, 1975; Thompson et al, 1987) and 43% of children (Meyerovitz and Fellows, 1984).

The technique involves heavy sedation, or general anaesthesia. A selective catheterization of the inferior and superior mesenteric arteries is usually done through the femoral artery. If that fails to provide a diagnosis, then selective catheterization of the colonic axis follows. Extravasation of the dye to the GI tract indicates an actively bleeding lesion, while a mucosal 'blush' represents a vascular lesion or an arteriovenous malformation (Sheedy et al, 1975; Best et al, 1979).

Angiography has also proven effective as a therapeutic procedure. Once a bleeding site is identified, the angiographic catheter can be left in position for therapy either by embolization of vascular malformations or local infusion of a vasoconstrictor such as Vasopressin (Baum and Nusbaum, 1971; Goldman et al, 1978; Athanasoulis, 1980).

Complications at the puncture site (bleeding, haematoma, pseudo-aneurysm, and arterial obstruction), from the catheter guidewire (breakage, embolism, vessel perforation), from the radiographic contrast (renal failure, and hypersensitivity reaction) and from cardiovascular reactions (vaso-vagal, arrhythmia) remain at about 1.7% (Mistretta et al, 1981; Gelfand et al, 1992).

Small intestinal endoscopy

It is defined as the endoscopic examination of the small intestine beyond the ligament of Treitz. This can be achieved either by using the enteroscopic techniques or by performing intraoperative endoscopy.

(a) Enteroscopy. It uses a paediatric colonoscope to reach the jejunum (jejunoscopy). However, a specially-made enteroscope ('sonde-type' small intestinal endoscope) has also been used. Essentially, it is a very long and passive fibreoptic bundle without biopsy capability, with a distensible balloon at the tip to let intestinal peristaltic movements carry it down toward the ileum. It was estimated that enteroscopy is able to identify a potential source of bleeding in approximately 33% of patients with chronic GI bleeding after all other investigations have been negative (Lewis and Waye, 1988). However, these figures apply to adults only. The paediatric experience is still in its infancy.

(b) Intraoperative endoscopy. It permits examination of the whole intestine. Three possible modes of access can be used: via the mouth; via a surgical enterotomy; or via the anus. After the instrument is introduced, the intestine is gradually telescoped over the endoscope by the surgeon. Bowen and colleagues were able to identify a real or potential bleeding site in 93% of patients presenting with GI bleeding of obscure aetiology (Bowden et al, 1979). Another report from Mayo Clinic (Ress et al, 1992) identified some type of mucosal abnormality in 70% of patients with obscure GI bleeding. However 52% of patients re-bled after resection of the identified lesion.

Contrast radiography

Barium radiography is still used in cases of GI bleeding. However, its use is limited by its lower sensitivity compared with endoscopy or angiography,

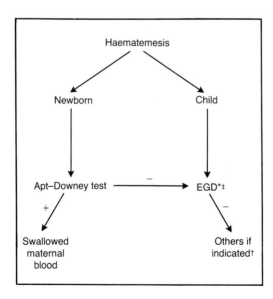

Figure 1. Diagnostic algorithm for patients with upper gastrointestinal bleeding. * After oropharyngeal source has been ruled out; † bleeding scan, or angiography; ‡ EGD—oeso-phagogastroduodenoscopy.

and by the inability to utilize other diagnostic modalities (endoscopy, angiography, radionuclide scanning, abdominal CT, etc.) once barium coats the GI tract. Enteroclysis (the rapid infusion of contrast directly into the small bowel through a catheter passed orally or nasally beyond the ligament of Treitz) continues to play a major role for ruling out structural defects in the small intestine such as tumours, strictures, and fistulae (Maglinte et al, 1984, 1985). It also detects Meckel's diverticula in some cases. However, this test will not identify arteriovenous malformations or other vascular lesions. The main disadvantage of enteroclysis is the need for intubation of the small intestine, and the resulting discomfort to the patient.

How to use the diagnostic tests

In order to provide proper and effective treatment for patients with GI bleeding, an accurate diagnosis is essential, helped by proper use of the different diagnostic modalities. A diagnostic scheme is provided as a general guidance to follow (Figures 1 and 2). Adjustments may need to be done depending on the clinical setting, and on many occasions observation might be the proper approach if the patient is stable and the clinical setting does not suggest ongoing bleeding.

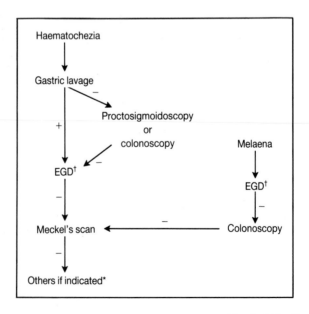

Figure 2. Diagnostic algorithm for patients with lower gastrointestinal bleeding. * Bleeding scan, angiography, small bowel enteroscopy, or intraoperative endoscopy; † EGD—oesophagogastroduodenoscopy.

THERAPEUTIC APPROACHES

Stabilizing the patient

Before any consideration is given to antacids, medications or therapeutic endoscopies, the primary concern is to stabilize the patient. Whether in the emergency room or at the bedside, one approach to the bleeding patient is for the physician to proceed with the history as the examination is being conducted, paying particular attention to the vital signs. Tachycardia, a thready pulse, orthostatism implicate large blood losses, and require prompt attention. Venous access is secured with large-bore catheters (two different sites in briskly bleeding patients) rather than butterfly needles which can easily dislodge. Laboratory studies, including blood typing and crossmatching, may be drawn at that time, and fluids and/or colloids may subsequently be infused. When UGI bleeding is suspected, a nasogastric tube is inserted for diagnostic and decompression purposes. When the patient is unstable, or brisk bleeding is evident, transfer to the intensive care unit is initiated, where proper observation and monitoring will be assured.

Hypovolaemia may be corrected with colloid or crystalloid, while haematocrit is restored with blood transfusions. When the bleeding does not alter the vital signs, we will often delay blood transfusions unless the patient has an underlying condition (such as cardiac disease) that may quickly decompensate. Urgent blood transfusion may be carried out with group O blood while waiting for type-specific blood, but only after typing and crossmatching to prevent subsequent difficulties. Group O packed red cells with low anti-A, anti-B titres reduce the risk of subsequent haemolysis. The only circumstance when typing may be omitted is when a sample of that patient's blood has been typed within 48 h; type-specific unmatched blood has been used without major problem in this circumstance (Gervin and Fischer, 1984). Information about the blood type of a patient obtained from the parent, the patient or a wallet card may be erroneous; a parent may mistakenly give the blood type of a sibling, or the patient may carry a wrong card (for whatever reason!). It takes only 15 min to do an immediate spin (saline) crossmatch; important ABO system antibodies are detected. A more complete crossmatching takes 45–90 min.

Hypothermia may follow transfusion of cool blood; a rewarming pump should be used as soon as possible. Certain clinical situations may dictate the use of platelets, fresh frozen plasma, or cryoprecipitates. Only when all the appropriate resuscitative manoeuvres have been in place, with adequate stabilization, should the patient be allowed to proceed with the indicated diagnostic tests.

Therapeutic modalities

The focus is on identifying, then neutralizing, the site of bleeding. Lavage of accumulated blood and clots will facilitate proper endoscopic visualization, and possibly therapy. If the returns from a nasogastric tube are bloody, saline or tap water at room temperature may be safely used by infusion and aspiration to clear the stomach. Iced saline lavage has not been shown to be superior to fluid at room temperature, and may even have deleterious effects, such as increasing the bleeding time and prothrombin time (Waterman and Walker, 1973), increasing the susceptibility of the mucosa to stress ulceration (Menguy and Masters, 1981), and may reduce tissue oxygenation due to a shift of the haemoglobin–oxygen dissociation curve to the left. For large clots, a large-bore orogastric tube should be used; it is passed with the patient in the left lateral decubitus position, after applying pharyngeal anaesthesia. A continuous bright red blood return from nasogastric lavage indicates acute bleeding and requires immediate intensive management. Variable shades of red returns in an otherwise stable patient could represent mixing of the lavage fluid with a clot. Coffee-ground material may imply a recent, but not current, bleeding event. Clear lavage fluid does not rule out an actively bleeding duodenal ulcer; parenthetically, large amounts of bright red blood from the rectum may indicate massive UGI bleeding, especially in a haemodynamically unstable patient. In preparation for urgent colonoscopy, rapid colonic lavage may be achieved with a nonabsorbable polyethylene glycol–electrolytes solution taken orally or via a nasogastric tube (20 ml/kg/h for 2–4 h).

Therapeutic manoeuvres

Until recently, identification of a bleeding lesion did not necessarily imply decreased blood transfusion requirements or improved survival, until the advent of therapeutic endoscopy. Now the gastroenterologist has the advantage of identifying a bleeding site, and of attempting to stop the bleeding at the same time. But when the bleeding is active, visualization of the bleeding site is not always possible, and temporizing methods will often permit a cleaner field.

1. *'Vasoactive' lavage*. For want of a better term, it refers to the addition of epinephrine (1 : 10 000 solution) (Gostout et al, 1992) or Levarterenol (8 mg/ 100 ml) (Ament, 1990) to the lavage solution, especially when directed endoscopically at the bleeding site; this has the potential of decreasing the bleeding even if only transiently, thus permitting a cleaner field of vision.

2. *Vasopressin, somatostatin (octreotide)*. The parenteral injection of these agents decreases the splanchnic blood flow with subsequent decreased GI bleeding. At first injected intra-arterially at the time of selective arteriography, vasopressin is now used almost exclusively intravenously, with as much effectiveness but less complications (Chojkier et al, 1979). Since it reduces cardiac output and arterial blood flow through the splanchnic bed, resulting in a fall in portal vein pressure, it is used particularly in bleeding from prehepatic portal hypertension, Mallory–Weiss tear, and stress-induced gastritis. The dose is 0.2–0.4 unit/1.73 m^2/min administered by continuous i.v. infusion. Careful monitoring of the patient is imperative since arrhythmias, hypertension, oliguria, and seizures from water retention (due to its antidiuretic hormone effect) have all been reported. Somatostatin and its synthetic analogue, octreotide both affect the haemodynamics of splanchnic circulation; the resistance of splanchnic arterioles is increased,

resulting in decreased flow to the portal system and its collaterals. Since the half-life of somatostatin is short, octreotide is used preferentially although it does not have a more prolonged effect on wedged hepatic venous pressure or intravariceal pressure (Jenkins, 1992). They are used intravenously (somatostatin 250 μg/h; octreotide 25 μg/h in adults) or by subcutaneous injection (octreotide 50 μg/h every 6 h). Their effectiveness in bleeding related to portal hypertension has been demonstrated in randomized studies (Hwang et al, 1992; Shields et al, 1992). Somatostatin affects the GI function, and some deleterious effects have been reported on the renal function in cirrhotics, and although continued attention to side-effects is imperative, their therapeutic use has not been curtailed (Dudley, 1992; Jenkins et al, 1993). Somatostatin has also been advocated for gastro-duodenal haemorrhage, because it reduces gastric acidity, gastrin pro-duction, and gastric blood flow (Reichlin, 1983), although this indication might still be controversial (Basso et al, 1986).

3. *Balloon tamponade.* Less used now but no less effective, the Sengstaken–Blakemore tube and its modifications (Sengstaken and Blakemore, 1950; Pitcher, 1971) provide a first-line approach to controlling bleeding in oesophageal–fundic variceal bleeding, and may also be used in Mallory–Weiss tears. It is not well tolerated without sedation, and the patient needs to be monitored carefully in the intensive care unit while the tube is in place, given the severe complications related to its use (gastric dilatation, aspiration, oesophageal ulcer). Its use is extensively reviewed elsewhere (Berry and Perrault, 1991).

4. *Therapeutic endoscopy.* The development of more sophisticated diagnostic instruments led to the elaboration of even more sophisticated therapeutic adaptations.

(a) Sclerotherapy. Although first described in 1939 (Crafoord and Frenckner, 1939), it was long abandoned until recently. The principle is to inject a sclerosing solution alongside, or more frequently directly into the varix; multiple sessions are required to achieve total obliteration of the variceal vessels (Lilly and Stellin, 1984; Donovan et al, 1986; Hassal et al, 1989; Hill and Bowie, 1991). The complications range from local (ulcer, pain, stricture) to systemic (fever, pleural effusion) effects (Howard et al, 1984; Van Stiegman and Stellin, 1985), to vascular events possibly related to the sclerosing solution (thoracic spinal cord paralysis) (Seidman et al, 1984). Endoscopic injection to achieve haemostasis is also used in other bleeding lesions (peptic ulcers, vascular malformations) with some success (Schuman, 1987; Lin et al, 1993).

(b) Oesophageal banding. Because of the local and systemic compli-cations associated with sclerosing solutions, a novel approach to controlling oesophageal variceal bleeding has been developed, mainly based on the experience with haemorrhoidal banding: endoscopic variceal ligation, or banding. The encircling of a segment of a varix with a tight elastic band seems to induce tissue sloughing by strangulation and tissue necrosis. Recent comparative studies with sclerotherapy indicate similar results, but less complications with banding in adult patients (Laine et al, 1993; Sivak and Catalano, 1993).

(c) Therapeutic endoscopy. More than just a diagnostic tool, endoscopy has opened the door to exciting therapeutic avenues, from thermal to electrocoagulation, to laser photocoagulation (Berry and Perrault, 1991), and soon to a microwave system (Kalabakas et al, 1993), applicable to bleeding lesions of both the upper and lower GI tract. The re-bleeding risk from an inactive visible vessel at the time of endoscopy is close to 60% (Swain et al, 1986); endoscopically directed treatment at that time may prevent further bleeding. Thermal and electrocoagulation depend on accurate pressure application before delivering the coagulation energy, whereas laser photocoagulation requires no contact with the bleeding site, which can be advantageous in acutely bleeding lesions, or in fragile lesions like vascular malformations. These techniques have been adapted to children (Noronha and Leist, 1988; Tedesco, 1988). Surrounding tissue injury, even perforation from full-thickness injury, especially in the caecum, are feared complications.

PROPHYLAXIS

In certain circumstances, it might be possible to prevent GI bleeding, and this applies in particular to critically ill children. The incidence of UGI bleeding in the paediatric intensive care unit is variable, but greater than in the general population (Lacroix et al, 1992; Lopez-Herce et al, 1992b). Even patients in a neonatal intensive care unit may be at increased risk for oesophageal and gastric lesions (Mäki et al, 1993). Prostaglandins provide protection to the gastroduodenal mucosa; the levels of prostaglandin E_2 in gastric juice and plasma of critically ill children were significantly lower in critically ill patients when compared to controls (Lopez-Herce et al, 1992b). Gastrointestinal bleeding usually becomes manifest in the first 3 days of hospitalization in the intensive care (Lacroix et al, 1992; Lopez-Herce et al, 1992a). H_2-blockers (ranitidine 1.5 mg/kg i.v. q.i.d.), antacids or sucralfate (0.5–1 g/nasogastric tube q.i.d.) were found to reduce significantly the incidence of UGI bleeding in critically ill children when compared to placebo (Lopez-Herce et al, 1992a). Driks et al (1987) raised a note of caution in the use of antacids or H_2-blocker in intubated patients; because of the changes in gastric pH, nosocomial pneumonia may be more frequent with these agents, when compared with sucralfate which does not raise the gastric pH. Enteral alimentation in mechanically ventilated adult patients provided as much, if not better, protection from bleeding when compared to antacids or cimetidine (Pingleton and Hadzima, 1983).

SUMMARY

This chapter on gastrointestinal (GI) bleeding is intended to provide a framework and practical approach to the diagnosis and treatment of this often frightening medical condition. A brief overview of the pathophysiology of GI bleeding is designed to permit a better understanding of the diagnostic and therapeutic measures. Four categories of lesions are then presented: mucosal, vascular, lesions associated with portal hypertension, and lesions associated with coagulopathies.

The section on causes of GI bleeding is discussed in an age-orientated manner, emphasizing the more common aetiologies in each age group, thereby allowing a proper approach to the patient.

Since the 'endoscopic revolution' has radically transformed the diagnostic and therapeutic approaches to the patient with GI bleeding, we review the methods and indications for newly emerging diagnostic endoscopic procedures such as enteroscopy and intraoperative endoscopy, as well as therapeutic endoscopic interventions.

The text is supported by two algorithms outlining a general practical approach for diagnosis, keeping in mind the need to individualize this approach in most cases.

REFERENCES

Abrahamson J & Shandling B (1973) Intestinal hemangiomata in childhood and a syndrome for diagnosis: a collective review. *Journal of Pediatric Surgery* **8:** 487–495.

Abramson DJ (1964) Curling's ulcer in childhood: review of the literature and report of five cases. *Surgery* **55:** 321–336.

Afshani E & Berger PE (1986) Gastrointestinal tract angiography in infants and children. *Journal of Pediatric Gastroenterology and Nutrition* **5:** 173–186.

Ahlquist DA & Beart RW (1985) Use of fecal occult blood tests in the detection of colorectal neoplasia. *Problems in General Surgery* **2:** 200–210.

Ahlquist DA, McGill DB, Schwartz S et al (1984) Hemoquant, a new quantitative assay for fecal hemoglobin. Comparison with hemoccult. *Annals of Internal Medicine* **101:** 297–302.

Allison MC, Howatson AG, Torrance CJ et al (1992) Gastrointestinal damage associated with the use of nonsteroidal anti-inflammatory drugs. *New England Journal of Medicine* **327:** 749–754.

Alvarez F, Bernard O, Brunelle F et al (1983) Portal obstruction in children. I. clinical investigation and hemorrhage risk. *Journal of Pediatrics* **103:** 696–702.

Ament ME (1990) Diagnosis and management of upper gastrointestinal tract bleeding in the pediatric patient. *Pediatrics Review* **12:** 107–116.

Ament ME, Berquist WE, Vargas J et al (1988) Fibreoptic upper intestinal endoscopy in infants and children. *Pediatric Clinics of North America* **35:** 141–155.

Apt L & Downey WS Jr (1955) 'Melena' neonatorum: the swallowed blood syndrome. *Journal of Pediatrics* **47:** 6–12.

Athanasoulis CA (1980) Therapeutic applications of angiography. *New England Journal of Medicine* **302:** 1117–1125.

Basso N, Bagarani M, Bracci F et al (1986) Ranitidine and somatostatin. Their effects on bleeding from the upper gastrointestinal tract. *Archives of Surgery* **121:** 833–835.

Baum S (1981) Pertechnetate imaging following cimetidine administration in Meckel's diverticulum of the ileum. *American Journal of Gastroenterology* **76:** 464–465.

Baum S & Nusbaum M (1971) The control of gastrointestinal hemorrhage by selective mesenteric arterial infusion of vasopressin. *Radiology* **98:** 497–505.

Beighton PH, Murdoch JL & Votteler T (1969) Gastrointestinal complications of the Ehlers–Danlos syndrome. *Gut* **10:** 1004–1008.

Berezin S, Newman L & Russe J (1986) Hemorrhage and shock due to intestinal malabsorption. *Pediatric Emergency Care* **2:** 91–92.

Berry R & Perrault J (1991) Gastrointestinal bleeding. In Walker WA, Durie PR et al (eds) *Pediatric Gastrointestinal Disease*, pp 111–131. Philadelphia: BC Decker.

Best EB, Teaford AK & Rader FH Jr (1979) Angiography in chronic/recurrent gastrointestinal bleeding: a nine year study. *Surgical Clinics of North America* **59:** 811–829.

Boley SJ, Brandt LJ & Mitsudo SM (1984) Vascular lesions of the colon. *Advances in Internal Medicine* **29:** 301–326.

Bornman PC, Theodorou NA, Shuttleworth RD et al (1985) Importance of hypovolaemic shock and endoscopic signs in predicting recurrent haemorrhage from peptic ulceration: a prospective evaluation. *British Medical Journal* **291:** 245–247.

Bowden TA Jr, Hooks VH III & Mansberger AR Jr (1979) Intraoperative gastrointestinal endoscopy in the management of occult gastrointestinal bleeding. *Southern Medical Journal* **72:** 1532–1534.

Byrn JR, Fitzgerald JF, Northway JD et al (1976) Unusual manifestations of Henoch–Schönlein syndrome. *American Journal of Diseases in Children* **130:** 1335–1337.

Cadranel S, Rodesch P, Peters JP et al (1977) Fibreendoscopy of the gastrointestinal tract in children. *American Journal of Diseases in Children* **131:** 41–45.

Callahan RJ, Forelich JW, McKusick et al (1982) A modified method for the in vivo labeling of red blood cells with Tc-99m: concise communication. *Journal of Nuclear Medicine* **23:** 315–318.

Chojkier M, Groszmann RJ, Atterbury CE et al (1979) A controlled comparison of continuous intra-arterial and intravenous infusions of vasopressin in hemorrhage from esophageal varices. *Gastroenterology* **77:** 540–546.

Coello-Ramirez P & Larrosa-Haro A (1984) Gastrointestinal occult hemorrhage and gastro-duodenitis in cow's milk protein intolerance. *Journal of Pediatric Gastroenterology and Nutrition* **3:** 215–218.

Conn HO & Blitzer BL (1976) Nonassociation of adrenocorticoid therapy and peptic ulcer. *New England Journal of Medicine* **294:** 473–479.

Cooney DR, Duszynski DO, Comboa E et al (1982) The abdominal technetium scan (A decade of experience). *Journal of Pediatric Surgery* **17:** 611–619.

Cox K & Ament ME (1979) Upper gastrointestinal bleeding in children. *Pediatrics* **63:** 408–413.

Crafoord C & Frenckner P (1939) New surgical treatment of varicose veins of the oesophagus. *Acta Otolaryngologica* **27:** 422–429.

Craner GE & Burdick (1976) Acute colitis resembling ulcerative colitis in the hemolytic–uremic syndrome. *Digestive Diseases* **21:** 74–76.

Cucchiara S, Guandalini S, Staiano A et al (1983) Sigmoidoscopy, colonoscopy and radiology in the evaluation of children with rectal bleeding. *Journal of Pediatric Gastroenterology and Nutrition* **2:** 667–671.

Datz FL, Thorne DA, Remley K et al (1986) Determination of bleeding rates necessary for imaging acute gastrointestinal bleeding with Tc-99m labeled red blood cells (Abstract). *Journal of Nuclear Medicine* **27:** 956.

Dewayne Andrews M & Papper S (1985) The kidneys and the urinary tract. In Berk JE, Haubrich WS, Kalser MH, Schaffner F (eds) *Bockus Gastroenterology*, 4th edn, pp 4613–4620. Philadelphia: WB Saunders.

Domschke S & Domschke W (1984) Gastroduodenal damage due to drugs, alcohol, and smoking. *Clinical Gastroenterology* **13:** 405–436.

Donovan TJ, Ward M & Shepherd RW (1986) Evaluation of endoscopic sclerotherapy of esophageal varices in children. *Journal of Pediatric Gastroenterology and Nutrition* **5:** 696–700.

Driks MR, Craven DE & Celli BR (1987) Nosocomial pneumonia in intubated patients given sucralfate as compared with antacids or histamine type 2 blockers. *New England Journal of Medicine* **317:** 1376–1382.

Dudley FJ (1992) Somatostatin and portal hypertensive bleeding: a safe therapeutic alterna-tive? *Gastroenterology* **103:** 1973–1977.

Fretzin DF & Potter B (1965) Blue rubber bleb nevus. *Archives of Internal Medicine* **116:** 924–929.

Fromm D (1978) Salicylate and gastric mucosal damage. *Pediatrics* **62:** 938–942.

Gelfand WD, Routh DW & Cowan JR (1992) Diagnostic imaging in gastrointestinal hemorrhage. In Sugawa G, Schuman B & Lucas C (eds) *Gastrointestinal Bleeding*, pp 205–221. New York: Igaku-Shoin Medical Publishers Inc.

Gervin AS & Fischer RP (1984) Resuscitation of trauma patients with type-specific uncross-matched blood. *Journal of Trauma* **24:** 327–331.

Gilbert DA (1990) Epidemiology of upper gastrointestinal bleeding. *Gastrointestinal Endoscopy* **36:** S8–S130.

Goldman ML, Freeny PC, Tallman JM et al (1978) Transcatheter vascular occlusion therapy with isobutyl 2-cyanoacrylate (bucrylate) for control of massive upper-gastrointestinal bleeding. *Radiology* **129:** 41–4978.

Gostout CJ, Wang KK, Ahlquist DA et al (1992) Acute gastrointestinal bleeding. Experience of a specialized management team. *Journal of Clinical Gastroenterology* **14:** 260–267.

Green M (1980) Rectal bleeding. In *Pediatric Diagnosis: Interpretation of Symptoms and Signs in Different Age Periods*, 3rd edn, p 435. Philadelphia: WB Saunders.

Grumbach MM & Conte FA (1985) Disorders of sexual differentiation. In Wilson JD & Foster DW (eds) *Textbook of Endocrinology*, 7th edn, p 341. Philadelphia: WB Saunders.

Gryboski JD (1981) The value of upper gastrointestinal endoscopy in children. *Digestive Diseases and Sciences* **26:** 17S–21S.

Halpin TC, Byrne WJ & Ament ME (1977) Colitis, persistent diarrhea and soy protein intolerance. *Journal of Pediatrics* **91:** 404–407.

Hassall E, Berquist WE, Ament ME et al (1989) Sclerotherapy for extrahepatic portal hypertension in childhood. *Journal of Pediatrics* **115:** 69–74.

Haubrich WS (1985) Proctosigmoidoscopy. In Berk JE, Haubrich WS, Kalser MH & Schaffner F (eds) *Bockus Gastroenterology*, 4th edn, p 581. Philadelphia: WB Saunders.

Hill ID & Bowie MD (1991) Endoscopic sclerotherapy for control of bleeding varices in children. *American Journal of Gastroenterology* **86:** 472–476.

Hoffmann J, Beck H & Jensen H-E (1984) Dieulafoy's lesion. *Surgery, Gynecology, Obstetrics* **159:** 537–540.

Holvoet J, Terriere L, Van Hee W et al (1991) Relation of upper gastrointestinal bleeding to non-steroidal anti-inflammatory drugs and aspirin: a case-control study. *Gut* **32:** 730–734.

Horton JW & Coln D (1985) Cardiovascular function and fluid compartments in newborn canine hemorrhagic shock. *American Journal of Physiology* **248:** R724–R731.

Howard ER, Stamatakis JD & Mowat AP (1984) Management of esophageal varices in children by injection sclerotherapy. *Journal of Pediatric Surgery* **19:** 2–5.

Hwang S-J, Lin HC, Chang C-F et al (1992) A randomised controlled trial comparing octreotide and vasopressin in the control of acute variceal bleeding. *Journal of Hepatology* **16:** 320–325.

Hyams JS, Leichtner AM & Schwartz AN (1985) Recent advances in diagnosis and treatment of gastrointestinal hemorrhage in infants and children. *Journal of Pediatrics* **106:** 1–9.

Jenkins SA (1992) Somatostatin in acute bleeding oesophageal varices. *Drugs* **44:** 36–55.

Jenkins SA, Sutton R, Kingsnorth AN & Shields R (1993) Somatostatin: safety in patients with variceal bleeding. *Gastroenterology* **105:** 642–649.

Kalabakas AA, Porter AJ, Mule L et al (1993) Design of a microwave system for endoscopy: an experimental study of energy, tissue contact, and hemostatic efficacy. *Gastroenterology* **104:** 680–689.

Kaplan B, Benson J, Rothstein F et al (1984) Lymphonodular hyperplasia of the colon as a pathologic finding in children with lower gastrointestinal bleeding. *Journal of Pediatric Gastroenterology and Nutrition* **3:** 704–709.

Katron RM (1981) Complications of upper gastrointestinal endoscopy in the gastrointestinal bleeder. *Digestive Diseases and Sciences* **26:** 47S–54S.

Kleinman PK, Brill PW & Winchester P (1986) Resolving duodenal–jejunal hematoma in abused children. *Radiology* **160:** 747–750.

Kline J (1986) Modification of the adult Blakemore tube for use in children with bleeding esophageal varices. *Journal of Pediatric Gastroenterology and Nutrition* **5:** 153–154.

Lacroix J, Infante-Rivard C, Gauthier M et al (1986) Upper gastrointestinal tract bleeding acquired in a pediatric intensive care unit: prophylaxis trial with cimetidine. *Journal of Pediatrics* **108:** 1015–1018.

Lacroix J, Nadeau D, Laberge S et al (1992) Frequency of upper gastrointestinal bleeding in a pediatric intensive care unit. *Critical Care Medicine* **20:** 35–42.

Laine L, El-Newihi HM, Migikovsky B et al (1993) Endoscopic ligation compared with sclerotherapy for the treatment of bleeding esophageal varices. *Annals of Internal Medicine* **119:** 1–7.

Lake AM, Whitington PF & Hamilton SR (1982) Dietary protein-induced colitis in breast fed infants. *Journal of Pediatrics* **101:** 906–910.

Levy M, Miller DR, Kaufman DW et al (1988) Major upper gastrointestinal tract bleeding. Relation to the use of aspirin and other nonnarcotic analgesics. *Archives of International Medicine* **148:** 281–285.

Lewis BS & Waye JD (1988) Chronic gastrointestinal bleeding of obscure origin: role of small bowel enteroscopy. *Gastroenterology* **94:** 1117–1120.

Lifton LJ & Kreiser J (1982) False-positive stool occult blood tests caused by iron preparations: a controlled study and review of the literature. *Gastroenterology* **83:** 860–863.

Lilly JR & Stellin G (1984) Variceal hemorrhage in biliary atresia. *Journal of Pediatric Surgery* **19:** 476–479.

Lin H-J, Perng C-L, Lee F-Y et al (1993) Endoscopic injection for the arrest of peptic ulcer hemorrhage: final results of a prospective, randomized comparative trial. *Gastrointestinal Endoscopy* **39:** 15–19.

Lopez-Herce J, Dorao P, Elola P et al (1992a) Frequency and prophylaxis of upper gastrointestinal hemorrhage in critically ill children: a prospective study comparing the efficacy of almagate, ranitidine, and sucralfate. *Critical Care in Medicine* **20:** 1082–1089.

Lopez-Herce J, Codoceo R, Delgado MA et al (1992b) Plasma and gastric juice levels of prostaglandins in critically ill children. *Journal of Pediatric Gastroenterology and Nutrition* **14:** 279–282.

Maddrey WC (1987) Hepatic vein thrombosis (Budd Chiari syndrome): possible association with the use of oral contraceptives. *Seminars in Liver Disease* **7:** 32–39.

Maeda M & Yamashiro Y (1986) Diagnostic red blood cell scintigraphy in GI tract bleeding from an intestinal hemangioma. *Journal of Pediatric Gastroenterology and Nutrition* **5:** 987–989.

Maglinte DDT, Hall R, Miller RE et al (1984) Detection of surgical lesions of the small bowel by enteroclysis. *American Journal of Surgery* **147:** 225–229.

Maglinte DDT, Elmore MF, Chernish SM et al (1985) Enteroclysis in the diagnosis of chronic unexplained gastrointestinal bleeding. *Diseases of the Colon and Rectum* **28:** 403–405.

Majd M (1985) Radionuclide imaging in pediatrics. *Pediatric Clinics of North America* **32:** 1573–1579.

Mäki M, Ruuska T & Kuusela A-L (1993) High prevalence of asymptomatic esophageal and gastric lesions in preterm infants in intensive care. *Critical Care in Medicine* **21:** 1863–1867.

Maxfield RG & Maxfield CM (1986) Colonoscopy as a primary diagnostic procedure in chronic gastrointestinal tract bleeding. *Archives of Surgery* **121:** 401–403.

McLaughlin WD, Kolts BE & Achem SR (1987) Nasogastric lavage compared with outcome in 101 patients seen in an emergency room for upper gastrointestinal hemorrhage. *Gastroenterology* **92:** 1529.

Menguy R & Masters YF (1981) Influence of cold on stress ulceration and on gastric mucosal blood flow and energy metabolism. *Annals of Surgery* **194:** 29–34.

Messer J, Reitman D, Sacks HS et al (1983) Association of adrenocorticosteroid therapy and peptic-ulcer disease. *New England Journal of Medicine* **309:** 21–24.

Mestre JR & Andres JM (1982) Hereditary hemorrhagic telangiectasia causing hematemesis in an infant. *Journal of Pediatrics* **101:** 577–579.

Meyer CT, Troncale FJ, Galloway S & Sheahan DG (1981) Arteriovenous malformations of the bowel: an analysis of 22 cases and a review of the literature. *Medicine* **60:** 36–48.

Meyerovitz MF & Fellows KE (1984) Angiography in gastrointestinal bleeding in children. *American Journal of Radiology* **143:** 837–840.

Michel L, Serrano A & Malt RA (1980) Mallory–Weiss syndrome. Evolution of diagnostic and therapeutic patterns over two decades. *Annals of Surgery* **192:** 716–721.

Mistretta CA, Crummy AB & Strother CM (1981) Digital angiography: a perspective. *Radiology* **139:** 273–276.

Morgan AA (1982) Recurrent gastrointestinal hemorrhage: an unusual cause. *American Journal of Gastroenterology* **77:** 925–928.

Nader PR & Margolin F (1966) Hemangioma causing gastrointestinal bleeding. *American Journal of Diseases in Children* **111:** 215–222.

Nord KS, Rossi TM & Lebenthal E (1981) Peptic ulcer in children. The predominance of gastric ulcers. *American Journal of Gastroenterology* **75:** 153–157.

Noronha PA & Leist MH (1988) Endoscopic laser therapy for gastrointestinal bleeding from congenital vascular lesions. *Journal of Pediatric Gastroenterology* **7:** 375–378.

O'Reilly RA (1985) Anticoagulant, antithrombotic and thrombolytic drugs. In Gilman AG, Goodman LS, Rall RW & Murad F (eds) *The Pharmacological Basis of Therapeutics*, 7th edn, p 1344. New York: Macmillan.

Peterson WL (1990) Clinical risk factors. *Gastrointestinal Endoscopy* **36:** S14–S15.

Pimpl W, Boeckl O, Waclawiczek HW & Heinerman M (1987) Estimation of the mortality rate of patients with severe gastroduodenal hemorrhage with the aid of a new scoring system. *Endoscopy* **19:** 101–106.

Pingleton SK & Hadzima SK (1983) Enteral alimentation and gastrointestinal bleeding in mechanically ventilated patients. *Critical Care in Medicine* **11:** 13–16.

Pinnell SR & Murad S (1983) Disorders of collagen. In Stanbury JB, Wyngaarden JB et al (eds) *The Metabolic Basis of Inherited Disease*, 5th edn, p 1434. New York: McGraw-Hill.

Pitcher JL (1971) Safety and effectiveness of the modified Sengstaken–Blakemore tube: a prospective study. *Gastroenterology* **61:** 291–298.

Powell GK (1978) Milk- and soy-induced enterocolitis in infancy. *Journal of Pediatrics* **93:** 553–560.

Powell TW, Herbst CA & Ulshen M (1984) Mallory–Weiss syndrome in a 10-month-old infant requiring surgery. *Journal of Pediatric Surgery* **19:** 596–597.

Price WH (1979) A high incidence of chronic inflammatory bowel disease in patients with Turner's syndrome. *Journal of Medical Genetics* **16:** 263–266.

Prolla JC, Diehl AS, Bemvenuti GA et al (1983) Upper gastrointestinal fiberoptic endoscopy in pediatric patients. *Gastrointestinal Endoscopy* **29:** 279–281.

Reichlin S (1983) Somatostatin. *New England Journal of Medicine* **309:** 1556–1563.

Ress AM, Benacci JC & Sarr MG (1992) Efficacy of intraoperative enteroscopy in diagnosis and prevention of recurrent, occult gastrointestinal bleeding. *American Journal of Surgery* **163:** 94–99.

Rosenthal P, Thompson J & Singh M (1984) Detection of occult blood in gastric juice. *Journal of Clinical Gastroenterology* **6:** 119–121.

Ross AJ, Siegel KR, Bell W et al (1987) Massive gastrointestinal hemorrhage in children with posterior fossa tumors. *Journal of Pediatric Surgery* **22:** 633–636.

Schmitt B, Posselt HG, Waag KL et al (1986) Severe hemorrhage from intestinal hemangiomatosis in Klippel–Trenaunay syndrome; pitfalls in diagnosis and management. *Journal of Pediatric Gastroenterology and Nutrition* **5:** 155–158.

Schuman BM (1987) Endoscopic injection therapy for nonvariceal upper gastrointestinal hemorrhage: is it too good to be true? *Gastrointestinal Endoscopy* **33:** 121–122.

Schuster DP, Rowley H, Feinstein S et al (1984) Prospective evaluation of the risk of upper gastrointestinal bleeding after admission to a medical intensive care unit. *American Journal of Medicine* **76:** 623–630.

Seidman E, Weber AM, Morin CL et al (1984) Spinal cord paralysis following sclerotherapy for esophageal varices. *Hepatology* **4:** 950–954.

Sengstaken RW & Blakemore AH (1950) Balloon tamponade for the control of hemorrhage from esophageal varices. *Annals of Surgery* **131:** 781–789.

Servelle M, Bastin R, Loygue J et al (1976) Hematuria and rectal bleeding in children with Klippel and Trenaunay syndrome. *Annals of Surgery* **183:** 418–428.

Sfakianakis GN & Conway JJ (1981) Detection of ectopic gastric mucosa in Meckel's diverticulum and in other aberrations by scintigraphy: II. Indications and methods—a 10-year experience. *Journal of Nuclear Medicine* **22:** 732–738.

Sheedy PF, Fulton RE & Atwell DT (1975) Angiographic evaluation of patients with chronic gastrointestinal bleeding. *American Journal of Radiology* **123:** 338–347.

Sherman MP & Cox KL (1982) Neonatal eosinophilic colitis. *Journal of Pediatrics* **100:** 587–589.

Sherman NJ & Clatworthy HW (1967) Gastrointestinal bleeding in neonates: a study of 94 cases. *Surgery* **62:** 614–619.

Shields R, Jenkins SA, Baxter JN et al (1992) A prospective randomised controlled trial comparing the efficacy of somatostatin with injection sclerotherapy in the control of bleeding oesophageal varices. *Journal of Hepatology* **16:** 128–137.

Silverman A & Roy CC (eds) (1983) Tumors of the peritoneum, gastrointestinal tract, liver and pancreas. In *Pediatric Clinical Gastroenterology*, 3rd edn, p 462. St. Louis: CV Mosby.

Sivak MV & Catalano MF (1993) Endoscopic ligation of esophageal varices. *Annals of Internal Medicine* **119:** 87–88.

Smith CR Jr, Bartholomew LG & Cain JC (1963) Hereditary hemorrhagic telangiectasia and gastrointestinal hemorrhage. *Gastroenterology* **44:** 1–6.

Smith R, Copely DJ & Bolen FH (1987) ^{99m}Tc RBC scintigraphy: correlation of gastrointestinal bleeding rates with scintigraphic findings. *American Journal of Radiology* **148:** 869–874.

Sunaryo FP, Boyle JT, Ziegler MM & Heyman S (1981) Primary nonspecific ileal ulceration as a cause of massive rectal bleeding. *Pediatrics* **68:** 247–250.

Swain CP (1990) Pathophysiology of bleeding lesions. *Gastrointestinal Endoscopy* **36:** S21–S22.

Swain CP, Storey DW, Brown SG et al (1986) Nature of bleeding vessel in recurrently bleeding gastric ulcers. *Gastroenterology* **90:** 595–608.

Sykes EM (1984) Colon perforation in Ehlers–Danlos syndrome. Report of two cases and review of the literature. *American Journal of Surgery* **147:** 410–413.

Tedesco FJ (1988) Endoscopic therapy for vascular lesions: new challenges. *Journal of Pediatric Gastroenterology* **7:** 321–322.

Tedesco FJ, Goldstein PD, Gleason WA et al (1976) Upper gastrointestinal endoscopy in the pediatric patient. *Gastroenterology* **70:** 492–494.

Tedesco FJ, Waye JD, Raskin et al (1978) Colonoscopic evaluation of rectal bleeding. A study of 304 patients. *Annals of Internal Medicine* **89:** 907–909.

Teitelbaum DH, Qualman SJ & Caniano DA (1988) Hirschsprung's disease. *Annals of Surgery* **207:** 240–244.

Teres J, Cecilia A, Bordas JM et al (1978) Esophageal tamponade for bleeding varices. *Gastroenterology* **75:** 566–569.

Testart J, LucMaupas J, Metayer J & Peillon C (1988) Rectal peptic ulceration—a rare cause of rectal bleeding. *Diseases of the Colon and Rectum* **31:** 803–805.

Thompson JN, Salem RR, Hemingway AP et al (1987) Specialist investigation of obscure gastrointestinal bleeding. *Gut* **28:** 47–51.

Treves S, Grand RJ & Eraklis AJ (1978) Pentagastrin stimulation of technetium-99m uptake by ectopic gastric mucosa in a Meckel's diverticulum. *Radiology* **128:** 711–712.

Van Stiegman G & Stellin GP (1985) Emergent and therapeutic upper gastrointestinal endoscopy in children. *World Journal of Surgery* **9:** 294–299.

Vase P & Grove O (1986) Gastrointestinal lesions in hereditary hemorrhagic telangiectasia. *Gastroenterology* **91:** 1079–1083.

Wara P & StØdkilde H (1985) Bleeding pattern before admission as guideline for emergency endoscopy. *Scandinavian Journal of Gastroenterology* **20:** 72–78.

Waterman NG & Walker JL (1973) The effect of gastric cooling on hemostasis. *Surgery, Gynecology, Obstetrics* **137:** 80–82.

Wesselhoeft CW, DeLuca FG & Luke M (1986) Positive ^{99m}Tc-pertechnetate scan in a child with intestinal arteriovenous malformation. *Journal of Pediatric Surgery* **21:** 71–72.

Wong SH & Lau WY (1982) Blue rubber-bleb nevus syndrome. *Diseases of the Colon and Rectum* **25:** 371–374.

Zuckerman GR, Cornette GL, Clouse RE et al (1985) Upper gastrointestinal bleeding in patients with chronic renal failure. *Annals of Internal Medicine* **102:** 588–592.

Index

Note: Page numbers of article titles are in **bold** type.

Abdomen, *see* Gastro- *aspects and also* Pain, abdominal; *see also* Stomach
Abdominal migraine, 791
Abdominal X-rays, for megarectum, 630–632
  see also X-ray investigations
Abetalipoproteinaemia, 654
Acute intermittent porphyria, 791
Age, and constipation, 626–628, 639–642
AIDS, 661, 677, 714, 718
Alagille syndrome, 674
L-Alanine, as ORS substrate, 615–616
Alkaline reflux, 779
  see also Gastro-oesophageal reflux *and also* pH, oesophageal; *see also* Oesophagus
Aluminium, 717
5-Aminosalicylate, *see* Mesalazine
Anal digital dilatation, 626–627
Anal fissures, *see under* Constipation
Anal stenosis, 626–627
Anaphylaxis, and food allergy, 729
Anderson's disease, 654
Angiography, 820
Anorectal function tests, 700–701
Anorectal manometry, 633, 701
  see also Manometry
Anorectal therapy, in constipation, 636–637
Anoscopy, 818
Antibody screening, 647
Anticholinergic therapy, 793–794
Antigens, food, 724–725
  see also Anaphylaxis, and food allergy
Apnoea, 772–774
Appendiceal colic, 790
Apt–Downey test, 813, 816
Arthritis, and IBD, 750
Aspiration, 772
Asthma, 731–732
  and gastro-oesophageal reflux, 772
Atopic dermatitis, 731
Autoimmune enteropathy, 660

Bacterial infections, 801–814
  and home parenteral nutrition, 714–715
  and IBD, 752

in liver transplants, 682
in ulcerative colitis, 757
Bacterial toxins, gut, 612–614
Balloon tamponade, 825
Barrett's oesophagus, 770–771
Barium, 821–822
  in gastro-oesophageal reflux, 774–775
Bases, in ORS, 616–617
Bernstein test, 776
Bethanechol, 780
Bicarbonate ion transport, in gut, 612
Bisacodyl, 636
Bleeding, gut, *see* Gastrointestinal bleeding
Blood-like agents, and 'gastrointestinal bleeding', 808
Blood testing, in IBD, 753
Bowel, *see* Gastro- *aspects*
Breath hydrogen analysis, 700
Breath testing, 647–648
Budd–Chiari syndrome, 812

Cancer, of liver, 673–674
Catheterization, for HPN, 707–708
  central line infections, 714–715
  line blockages, 715–716
Cevelac, 636
Charcoal, activated, 804
Chloride ions, gut transport, 612
Cholera, 612–614
Cirrhosis, *see* Liver disease
Cisapride, 780, 803–804
Coagulopathies, 812
Coeliac disease, 653
Colonic function tests, 700–701
Colonoscopy, 818
Colyte, 818
Constipation, **625–644**
  development of, 626–628, 640
    late infancy, 627, 639, 641
    neonatal, 626–627, 639
    older children, 628, 641–642
    toddlers, 627–628, 641
  diet and, 633–634
  factors causing, 625

Constipation—(cont.)
  laxatives in, 634–636
    maintenance, 635–636
    stool softeners, 634–635
  psychological treatment, 638–639
  surgery for, 637–638
  treatment of, 633–642
    psychiatric, 636–637
    rectal, 636–637
Contrast radiography, for gut bleeding, 821–822
  see also X-ray investigations
Corticosteroids, and gastrointestinal bleeding, 810
Cow's milk, see under Food allergies
Cow's milk sensitive enteropathy, 654
Crigler–Najjar type I syndrome, 673
Crohn's disease, 747–748
  diagnosis of, 753, 755
  nutritional support, 759–760
  presentation, 749
  prognosis, 761
  surgery for, 760–761
  therapy of, 758–759
  vs. ulcerative colitis, 747
  see also Inflammatory bowel disease and Ulcerative colitis
Cryptosporidiosis, 657–658
Cyclospora spp., 658
Cyclosporins, 675, 682, 757
Cystic teratoma, 791
Cytomegalovirus, 682, 796, 797

Delivery systems, for HPN, 708
Developing countries, ORT in, 617–619
  and developed countries, 619
Diarrhoea, 612–614, 655–659
  oral rehydration therapy and, see under Oral rehydration therapy (ORT)
Dicyclomine, 793
Diets—
  and constipation, 633–634
  Crohn's disease, 759–760
  elimination, in food allergy, 737–739
  and liver transplant, 678
  and paroxysmal abdominal pain, 793
  and ulcerative colitis, 759
  see also Parenteral nutrition, at home
Dioctyl, 634
Disodium cromoglycate, 739
Dissecting microscopy, 650–652
Docusate sodium, 634, 641
Down's syndrome, 647
Dysmenorrhoea, 791
Dyspepsia, pain associated with, 794–800
  diagnosis, 797–798
  differential diagnosis, 794–797
  endoscopy in, 798–799
  treatment of, 799–800

Eczema, 731
Ehlers–Danlos syndrome, 811
Electrical impedance tomography, 697
Electrogastrography, 698
Electrolytes, in the gut, 612
Electronmicroscopy, 651, 653
Endoanal sonography, 633
Endoscopy, 752, 825–826
  avulsion biopsy, 649–650
  of Crohn's disease, 755
  in dyspepsia, 798–799
  for gastrointestinal bleeding, 817–820
    lower, 818
    upper, 817–818
  and gut pain, **787–806**
  IBD and, see Inflammatory bowel syndrome
  small intestinal bleeding, 820–821
    enteroscopy, 820–821
    intraoperative, 821
Enteroaggregative E. coli, 657
Enterocytozoon bieneusi, 661
Enteropathogenic E. coli, 655–657
Eosinophilic gastroenteritis, 796–797
Epilepsy, 791
Epstein–Barr virus, 683
Escherichia coli, 612–614, 646, 655–657
Evacuants, 635
Ex-Lax chocolate, 636
Eyes, and IBD, 752

Faeces, see Stool aspects
FK506, 681
Food allergies, **723–746**
  arthralgia, 732
  challenge tests, 732–735
    skin, 735–736
  clinical features, 728–732
  colitis, 730
  definition of, 723–724
  delayed-onset, 727–728
  enteropathy, 729–730
  epidemiology, 723–724
  immediate-onset, 726–727
  immune-complex-mediated, 727
  immunology of, 724–728
  lungs and, 731–732
  management of, 727–729
  neurological effects of, 732
  prevention of, 739–740
  prognosis in, 741
  shock in, 729
  the skin and, 730, 731, 735–736
Food antigens, 724–725
Fulminating hepatitis, 672
Fundoplication, 781
Fungal infections, and liver transplant, 682

Gastric emptying, 696

Gastroccult, 817
Gastrointestinal bleeding, **807–832**
  age and, 812–816
    in neonates, 812–814
    over 2 years, 815–816
    under 2 years, 814–815
  assessment of, 816–822
  causes of, 812–816
  coagulopathies, 812
  confirmation of, 816–817
  diagnostic algorithm for, 822
  hypothermia in, 823
  hypovolaemia in, 823
  localization of, 817–822
    by angiography, 820
    by contrast radiography, 821–822
    by endoscopy, 817, 818, 820, 821
    using nasogastric tubes, 817
    using scintigraphy, 819–820
  lower, differential diagnosis, 813
  mucosal lesions in, 809–811
    inflammation, 810
    polyps, 810
    trauma, 811
    ulcers, 809–810
  pathophysiology of, 809–812
  patient stabilization in, 823
  portal hypertension, 811–812
  presentation, 807–808
  prophylaxis, 826
  therapy, 823–826
  upper, differential diagnosis, 813
  vascular lesions, 811
    haemangiomas, 811
    telangiectasias, 811
Gastrointestinal electrolyte transport, 612
Gastrointestinal food allergy, see Food
  allergies
Gastrointestinal motility tests, **689–703**
  ambulatory studies, 692–693
  anorectal function, 700–701
  colonic function, 700
  manometry, 691; see also Manometry
  oesophagus and, 693–696
  radiology and, 690–691
  scintiscanning, 691
  small intestines, 698–700
  stomach, 696–698
Gastrointestinal pain, **787–806**
Gastrointestinal water transport, 612
Gastro-oesophageal reflux, 694–696, **767–785**, 795
  evaluation in, 774–779
  gastric emptying, 696
  hiatus hernia and, 695
  hoarseness and, 774
  management of, 779–782
    acid reduction, 780–781
    by drug treatment, 779–780

  by surgery, 781–782
  oesophagitis, 770–772
  pH monitoring, 776–779
  regurgitation in, 769–770
  respiratory disorders, 772–774
Gastrostomy, 781
Giardiasis, 657–658
Glucose, as ORS substrate, 614–615
Glucose–galactose malabsorption, 659
Glycyl–glycine, 616
Golytely, 635, 641, 818
GOR, see Gastro-oesophageal reflux
Growth, and IBD, 750–751
Gut, see Gastro- aspects, Small bowel biopsy,
  Stomach and specific gut areas
Gut-associated lymphoid tissue (GALT),
  725–726

Haematemesis, 807
Haematochezia, 807, 814, 816
Hafnea alvei, 656
Heart, and liver transplant, 674
Heiner's syndrome, 732
Helicobacter pylori, 796–799
HemoQuant, 817
Henoch–Schönlein purpura, 796
Hiatus hernia, 695
Hickman–Broviac catheter, 707
Hirschsprung's disease, 626, 632–633, 639,
  693, 701, 814
HIV, see AIDS
Hoarseness, 774
Home parenteral nutrition, see Parenteral
  nutrition, at home; see also Diet and
  also Nutritional deficiency
HPN, see Parenteral nutrition, at home
H_2-receptor blockers, 780–781, 800, 826
Hyoscyamine, 793
Hypertriglyceridaemia, 654
Hypobetalipoproteinaemia, 654

Idiopathic enteropathy, 661
Idiopathic intussusception, 814–815
Immunization, in liver transplant, 677–678
Immunosuppression, 757
  and liver transplant, 680–681
Infectious diarrhoea, 612–614
Inflammatory bowel disease (IBD), **747–765**,
  815–816
  arthralgia in, 750
  diagnosis in, 752–755
  endoscopy, 802–803
  epidemiology of, 748
  eyes and, 752
  fever in, 750
  growth and, 750–751
  hepatobiliary disease and, 752
  kidneys and, 751–752
  mucocutaneous lesions, 751

Inflammatory bowel disease (IBD)—(*cont.*)
  pain in, 800–804
  nutritional support, 759–761
  presentation, 749–752
  prognosis in, 761
  sexual maturation and, 750–751
  weight loss in, 750
  see also Crohn's disease *and also* Ulcerative
    colitis
Intestinal permeability testing, 648
Intestines, *see* Gastro- *aspects and also
    specific areas of the gut*
Intravenous infusions, 707–708
  pumps for, 708
  see also Catheterization, for HPN
Isolated paroxysmal abdominal pain, 788–
    794
  diagnosis, 792
    differential, 789–792
  endoscopy for, 792
  treatment of, 793–794

Kidney—
  and IBD, 751–752
  and liver transplants, 675
Klean-Prep, 635, 641, 642
Klippel–Trenaunay syndrome, 811
Kock pouch, 760

Lactose intolerance, 802
Lactulose, 636, 641
Laxatives, 634–636
Light microscopy, 651
Lipoprotein disorders, 654–655
Liver disease, 669–673
  acute, 672–673
  chronic, 669–671
  home parenteral nutrition, 716
  metabolic, 673
Liver, and IBD, 752
Liver, portal vein hypertension and, 811–
    812
Liver transplants, **667–687**
  acute liver failure, 672–673
  blood evaluation in, 675–676
  chronic liver disease and, 669–671
    at age over 2 years, 670
    neonatal, 669–670
  contraindications, 677
  dental assessments, 675
  fulminant hepatitis, 672
  heart assessment in, 674
  hepatic complications, 678
  immunization in, 677–678
  indications for, 668–674
  inherited disorders, 673
  kidney assessment, 675
  liver function and, 675
  lungs and, assessment of, 674

metabolic liver disease and, 673
  neurological assessment, 675
  nutritional support, 678
  operative technique, 679–680
  paracetamol poisoning, 672–673
  patient evaluation, 674–679
  postoperative management and, 680–684
    early complications, 681–682
    late complications, 682–683
    quality of life and, 683–684
    retransplantation and, 682
    survival, 683
  preparation for, 677–679
  psychological aspects in, 678–679
  radiology and, 676–677
  sepsis, 682
  timing of, 671, 673
    chronic liver disease, 671
    inherited disorders, 673
  tumours, 673–674
  tyrosinaemia type I, 670
  Wilson's disease, 670–671
Liver tumours, 673–674
Loperamide, 803
Lungs—
  and food allergies, 731–732
  and gastro-oesophageal reflux, 772–774
  and liver transplants, 674
Lymphangiectasia, 654

Manometry, 633, 691–692, 694–695, 698–701,
    775
Meckel's diverticulum, 814–815
Megarectum, 628–633
  investigations into, 629
    anorectal anomanometry, 633
    histochemistry, 632–633
    rectal biopsy, 632–633
    X-ray, 630–632
Melaea, 807
Ménétrier's disease, 796
6-Mercaptopurine, 757, 759
Mesalazine, 756–759
Methyl cellulose, 636, 641
Metoclopramide, 779–780
'Microscopic' colitis, 802
Microscopy, in small bowel biopsy, 650–653
  dissecting, 650–652
  electron, 651, 653
  light, 651
Microvillous atrophy, 659, 660
Migrating motor complex, 699
Milk protein hydrolysates, 738, 740
Münchausen's syndrome by proxy, 724
Muscle pain, 791

Nonsteroidal anti-inflammatory drugs, 796,
    810
Noonan's syndrome, 699

Nutrition, for HPN, 708–709
  see also Diet *and also* Parenteral nutrition, at home
Nutritional deficiencies, and HPN, 716–717

Octreotide, 824–825
Oesophageal banding, 825
Oesophageal biopsy, 775
Oesophageal manometry, 694, 695
Oesophagitis, 770–772
  Barrett's oesophagus, 770–771
  histology of, 770
  symptoms of, 771–772
Oesophagus, 693–696
  gastro-oesophageal reflux, *see under* Gastro-oesophageal reflux
  manometry, 694–695
  pH monitoring, 694–695
  swallowing disorders, 693
Omeprazole, 781
Oral rehydration therapy (ORT), **611–624**
  American Academy of Pediatrics' recommendations, 618
  basis of, 612–614
    electrolyte/water transport and, 612
    infectious diarrhoea and, 612–624
  developed countries and, 619
  ESPGAN recommendations, 618
  history of use, 614
  recommendations, 619–620
  solution composition (ORS), 614–615
    bases in, 616–617
      sodium content, 616
      substrates, 615–616
    success of, 617–618
    use of, 617–619
      in developed countries, 619
      in developing countries, 617–618
      under-, 618–619
ORS, *see* Oral rehydration therapy (ORT)
ORT, *see* Oral rehydration therapy
Osler–Weber–Rendu syndrome, 811
Osmolality, of ORS, 616
Oxalosis, 673

Pain, abdominal, **787–806**
  bowel pattern alterations, 800–804
    differential diagnosis, 800–802
    endoscopy and, 802–803
    treatment, 803–804
    see also Inflammatory bowel disease; *see also* Crohn's disease *and* Ulcerative colitis
  dyspepsia, 794–800
  isolated paroxysmal, 788, 794
Paracetamol poisoning, 672–673
Parasitic infections, 801
Parenteral nutrition, at home (HPN), **705–721**

catheter line blockages, 715–716
  complications of, 714
  delivery systems, 708–712
  indications for, 705–707
  infections and, 714–715
  liver disease and, 716
  nutritional deficiencies, 716–717
  organization of, 710–713
    funding in, 711
    training for, 711–712
  outcome of, 713–714
  venous access, 707–708
  see also Diet
Peptic ulcers, 809–810, 814
Periodic acid–Schiff staining, 659
pH, oesophageal, 776–779
  age and, 777–778
  alkaline, 779
  food and, 778
  quantification, 694–695, 777
  sleep and, 778
Picolax, 635
Pneumocystic carinii, 682
Polyethyleneglycol, 635
Polyps, 810, 815
Port-A-Cath catheter, 707
Portal vein hypertension, 811–812
Proctocolectomy, and ulcerative colitis, 760
Proctosigmoidoscopy, 818
Prostaglandins, 826
Provocative testing, 682–693, 701
Pseudoxanthoma elasticum, 811
Psychiatry, in constipation therapy, 638–639
Psychological testing, 675
Psychology—
  in constipation therapy, 638–639
  in liver transplant, 678–679

Radiology, *see* X-ray investigations
Rectal biopsy, 632–633
Rectal manometry, 633
  see also Manometry
Rectal therapy, in constipation, 636–637
Recurrent abdominal pain, *see* Pain, abdominal
Regurgitation, 769–770
Rehydration, *see* Oral rehydration therapy (ORT)
RET proto-oncogene, 626

Sandifer's syndrome, 772
Scintigraphy, 775
  for gastrointestinal bleeding, 819–820
Scintiscanning, 691, 697
Sclerotherapy, 825
Selenium, 717
Sengstaken–Blakemore tube, 817, 825
Senna, 635–636, 641
Sexual maturation, and IBD, 750–751
Simethicone, 804

Skin—
    and food allergies, 730–731
        tests for, 735–736
    and IBD, 751
Sleep, and gut pH, 778
Small bowel biopsy, **645–666**
    AIDS and, 661
    antibody screening, 647
    autoimmune enteropathy, 660–661
    biochemical tests, 649
    breath tests and, 647–648
    coeliac disease, 653
    cow's milk sensitive enteropathy, 654
    cryptosporidiosis and, 657
    Cyclospora spp., 658
    dissecting microscopy in, 650–652
    electronmicroscopy in, 651, 653
    enteroaggregative *E. coli* and, 657
    enteropathogenic *E. coli* and, 655–657
    food-related disorders, 653–655
    giardiasis and, 657–658
    idiopathic enteropathy, 661
    immune deficiency, 661
        AIDS, 661
    indications for, 645–646
    intractable diarrhoea and, 659–661
    light microscopy in, 651
    lipoprotein disorders, 654–655
    lymphangiectasis, 654, 656
    microvillous atrophy, 659–660
    permeability tests, 648
    results interpretation, 650–653
    sample handling, 650
    stool microbiology, 648
    technique of, 649–650
        suction vs. endoscopic avulsion, 649–650
    Whipple's disease, 657
Small intestines, motility of, 698–700
    breath hydrogen analysis, 700
    manometry, 699–700
Sodium, in ORS, 616
Sodium ion transport, gut, 612
Sodium picosulphate, 635, 641
Solutions, parenteral nutrient, 709–710, 712
Somatostatin, 824–825
Sonography, *see* Ultrasound
Soy formulas, 738
Stomach, 696–698
    barostat manometry, 698
    electrical impedance tomography, 697
    electrogastrography, 698
    emptying, 696
    radiology of, 697
    ultrasound and, 697
    see also Gastro- *aspects*
Stool microbiology, and gut biopsy, 648
Stool softeners, 634
    maintenance therapy, 636
Sturge–Weber syndrome, 647

Substrate, in ORS, 615–616
Sucralfate, 780–781
Sucrase–isomaltase deficiency, 659
Suction biopsy (small bowel), 649–650
Sulphasalazine, 756–759
Surgery—
    for constipation, 637–638
    for Crohn's disease, 760–761
    for gastro-oesophageal reflux, 781–782
    for ulcerative colitis, 760
Swallowing disorders, 693

Teeth, 675
Telangiectasias, 811
Toxins, bacterial, 612–614
Turner's syndrome, 699, 811
Tyrosinaemia type I, 670

Ulcerations, 809–810
    see also Peptic ulcers
Ulcerative colitis—
    vs. Crohn's disease, 747–748
    diagnosis of, 752–753
    food allergies, 730
    nutritional support, 759
    presentation, 749
    prognosis, 761
    surgery for, 760
    therapy of, 756–758
        mild form, 756
        moderate form, 757
        severe form, 757–758
    see also Crohn's disease *and also* Inflammatory bowel disease
Ultrasound, 633, 676–677, 697, 775
Ureteropelvic junction, 790–791
Urticaria, 731

Varioloform gastritis, 796
'Vasoactive' lavage, 824
Vasopressin, 824–825
Verotoxin, 656
Vibrio cholerae, 612–613
    see also Bacterial infections
Video fluoroscopy, 693
VIP-omas, 659

Water transport, in gut, 612
Whipple's disease, 657
WHO-ORS, *see under* Oral rehydration therapy
Wilson's disease, 670–671

X-ray investigations, 676–677, 690–691, 697, 700, 753
    Crohn's disease, 755
    gastrointestinal tract, 630–632

Zinc, 717